Recent Results in Cancer Research 76

Fortschritte der Krebsforschung
Progrès dans les recherches sur le cancer

Edited by

V. G. Allfrey, New York · M. Allgöwer, Basel
I. Berenblum, Rehovot · F. Bergel, Jersey
J. Bernard, Paris · W. Bernhard, Villejuif
N. N. Blokhin, Moskva · H. E. Bock, Tübingen
W. Braun, New Brunswick · P. Bucalossi, Milano
A. V. Chaklin, Moskva · M. Chorazy, Gliwice
G. J. Cunningham, Richmond · G. Della Porta, Milano
P. Denoix, Villejuif · R. Dulbecco, La Jolla
H. Eagle, New York · R. Eker, Oslo
R. A. Good, New York · P. Grabar, Paris
R. J. C. Harris, Salisbury · E. Hecker, Heidelberg
R. Herbeuval, Vandoeuvre · J. Higginson, Lyon
W. C. Hueper, Fort Myers · H. Isliker, Lausanne
J. Kieler, Kobenhavn · W. H. Kirsten, Chicago
G. Klein, Stockholm · H. Koprowski, Philadelphia
L. G. Koss, New York · R. A. Macbeth, Toronto
G. Martz, Zürich · G. Mathé, Villejuif
O. Mühlbock, Amsterdam · L. J. Old, New York
V. R. Potter, Madison · A. B. Sabin, Charleston, S.C.
L. Sachs, Rehovot · E. A. Saxén, Helsinki
C. G. Schmidt, Essen · S. Spiegelman, New York
W. Szybalski, Madison · H. Tagnon, Bruxelles
A. Tissières, Genève · E. Uehlinger, Zürich
R. W. Wissler, Chicago

Editor in Chief: P. Rentchnick, Genève
Co-editor: H. J. Senn, St. Gallen

New Drugs
in Cancer Chemotherapy

Edited by
S. K. Carter Y. Sakurai H. Umezawa

With 133 Figures and 170 Tables

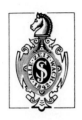

Springer-Verlag
Berlin Heidelberg New York 1981

U.S. Japan Joint Agreement on Cancer Research
5th Annual Program Review Symposium
San Francisco (USA), May 21−22, 1979

Dr. Stephen K. Carter
Northern California Cancer Program,
1801 Page Mill Road, Suite 200,
Building B, Palo Alto, CA 94304 (USA)

Dr. Yoshi Sakurai
Cancer Chemotherapy Center, Japanese
Foundation for Cancer Research,
Kami-Ikebukuro 1-37-1, Toshima-ku,
Tokyo 170 (Japan)

Dr. Hamoa Umezawa
Institute of Microbial Chemistry,
14−23 Kamiosaki 3-Chome, Shinagawa-ku,
Tokyo 141 (Japan)

Sponsored by the Swiss League against Cancer

ISBN 3-540-10487-9 Springer-Verlag Berlin Heidelberg New York
ISBN 0-387-10487-9 Springer-Verlag New York Heidelberg Berlin

Library of Congress Cataloging in Publication Data. Main entry under title: New drugs in cancer chemotherapy. (Recent results in cancer research; 76) "U.S. Japan Joint Agreement on Cancer Research, 5th Annual Program Review Symposium, San Francisco (USA), May 21−22, 1979. Sponsored by the Swiss League against Cancer." Includes bibliographical references and index. 1. Cancer − Chemotherapy − Congresses. 2. Anti-neoplastic agents − Congresses. I. Carter, Stephen K. II. Sakurai, Yoshio. III. Umezawa, Hamao, 1914− IV. Schweizerische Nationalliga für Krebsbekämpfung und Krebs-forschung. V. Series. [DNLM: 1. Antineoplastic agents − Therapeutic use − Congresses. 2. Neoplasms − Drug therapy − Congresses. W1 RE106P v. 76 / QZ 267 N532 1979] RC261.R35 vol. 76 [RC271.C5] 616.99′4s 80-39739 [616.99′4061]

© Springer-Verlag Berlin Heidelberg 1981
Printed in Germany

The use of registered names, trademarks, etc. in the publication does not imply, even in the absence of a specific statement, that such names are exempt from the relevant protective laws and regulations and therefore free for general use.

Typesetting and printing: Carl Ritter-GmbH & Co.KG., Wiesbaden
Binding: J. Schäffer OHG, Grünstadt

2125/3140−5 4 3 2 1 0

Contents

List of Contributors

J. L. Au
School of Pharmacy and Department of Pharmaceutical
Chemistry, University of Carlifornia,
San Francisco, CA (USA)

L. H. Baker
Wayne State University, Detroit, MI (USA)

R. H. Blum
Sidney Farber Cancer Institute, Harvard Medical School,
Boston, MA (USA)

M. Boiron
Hopital ST. Louis, Paris (France)

W. T. Bradner
Bristol Laboratories, Syracuse, NY (USA)

R. Brunet
Fondation Bergonie, Bordeaux (France)

G. P. Canellos
Sidney Farber Cancer Institute, Harvard Medical School,
Boston, MA (USA)

S. K. Carter
Northern California Cancer Program, Palo Alto, CA (USA)

R. Catane
National Cancer Institute, Bethesda, MD (USA)

L. M. Charles, Jr.,
National Cancer Institute, Bethesda, MD (USA)

R. L. Comis
State University of New York Upstate Medical Center,
Syracuse, NY (USA)

S. T. Crooke
Bristol Laboratories, Syracuse, NY (USA)

H. L. Davis
University of Wisconsin, Wisconsin Clinical Cancer Center,
Madison, WI (USA)

J. Douros
National Cancer Institute, Bethesda, MD (USA)

E. Frei III
Sidney Farber Cancer Institute, Harvard Medical School,
Boston, MA (USA)

M. A. Friedman
Cancer Research Institute, University of California,
San Francisco, CA (USA)

S. Fujimoto
Cancer Chemotherapy Center, Tokyo (Japan)

M. B. Garnick
Sidney Farber Cancer Institute, Harvard Medical School,
Boston, MA (USA)

S. J. Ginsberg
State University of New York Upstate Medical Center,
Syracuse, NY (USA)

C. Gisselbrecht
Hopital St. Louis, Paris (Fance)

A. Goldin
National Cancer Institute, Bethesda, MD (USA)

J. Hannigan
Cancer Research Institute, University of California,
San Francisco, CA (USA)

S. Hattori
The Center for Adult Diseases, Osaka (Japan)

I. C. Henderson
Sidney Farber Cancer Institute, Harvard Medical School,
Boston, MA (USA)

G. A. Higgins
Veterans Administration Medical Center,
Washington, DC (USA)

T. Horai
The Center for Adult Diseases, Osaka (Japan)

D. F. Hoth
Georgetown University School of Medicine,
Washington, DC (USA)

S. Ikeda
Saitama Medical School, Moroyama-cho, Saitama Prefecture
(Japan)

H. Ikegami
The Center for Adult Diseases, Osaka (Japan)

M. Israel
Sidney Farber Cancer Institute, Harvard Medical School,
Boston, MA (USA)

C. Jacobs
Stanford University School of Medicine,
Palo Alto, CA (USA)

M. S. Jensen-Akula
National Cancer Institute, Bethesda, MD (USA)

K. Katayama
University of Tokyo Faculty of Medicine, Tokyo (Japan)

K. Kimura
National Nagoya Hospital, Nagoya (Japan)

K. W. Kohn
National Cancer Institute, Bethesda, MD (USA)

H. Koyama
The Center for Adult Diseases, Osaka (Japan)

C. Lagarde
Fondation Bergonie, Bordeaux (France)

R. B. Livingston
University of Texas Health Science Center,
San Antonio, TX (USA)

J. S. Macdonald
Georgetown University School of Medicine,
Washington, DC (USA)

T. Miura
University of Tokyo Faculty of Medicine, Tokyo (Japan)

H. Miyasato
Saitama Medical School, Moroyama-cho,
Saitama Prefecture (Japan)

F. M. Muggia
National Cancer Institute, Bethesda, MD (USA)

H. Nakayama
Saitama Medical School, Moroyama-cho,
Saitama Prefecture (Japan)

M. Ogawa
Cancer Chemotherapy Center, Tokyo (Japan)

S. Oka
Institute of Microbial Chemistry, Tokyo (Japan)

T. Oki
Central Research Laboratories, Sanraku-Ocean Co., Ltd.,
Fujisawa (Japan)

J. S. Penta
National Cancer Institute, Bethesda, MD (USA)

A. W. Prestayko
Bristol Laboratories, Syracuse, NY (USA)

S. D. Reich
State University of New York Upstate Medical Center,
Syracuse, NY (USA)

W. Sadée
School of Pharmacy and Department of Pharmaceutical
Chemistry, University of California, San Fracisco, CA (USA)

Y. Sakurai
Cancer Chemotherapy Center, Tokyo (Japan)

A. Sato
Saitama Medical School, Moroyama-cho,
Saitama Prefecture (Japan)

P. S. Schein
Georgetown University School of Medicine,
Washington, DC (USA)

A. Schlein
Bristol Laboratories, Syracuse, NY (USA)

J. Schurig
Bristol Laboratories, Syracuse, NY (USA)

F. P. Smith
Georgetown University School of Medicine,
Washington, DC (USA)

M. E. Smulson
Georgetown University School of Medicine,
Washington, DC (USA)

J. E. Strong
Bristol Laboratories, Syracuse, NY (USA)

M. Suffness
National Cancer Institute, Bethesda, MD (USA)

T. Takeuchi
Institute of Microbial Chemistry, Tokyo (Japan)

K. Tajima
Saitama Medical School, Moroyama-cho,
Saitama Prefecture (Japan)

T. Terasawa
The Center for Adult Diseases, Osaka (Japan)

K. D. Tew
Georgetown University School of Medicine,
Washington, DC (USA)

H. Umezawa
Institute of Microbial Chemistry, Tokyo (Japan)

J. M. Venditti
National Cancer Institute, Bethesda, MD (USA)

T. Wada
The Center for Adult Diseases, Osaka (Japan)

T. Wada
University of Tokyo Faculty of Medicine, Tokyo (Japan)

R. E. Wittes
Memorial-Sloan-Kettering Cancer Center,
New York, NY (USA)

P. V. Wooley
Georgetown University School of Medicine,
Washington, DC (USA)

K. Yamada
Nagoya University School of Medicine, Nagoya (Japan)

Introduction

The Analog Potential in Cancer Chemotherapy in the United States and Japan

S. K. Carter

Northern California Cancer Program, 1801 Page Mill Road, Building B, Suite 200, USA – Palo Alto, CA 94304

The bilateral collaborative program in cancer research between Japan and the United States is one of the oldest programs of this type. It is sponsored in the United States by the National Cancer Institute [1], while in Japan the sponsoring organization is the Japan Society for the Promotion of Science. Annual symposia concerning treatment have been held and in recent years they have been published [2, 3].

Drug development in both Japan and the United States has evolved over the years to an increasing emphasis on second generation compounds. This has come about as a result of the initial successes of chemotherapy development. Many active structures have been uncovered and the armamentarium of the medical and pediatric oncologist has grown dramatically. The uncovering of an active structure provides an opportunity for analog synthesis and attempts at elucidating structure-activity relationships. It is hoped that the therapeutic index of active structures can be improved so as to achieve superior clinical results. This increase in therapeutic index can be achieved in a variety of ways: (1) by increasing the response rate in tumors previously sensitive; (2) by achieving response in patients resistant to the parent structure – a resistance that can be either primary (broader spectrum) or secondary (cross resistance); and (3) by diminished toxicity, which can be either acute or chronic.

Analog development in Japan and the United States has attempted to improve the therapeutic indices of active structures in all of the above ways. Four major drug classes have received particular emphasis in the United States–Japan cancer research agreement that is now in its 6th year. These drug classes are: (1) anthracyclines, (2) bleomycins, (3) nitrosoureas, and (4) fluorinated pyrimidines.

The anthracyclines, as exemplified by adriamycin, are among the most active of the anticancer agents with a broad spectrum of antitumor activity [4]. Analog development in this area has gone on in many countries (Table 1). One of the major limiting factors in the use of the anthracyclines is the development of cardiomyopathy clinically expressed as congestive heart failure.

The chronic toxicity of drug-induced cardiomyopathy can produce significant morbidity and mortality. This "pump" failure is dose-dependent, but shows no apparent relationship to preexisting heart disease. The clinical presentation and pathophysiology of cardiac damage caused by adriamycin are indistinguishable from other known cardiomyopathies. Although the speed of the clinical course varies, it is usually a rapidly progressing syndrome of congestive heart failure and cardiorespiratory decompensation including dilation of the heart, pleural effusion, and venous

Table 1. Adriamycin: Analogues under clinical study

Drug	Country of origin
Daunomycin[a]	Italy
Aclacinomycin-A	Japan
Adriamycin trifluoro valerate (AD-32)	U.S.A.
Rubidazone	France
Carminomycin	U.S.S.R.
Quelamycin	Spain
4'-epiadriamycin	Italy
14-DEA adriamycin	France
Adriamycin-DNA	Belgium
Daunomycin-DNA	Belgium

[a] First anthracycline clinically studied

congestion. Reversibility of the heart failure does not appear to be a function of the therapeutic intervention.

The overall incidence of congestive heart failure caused by drug-induced cardio-myopathy is 1%, although this is deceptive since the toxicity is related to the total dose administered. If the total dose is kept below 450 mg/m^2, cardiomyopathy is rarely observed [4]. Unfortunately, this limits the amount and the duration of drug therapy. The frequency of cardiomyopathy is markedly increased at total doses above 550 mg/m^2, so that a clinician who exceeds these dose levels must be aware of the high risk and must balance it against the risk of discontinuing therapy in a rapidly growing tumor.

The Stanford group [5] has studied right ventricular endomyocardial biopsy, right heart catheterization, and systolic time interval determination in patients treated with adriamycin. Their results in 33 adult patients indicate that adriamycin administration is associated with a dose-related increase in the degree of myocardial necrosis. In 29 patients who received total doses equal to or greater than 240 mg/m^2, they found 27 with degenerative changes that could be identified on biopsy. The preejection period to left ventricular ejection time ratio (PEP/LVET) exhibited a threshold phenomenon and did not begin to increase until a total dose of 400 mg/m^2 had been reached. Seven patients had catheterization-proven heart failure. These seven had a significantly greater amount of myocardial necrosis on biopsy than dose-matched controls ($p < 0.01$). Previous mediastinal radiation appears to poten-tiate the adriamycin-associated degenerative process. Mediastinal radiation, age over 70 years, and concurrent cyclophosphamide administration appeared to be the three risk factors for adriamycin-associated heart failure. It is the feeling of the Stanford group that dose limitation by combined clinical, noninvasive, invasive, and morphological criteria offers an advantage over empirical dose limitation or dose limitation by PEP/LVET alone.

Human right ventricular endomyocardial biopsies are obtained by a transvenous intracardiac catheter technique. A flexible biotome is introduced percutaneously through the right internal jugular vein and advanced across the tricuspid valve to the apical portion of the right ventricular septum where four cardiac muscle specimens from 0.15–0.30 cm in diameter are taken serially.

The biopsy tissue is fixed immediately in 10% buffered formalin and processed in a conventional manner for light microscopy. Tissue for electron microscopy is fixed immediately in 2.5% glutaraldehyde in 0.1 M sodium cacodylate buffer pH 7.2. Although severe cardiotoxic changes can be detected by light microscopy, electron microscopy is required to score accurately the severity of cardiac toxicity. Two types of damage caused by adriamycin have been observed. The first is a cell totally or partially devoid of myofibrillar content even though the nucleus and mitochondria might be intact. The second type of myocyte damage is vacuolar degeneration. A biopsy score on a scale of 0−3 has been developed at Stanford:

0 = No change from normal.
1 = Scanty cells showing early myofibrillar drop out and/or swelling of the sarcoplasmic reticulum.
2 = More widespread changes with groups of cells showing definite myofibrillar drop out, cells showing definite cytoplasmic vacuolization, or both.
3 = Diffuse myocyte damage with more marked cellular changes and frank necrosis.

The guidelines developed at Stanford for stopping adriamycin because of potential cardiac risk are as follows. A 3+ biopsy score is an absolute indication for stopping the therapy. A second indication is a PEP/LVET ratio of ≥ 0.45 or an increase of ≥ 0.10 over the pretreatment value if combined with a 2+ biopsy change or a catheterization abnormality consistent with myocardial dysfunction. It is seen that PEP/LVET ratio increase alone without any other evidence of myocardial dysfunction, such as biopsy change or catheterization change, is not an indication for stopping therapy.

In the past, the clinical evaluation of new adriamycin analogs would have required determination of the cumulative dose and the number of courses needed to reach that dose which resulted in cardiomyopathy, and then comparing these results to those obtained with adriamycin. This would have required large numbers of patients, would have suffered from the faults inherent in the use of historical controls, and would have been questionable in ethical terms. The endomyocardial biopsy techniques enable one safely to determine a dose level that causes pathologic changes at a preclinical level. It gives both an objective and quantifiable end-point without having to wait for the patient to develop a life-threatening clinical situation. This technique should now play a major role in the clinical trial strategy for any new analogs.

Schedule is a variable in the use of adriamycin which may have an impact on cardiac toxicity. The Central Oncology Group in a study reported by Weiss [6] indicates that weekly adriamycin may be less toxic. Benjamin [7] in a more stringent analysis than that used by Weiss, has calculated that cardiomyopathy occurred in only 2 of 31 patients who received over 1 000 mg/m^2 and in 4 of 68 who received more than 600 mg/m^2 total dose. The Western Cancer Study Group [cit. by 7] also used a weekly schedule and reported cardiomyopathy in only 1 of 23 patients who received more than 500 mg/m^2 total dose. The activity on the weekly schedule appears comparable. The Northern California Oncology Group is starting a study in breast cancer that will evaluate a weekly dose of 17 mg/m^2 for efficacy and cardiac toxicity as measured by the endomyocardial biopsy.

Bleomycin has become an integral part of the successful combination chemotherapy of testicular cancer, the malignant lymphomas, and squamous cell carcinoma of the head and neck [8]. It is highly attractive for its lack of myelosuppression. It is limited by skin toxicity, stomatitis, and pulmonary toxicity. Analog development has been ongoing in both Japan and the United States (Table 2). The aim is both to broaden the spectrum and to diminish the pulmonary toxicity. Both PEP-bleomycin from Japan and tallysomycin from the United States give experimental results that are encouraging in that direction. The former drug is already under clinical study in Japan while tallysomycin is approaching clinical study in the United States.

PEP-bleomycin is one of more than 300 bleomycins obtained by precursor-fed fermentation or chemical derivation. PEP-bleomycin was selected for clinical trials, according to Matsuda of Nippon Kayaku, for the following reasons: (1) it had superior antitumor activity, compared to bleomycin, in Ehrlich carcinoma (solid), AH66 ascites hepatoma, HeLaS$_3$ cells, and in chemically induced gastric adenocarcinoma in rats; (2) organ distribution studies in mice showed concentrations 2−3 times higher than bleomycin in skin, lung, stomach, brain, and tumor; (3) the pulmonary toxicity was only one-quarter that of bleomycin in studies in old mice and dogs.

Ikeda has presented data on PEP-bleomycin indicating significant activity in skin cancer. The schedule used was 10 mg three times weekly to a total of 200 mg. Activity in squamous cell lesions was high (4 of 5) as well as in malignant lymphoma (2 of 2) and a variety of other skin lesions. Toxicity observed included anorexia, alopecia, fever, scratch dermatitis, hyperkeratosis of the skin, and stomatitis. No cases of pulmonary toxicity were seen.

The nitrosoureas have been among the most studied group of compounds as regards clinical analog studies (Table 3). Beginning with the brief clinical trial of MNNG, six

Table 2. Bleomycin analogs under clinical study

Drug	Country of origin
PEP-bleomycin	Japan
Tallysomycin[a]	U.S.A.

[a] Approaching clinical trials

Table 3. Nitrosoureas ("parent" drug − BCNU[a]): Analogs under clinical study

Drug	Country of origin
CCNU	U.S.A.
MeCCNU	U.S.A.
Streptozotocin	U.S.A.
Chlorozotocin	U.S.A.
PCNU	U.S.A.
ACNU	Japan
GANU	Japan
MCNU	Japan
RPCNU	France
RPFNU	France
MNU	U.S.S.R.

[a] An "analog" of MNNG which had brief clinical study in the United States

additional structures are still under clinical study today. The first was BCNU and this was followed by streptozotocin, CCNU, methyl CCNU, chlorozotocin, and now PCNU. In Japan three structures have been studied; ACNU, GANU, and MCNU. The international picture becomes rounded out by MNU in the Soviet Union and the sugar-containing analogs under study in France. The nitrosoureas are active but toxic drugs. Their activity range includes brain tumors, gastrointestinal cancer, oat cell lung cancer, Hodgkin's disease, and malignant melanoma [9]. With the exception of streptozotocin, all the fully evaluated drugs are limited by delayed myelosuppression, which is cumulative with repeated exposure. Nausea and vomiting are prominent, and now evidence of delayed pulmonary fibrosis and renal damage is coming to the fore with long-term administration. Streptozotocin, which is not myelosuppressive, is dose limited by renal toxicity, which along with severe nausea and vomiting makes it a difficult drug to use.

The nitrosoureas are highly active structures in experimental tumor systems. They are curative to such a degree in some predictive systems that elucidation of analogs becomes difficult from an efficacy point of view. The current emphasis in analog study is to try to develop less myelosuppressive compounds. It was hoped that study of relative alkylating versus carbamoylating activity would aid in the choice of drugs with so improved therapeutic indexes. This had not been accomplished to date, but the available clinical correlations with the experimental data will soon be extensive. One of the exciting aspects of the United States–Japan agreement has been the exchange of the nitrosourea compounds under study in both countries. This has led to the ability to devise extensive correlations between the experimental data and the ultimate clinical fate of the newer compounds such as chlorozotocin and GANU.

5-Fluorouracil (5-FU) has long been the mainstay drug for the treatment of gastrointestinal adenocarcinoma and an important component in the successful drug treatment of breast cancer. The drug, as usually administered, is dose limited by myelosuppression. Other toxicities include gastrointestinal damage and occasional cerebellar ataxia. An analog which would not have bone marrow toxicity would have the distinct advantage of making possible easier combination with other myelosuppressive drugs (Table 4). One approach to achieving this involves the concept of a prodrug that is metabolized in vivo to 5-FU and so achieves the equivalent of a continuous infusion. The first attempt to be clinically evaluated involved the use of ftorafur. This compound was synthesized in the Soviet Union and extensively studied in Japan. In the United States, when used on a high dose intermittent intravenous schedule, ftorafur has shown equivalent activity to 5-FU and has a lack of myelosuppression. Unfortunately, significant CNS toxicity has been observed. The

Table 4. Fluorinated pyrimidines ("parent" drug − 5 Fluorouracil): Analogs under clinical study

Drug	Country of origin
5-FUDR	U.S.A.
F_3TDR	U.S.A.
Ftorafur	U.S.S.R.
FD-1	Japan
HCFU	Japan

required attenuation of the intensity of drug administration because of the CNS toxicity appears to diminish the activity as well. In Japan ftorafur is used orally on a more chronic schedule and is well tolerated. Studies on the oral formulation are just beginning in the United States. Newer analogs utilizing the prodrug approach are under study in Japan. These include FD-1 and HCFU, and the latter is discussed in the paper by Sakurai.

References

1. Goldin A, Muggia FM, Rozencweig M (1979) International activities of the division of cancer treatment. Natl Cancer Inst Monogr 2: 29–35
2. Carter SK, Umezawa H, Douros J, Sakaurai Y (eds) (1978) Antitumor antibiotics. Recent Results Cancer Res 63: 303
3. Carter SK, Sakarai Y, Muggia FM, Umezawa H (eds) (to be published) Phase I and phase II trials. Recent Results Cancer Res
4. Carter SK (1975) Adriamycin. Rev J Natl Cancer Inst 55: 1265–1274
5. Bristow MR, Mason JW, Billingham ME, Daniels JR (1978) Adriamycin cardiomyopathy: Evaluation by phonocardiography, endomyocardial biopsy and cardiac catheterization. Ann Intern Med 88: 168–175
6. Weiss AJ, Metter GE, Fletcher WS, Wilson WL, Grage TB, Ramirez G (1976) Studies on adriamycin using a weekly regimen demonstrating its clinical expectancies and lack of cardiac toxicity. Cancer Treat Rev 60: 813–822
7. Benjamin RS (1978) Adriamycin and other anthracycline antibodies under study in the United States. Recent Results Cancer Res 62: 230–240
8. Carter SK (1978) The current role of bleomycin in cancer therapy. In: Carter SK, Crooke ST, Umezawa H (eds) Bleomycin: Current status and new developments. Academic Press, New York San Francisco London, pp 9–15
9. Wasserman TH, Slavik M, Carter SK (1975) Clinical comparisons of the nitrosoureas. Cancer 36: 1258–1268

Preclinical Rationale and Phase I Clinical Trial of the Adriamycin Analog, AD 32*

R. H. Blum, M. B. Garnick, M. Israel, G. P. Panellos,
I. C. Henderson, and E. Frei III**

Division of Medical Oncology and Pharmacology, Sidney Farber Cancer Institute,
Havard Medical School, USA – Boston, MA 02115

Introduction

The preclinical and clinical data for the adriamycin analog (AD 32) will be reviewed and compared to adriamycin. Emphasis will be placed on demonstrated biologic differences that may make AD 32 the better compound for clinical use.

Biochemistry

In attempts to synthesize adriamycin analogs with greater therapeutic efficacy and with less toxicity, Israel and co-workers at the Sidney Farber Cancer Institute have identified over 180 adriamycin analogs. N-trifluoroacetyladriamycin-14-valerate (AD 32, NSC-246131), the 32nd analog, was selected for clinical trial. AD 32 differs from adriamycin both at the C-14 function and at the substitution on the aminoglycoside (Fig. 1). The C-14 sidechain of AD 32 has a 5 carbon straight-chain valerate substituent, while adriamycin has a hydroxy group and daunorubicin a hydrogen group. The aminoglycoside of AD 32 has a trifluoroacetyl substitution, while adriamycin has no substitution of the amino sugar. AD 32 has a molecular weight of 724, is insoluble in water but soluble in a wide variety of organic and lipophilic solvents and surfactant. For biologic testing, AD 32 was formulated in either a 10% aqueous Tween 80 solution or in an Emulphor-ethanol-saline solution [19].

Biologic Effects

The comparative in vitro effects of AD 32 and adriamycin have been studied (Table 1). The trifluoroacetyl substitution significantly alters DNA binding properties. Sengupta and co-workers, using isolated calf thymus DNA, demonstrated that while adriamycin binds strongly to DNA, AD 32 does not bind [20]. Differences in DNA binding were

 * Supported in part by Contract N01-CM-53839 (Division of Cancer Treatment), and Public Health Service Grant CA-19118 from the National Cancer Institute
** The authors wish to acknowledge the invaluable assistance of Ms. Carol McCormick for her data management, and Ms. Martha J. Sack for manuscript preparation

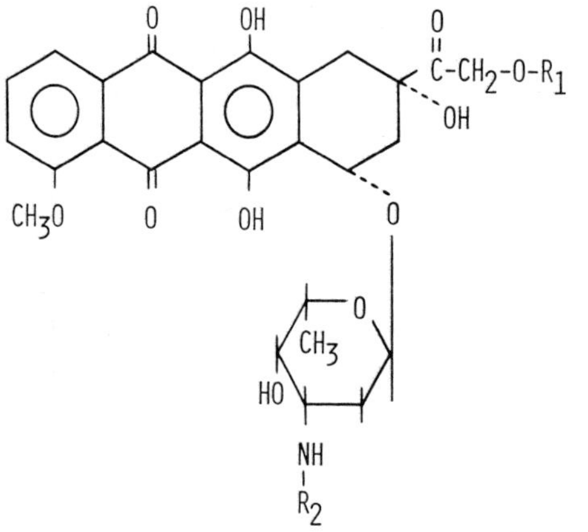

	R_1	R_2
ADRIAMYCIN	H	H
AD 32	$CO(CH_2)_3CH_3$	$COCF_3$

Fig. 1. The structural differences between adriamycin and AD 32 (*N*-trifluoroacetyladriamycin-14-valerate)

Table 1. A comparison of the various biologic properties of adriamycin and AD 32, as determined from multiple in vitro investigations

	Adriamycin	AD 32
DNA binding		
Isolated DNA	Significant	Negligible
Propidium-iodide fluorescence	Quenched	Enhanced
DNAase I inhibition	Yes	No
Cellular uptake		
Rate	Slow	Rapid
Localization	Nucleus	Cytoplasm
Cycle specificity		
Block	G_2	G_2
Phase	$S > G_1$	$S = G_1$
Log vs. plateau	$> \log$	Equal
Precursor uptake		
DNA inhibition	Yes	Yes
RNA inhibition	Yes	Yes
Protein inhibition	Yes	Yes

also shown by Krishan and co-workers who studied propidium-iodide stained cells. The fluorescent properties of propidium, an analog of ethidium bromide, depend on the degree and character of DNA intercalation. Anthracyclines alter the propidium-DNA intercalation. Differences in DNA binding between AD 32 and adriamycin have been demonstrated. AD 32 enhances propidium fluorescence, but adriamycin quenches fluorescence. This observed difference implies that AD 32 or a metabolite enters the nucleus and interacts with DNA in a manner different than adriamycin [15].

DNA binding can also be studied by measuring DNAase I inhibition. Facchinetti and co-workers demonstrated that adriamycin, but not AD 32, inhibits DNAase I. By correlating DNA-anthracycline binding and DNAase I inhibition, they demonstrated that the enzyme inhibition was due to drug-induced DNA substrate change, and not a direct drug effect of the enzyme [4]. These studies are consistent with the assumption that, in contrast to adriamycin, the cytotoxic effect of AD 32 is not mediated by DNA intercalation and/or inhibition of DNAase I.

AD 32 and adriamycin differ in their cellular transport properties. Meriwether and Bachur have shown that adriamycin is slowly transported across the cellular membrane [18]. By using the semiquantitative technique of cytofluorescence, Krishan and co-workers demonstrated that AD 32 rapidly enters cells with fluorescence localized in the cytoplasm. In contrast to this system, adriamycin uptake is slower, with cytofluorescence localization only in the nucleus [16]. Although these studies imply differences in cellular distribution, relatively smaller accumulations of AD 32 cannot be ruled out.

Using laser flow-cytometry, Krishan and co-workers demonstrated that both AD 32 and adriamycin prevent cell cycle traverse at the S-G_2 interface. Differences in cell cycle specificity were apparent with CCRF-CEM human lymphoblasts. AD 32 was equally effective in both S and G_1 cycle phases, but adriamycin demonstrated greater cytotoxicity in S compared to G_1. This observation is supported by the greater sensitivity of adriamycin to log growth phase compared to plateau, while AD 32 showed no such differential cytotoxicity [14]. Regardless of these differences, adriamycin and AD 32 inhibit incorporation of radiolabeled precursors, documenting inhibition of DNA, RNA, and protein synthesis [17].

Pharmacology

Pharmacokinetic and metabolic degradation pathways have been characterized for AD 32 and compared to adriamycin in the mouse, rat, rabbit, monkey, and human. The use of high performance liquid chromatography (HPLC) with continuous flow fluorescence allows highly specific separation of the parent anthracycline and metabolites with sensitivity in the picomole range [10]. The major metabolic pathways for AD 32 have been similar in all the species studies (Fig. 2). The hepatobiliary system is the major metabolic and excretory pathway for AD 32. In the species studied, combined biliary and urinary metabolites accounted for approximately 50% of the administered AD 32 dose. AD 32 undergoes esterase cleavage to the N-trifluoro-acetyladriamycin (AD 41), which in turn undergoes further reduction with an aldoketo reductase to the N-trifluoroacetyladriamycinol (AD 92). Both these compounds undergo glucuronide conjugation or cleavage to aglycones [11−13].

Human pharmacokinetic studies demonstrate that AD 32, when given by continuous infusion, reaches plateau levels within 1−2 h and rapidly disappears from plasma after completion of the infusion. The metabolism and elimination of AD 32 paralleled that seen in the other species. Plasma levels of adriamycin and adriamycinol have been detected, but at insignificant levels, in patients receiving AD 32 [6, 8]. One patient with biliary obstruction but normal liver function underwent hepatobilliary pharmacokinetic studies. Approximately 3% of the total amount of administered AD 32 in bile was accounted for as adriamycin and adriamycinol. This component did not

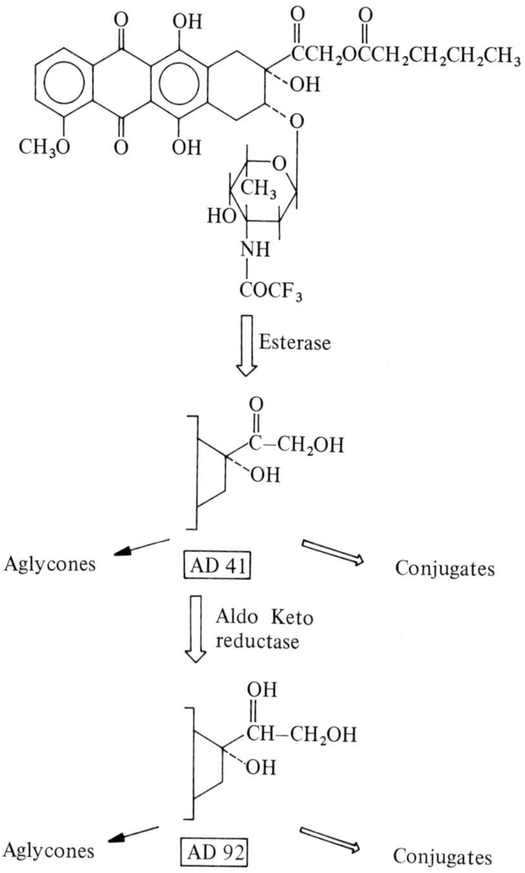

Fig. 2. Metabolic schema for AD 32. Code number AD 41 refers to N-trifluoroacetyladriamycin; code number AD 92 refers to N-trifluoroacetyladriamycinol

undergo an entrohepatic recirculation and no adriamycin was detected in the plasma [6]. The significance of this observation is not known.

Preclinical Testing

Initially, AD 32 was selected for further trial because of its superior activity compared to adriamycin in both the L1210 and P388 leukemia [9]. In subsequent studies by Parker [19], Vecchi and co-workers [21], it was demonstrated that AD 32 was significantly more effective than adriamycin in early and advanced L1210 leukemia intravenously administered. Only AD 32 produced long-term survivors. Neither adriamycin nor AD 32 were active against the intracranially implanted L1210. In the Lewis lung carcinoma, AD 32 was significantly more effective in increasing the life span and in reducing the percentage of pulmonary metastases at death on day 23 [21].
AD 32 was compared to adriamycin in a rabbit model. Both drugs induced dose-limiting myelosuppression. At equally myelosuppressive doses, the AD 32-treated animals, compared to adriamycin-treated animals, had less alopecia, greater weight gain, less local skin damage at the infusion site, less azotemia, and less

clinical and pathologic evidence of anthracycline cardiomyopathy [7]. These results were confirmed with appropriate vehicle and schedule controls.

Clinical Trial

Drug Administration

The AD 32 used in the clinical trial was manufactured in bulk by Farmatalia S.p.A., Milan, Italy through a joint agreement between the Sidney Farber Cancer Institute, Adria Laboratories, and the National Cancer Institute. AD 32 was formulated as a lyophilized powder in 200-mg vials. As AD 32 is insoluble in aqueous phase, a lipophilic solvent media of equal volumes of absolute ethanol and polyethoxylated vegetable oil (Emulphor EL620) is used to solubilize the drug. This solution is then diluted in aqueous medium, yielding a final clinical formulation of 0.35 mg AD 32/ml, in 0.5% alcohol, 0.5% Emulphor and 99.0% aqueous medium. AD 32 was administered by IMED pumps (San Diego, CA) as a 24-h continuous infusion. Treatments were repeated at 21 day intervals [2].

Patient Selection

Sixty-one patients with advanced metastatic disease, for which no therapy of proven benefit was available, have been entered. Only ambulatory patients with normal bone marrow, renal, hepatic, and cardiac functions were eligible. Twelve patients (20%) could not be evaluated for response because they were treated at low dose levels (five patients), or had lack of serial documentation of extent of disease (six patients). One patient had drug-induced pancytopenia, which led to a fatal septic episode 10 days from the start of AD 32. The remaining 49 patients (80%) were evaluable for response. The median age was 56 with a range of 15−78 years. Only 12 patients (24.5%) had not received prior chemotherapy or radiation. Twenty-six patients (53%) had either chemotherapy or radiation and an additional ten patients (20%) had both prior radiotherapy and chemotherapy.

Results

A starting dose of 100 mg/m^2 was extrapolated as a fraction of the maximally tolerated doses of AD 32 in preclinical evaluation and as an extrapolation from previous adriamycin comparative studies. Two hundred and thirty courses of AD 32 have been administered over a dose range of 100−900 mg/m^2. No significant toxicity was encountered until the 400 mg dose level. The highest maximally tolerated but safe starting dose was found to be 600 mg/m^2. Escalation above this dose level was accomplished in those patients who had minimal toxicity from the previous course. Only two patients have tolerated the highest dose of 900 mg/m^2.
Leukopenia is dose limiting. At 600 mg/m^2, the median total white count in 47 patients was 1 500 cells/mm^3 with a mean of 1 900 cells/mm^3 and a range of 100−5 400 cells/mm^3. The white count nadir occurred between 12 and 14 days after treatment with recovery to normal counts by 21 days. This degree of leukopenia is approximately

equal to that reported for 90 mg/m^2 of adriamycin [5]. Drug-induced thrombocytopenia was minimal with only 17% of patients having platelet nadirs below 100 000/mm^3, and only one patient with thrombocytopenia below 20 000/mm^3. Drug induced anemia requiring transfusion was rarely encountered. Myelosuppression has not been cumulative.

At a dose level of 600 mg/m^2 58% of patients had no gastrointestinal toxicity, but 36% of patients reported some effect and 6% had moderate toxicity. No patient had acute gastrointestinal toxicity lasting longer than 24 h.

An acute systemic reaction was encountered in five of the initial eight courses given at 400 mg/m^2. Within the initial 12−16 h of initiating the infusion, patients developed moderate to severe chest pain, bronchospasm, fever to 103° F, and hypotension. This reaction was thought to be vehicle-related. Corticosteroids reversed all manifestations of this reaction [2]. In all subsequent courses, 100 mg hydrocortisone was given as a rapid intravenous infusion beginning just prior to AD 32 infusion and at 6-h intervals for a total of five doses. With steroid prophylaxis, no acute systemic reactions have occurred.

No other clinically significant toxicities have been encountered, except partial to total alopecia. Hepatic, renal, neurologic or pulmonary toxicities have not been observed. No subcutaneous ulcers have developed when AD 32 was inadvertently extravasated.

Evaluation of anthracycline analogs for cardiac toxicity is essential but problematic. In the initial clinical trials of new drugs, patients with advanced disease and a lower probability of prolonged survival are studied, making the evaluation of chronic toxicity more difficult. Preliminary observations for AD 32 can be reported if the following assumptions are made: (1) the histopathologic lesions are similar for anthracycline analogs; (2) 600 mg/m^2 of AD 32 and 90 mg/m^2 of adriamycin are equally myelosuppressive [5]; (3) cardiac toxicity can be expected if cumulative doses of greater than 450 mg/m^2 of adriamycin are given; (4) when AD 32 is equally toxic, cardiotoxicity can be expected to occur at doses of greater than 3 g/m^2. To date, a total of ten patients, eight of whom are still receiving treatments, have achieved cumulative doses of AD 32 greater than 3 g/m^2 (Table 2). No patient has had any clinical evidence of anthracycline cardiomyopathy. Although the number is small and the time of risk is limited, this lack of toxicity is corroborated by data on three patients who underwent endomyocardial biopsy to assess histologic evidence of anthracycline damage [3]. Billingham, unaware of cumulative doses of AD 32, graded material from 0 (no damage) to 3 (severe anthracycline damage) [1]. These grades were compared to that expected from equivalent cumulative doses of adriamycin (Table 3). The scores of two patients were at least one standard deviation below what would have been expected from equivalent doses of adriamycin. One patient who accumulated 9.8 g/m^2 of AD 32 had no histologic evidence of anthracycline cardiac damage. Additional patients will be studied as they accumulate doses of AD 32.

Preliminary therapeutic data is available for 49 evaluable patients (Table 4). According to the previously defined criteria, six have demonstrated objective response [2]. Two of the evaluable patients with nonsmall cell lung cancer have responded. After 12 months, one patient continues to have a partial response of a pulmonary lesion. The other patient had regression of pulmonary disease for 1 year. Two of four patients with breast cancer have responded. One patient, who had not responded to adriamycin, has a regression of *en curasse* soft tissue disease lasting more than 2 months. One of three patients with bladder cancer had regression of pulmonary

Table 2. Current dose schedules of the Phase I/Phase II clinical study of AD 32[a]

AD 32 g/m^2	ADR eqv. mg/m^2	No.	Alive
3–4	450– 600	4	3
4–6	600– 900	3	2
6–8	900–1200	2	2
13	1950	1	1
		10	8

[a] Only patients who have received more than 3 g/m^2 of AD 32 are induced

Table 3. Cumulative dose of AD 32 received with the resultant histopathologic score based on endomyocardial biopsy (Billingham, unpublished data)[a]

g/m^2	Score	Expected
3.2	0	1.9 ± .72
3.5	1	1.9 ± .72
9.8	0	> 2.4 ± .52

[a] The expected value refers to that score which would be anticipated if an equivalent cumulative dose of adriamycin had been administered. In all instances, the AD 32 score was significantly less than expected from a comparable adriamycin score

Table 4. Response data according to histopathologic cell type

	No.	PR[a]	No Δ[b]	PD[c]
Lung (non small)	8	2	2	4
Breast	4	2	1	1
Bladder	3	1	1	1
Adeno (unknown)	3	1	0	2
Colon	7	0	0	7
Sarcoma	7	0	1	6
Renal	4	0	0	4
Melanoma	3	0	0	3
Head and Neck	3	0	0	3
Hepatoma	2	0	1	1
Miscellaneous	5	0	2	3
	49	6	8	35

[a] PR, partial response
[b] No Δ, no change or stabilization of disease
[c] PD, progressive disease

metastases lasting 5 months. One of three patients with an adenocarcinoma of an unknown origin continues to respond after 5 months of AD 32 therapy. Although no other objective responses have been observed, no histologic category has accrued enough patients to draw definitive therapeutic conclusions.

Discussion

Currently, the experimental and clinical data justify further development of AD 32. It was rationally synthesized as an analog of adriamycin; yet there are significant in vitro and in vivo differences. Compared to adriamycin in vitro, AD 32 demonstrated different cellular uptake and DNA binding. Differences are also seen in synchronized cell populations with AD 32 being cycle-specific but not phase-specific, while cytotoxicity of adriamycin is both cell cycle-specific and phase-specific. These data imply that adriamycin and AD 32 have different mechanisms of cytotoxicity.

The pharmacokinetic and metabolic degradation pathways of both adriamycin and AD 32 have been studied in a number of experimental species, with little difference among the species. Both drugs are metabolized and excreted via the biliary system with initial esterase cleavage and further reduction via an aldoketo reductase. AD 32 does not appear to be a prodrug of adriamycin. Also, there are the differences between AD 32 and adriamycin, both in their biologic effect in vitro and their therapeutic index in vivo.

AD 32 was selected for clinical trial based on both greater antitumor activity and less toxicity. Comparative studies of AD 32 and adriamycin consistently demonstrated that AD 32 is more effective than adriamycin in animal tumor models, producing a greater percent increase in survival and long-term cures. In direct comparative animal toxicity studies, using identical rapid-infusion schedules without steroids, AD 32 was less toxic than adriamycin. Myelosuppression was the limiting acute toxicity of both compounds, but at equally myelosuppressive doses, AD 32 induced less gastrointestinal toxicity (reflected by more weight gain), less skin toxicity, less nephrotoxicity, and significantly less cardiac toxicity.

The experimental assumptions made during the preclinical development of AD 32 are valid in humans. In the initial clinical studies, the preclinical tests of AD 32 were predictive of less gastrointestinal toxicity, less skin toxicity, and, in a preliminary way, less cardiac toxicity. Although at the present time inadequate data are available to make relative assessment of antitumor activity of AD 32 compared to adriamycin, AD 32 demonstrates antineoplastic activity. Further clinical testing of AD 32 is ongoing.

References

1. Billingham ME, Mason JW, Bristow MR, Daniels JR (1978) Anthracycline cardiomyopathy monitored by morphologic changes. Cancer Treat Rep 62: 865−872
2. Blum RH, Garnick MB, Israel M, Canellos GP, Henderson IC, Frei III E (to be published) Initial clinical evaluation of N-trifluoracetyladriamycin-14-valerate (AD 32), and adriamycin analog. Cancer Treat Rep 63
3. Bristow MR, Mason JW, Billingham ME, Daniels JR (1978) Duxorubicin cardiomyopathy: Evaluation by phonocardiography, endomyocardial biopsy and cardiac catheterization. Ann Intern Med 88: 168−175

4. Facchinetti T, Mantovani A, Cantoni L, Cantoni R, Salmona M (1978) Intercalation with DNA is a prerequisite for daunomycin, adriamycin and its congeners in inhibiting DNAase I. Chem Biol Interact 20: 97–102
5. Frei III E, Luce JK, Middleman E (1972) Clinical trials of adriamycin. In: Carter SK, DiMarco A, Ghione M, Krakoff IH, Mathe G (eds) International symposium of adriamycin. Springer, Berlin Heidelberg New York, pp 153–160
6. Garnick MB, Israel M, Pegg WJ, Blum RH, Smith E, Frei III E (1979) Hepatobiliary pharmacokinetics of AD 32 in man. Proc Am Assoc Cancer Res 20: 206
7. Henderson IC, Billingham M, Israel M, Krishan A, Frei III E (1978) Comparative cardiotoxicity studies with adriamycin (ADR) and AD 32 in rabbits. Proc Am Assoc Cancer Res 19: 158
8. Israel M, Garnick MB, Pegg WJ, Blum RH, Frei III E (1978) Preliminary pharmacology of AD 32 in man. Proc Am Assoc Cancer Res 19: 160
9. Israel M, Modest EJ, Frei III E (1975) N-trifluoroacetyladriamycin-14-valerate, an analog with greater experimental antitumor activity and less toxicity than adriamycin. Cancer Res 35: 1365–1368
10. Israel M, Pegg WJ, Wilkinson PM, Garnick MB (1979) HPLC applications in the analysis of adriamycin and analogs in biological fluids. In: Hawk GL (ed) Biological-biomedical applications of liquid chromatography. Dekker, New York, pp 413–428
11. Israel M, Pegg WJ, Wilkinson PM (1978) Urinary anthracycline metabolites from mice treated with adriamycin and N-trifluoroacetyladriamycin-14-valerate. J Pharmacol Exp Ther 204: 696–701
12. Israel M, Wilkinson PM, Osteen RT (1978) Comparative pharmacology of adriamycin and N-trifluoroacetyladriamycin-14-valerate in the monkey. Int Cancer Congr (Abstr) 1: 279
13. Israel M, Wilkinson PM, Pegg WJ, Frei III E (1978) Hepatobiliary metabolism and excretion of adriamycin and N-trifluoroacetyladriamycin-14-valerate in the rat. Cancer Res 38: 365–370
14. Krishan A, Dutt K, Israel M Personal communication
15. Krishan A, Ganapathi RN, Israel M (1978) Effect of adriamycin and analogs on the nuclear fluorescence of propidium iodide-stained cells. Cancer Res 38: 3656–3662
16. Krishan A, Israel M, Modest EJ, Frei III E (1976) Differences in cellular uptake and cytofluorescence of adriamycin and N-trifluoroacetyl-adriamycin-14-valerate. Cancer Res 36: 2114–2116
17. Lazarus H, Yuan G, Tan E, Israel M (1978) Comparative inhibitory effects of adriamycin, AD 32, and related compounds on in vitro cell growth and macromolecular synthesis. Proc Am Assoc Cancer Res 19: 159
18. Meriwether WD, Bachur NR (1972) Inhibition of DNA and RNA metabolism by daunorubicin and adriamycin in L-1210 mouse leukemia. Cancer Res 32: 1137–1142
19. Parker LM, Hirst M, Israel M (1978) N-trifluoroacetyladriamycin-14-valerate: Additonal mouse antitumor and toxicity studies. Cancer Treat Rep 62: 119–127
20. Sengupta SK, Seshadri R, Modest EJ, Israel M (1976) Comparative DNA-binding studies with adriamycin (ADR), N-trifluoroacetyladriamycin-14-valerate (AD 32) and related compounds. Proc Am Assoc Cancer Res 17: 109
21. Vecchi A, Cairo M, Mantovani A, Sironi M, Spreafico F (1978) Comparative antineoplastic activity of adriamycin and N-trifluoroacetyladriamycin-14-valerate. Cancer Treat Rep 62: 111–117

Available Data from Carminomycin Studies in the United States: The Acute Intermittent Intravenous Schedule

R. L. Comis, S. J. Ginsberg, S. D. Reich, L. H. Baker, and S. T. Crooke

The Department of Medicine, Suny Upstate Medical Center, USA – Syracuse, NY

Introduction

Carminomycin is an anthracycline antitumor antibiotic isolated from the mycelia of *Actinomadura carminata* [5]. The structure of carminomycin is presented in Fig. 1. Carminomycin is steriochemically quite similar to daunorubicin. The molecule differs from daunorubicin in the aglycone, being a desmethyl daunomycin. Carminomycin is active in a variety of animal tumor systems including L1210 and sarcoma 180 [9]. Antitumor activity does not appear to be schedule dependent in L1210 [2]. Carminomycin is orally absorbed, and the ratio of the LD_{50} of oral to intravenous administration is 2 : 1 in mice.

In animal toxicology systems including the mouse, beagle dog, and monkey, gastrointestinal, hematopoietic, and lymphoid toxicities predominate [3, 10, 12]. Cardiac effects, as measured by the Zbinden [11] rat cardiac toxicity model and the acute cardiac toxicity model proposed by Merski et al. [6], appear to be less than those observed with adriamycin.

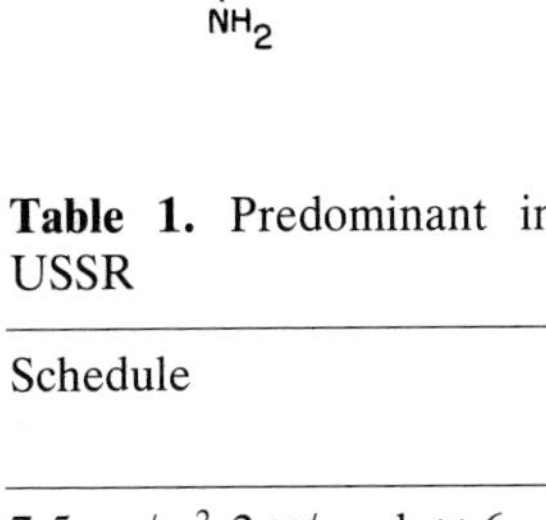

Fig. 1. The structure of carminomycin

Table 1. Predominant intravenous schedules in studies from the USSR

Schedule	dose/course	Treatment interval
7.5 mg/m² 2 ×/week × 6	35–45 mg/m²	4 weeks
5.5 mg/m²/day × 5	23–30 mg/m²	3 weeks

More than 300 patients have been treated with carminomycin in the Soviet Union. The predominant dose schedules which have been employed are presented in Table 1. The toxicities encountered included nausea and vomiting (18.3%), leukopenia (less than 3 000 cell/mm^3) (43.4%), and thrombocytopenia (8.4%). Less than 10% of the patients experienced alopecia, and no patient developed congestive heart failure. A spectrum of antitumor activity comparable to that of adriamycin has been reported [7, 8].

In order to initiate clinical trials within the United States the drug was obtained from the U.S.S.R. by Bristol Laboratories. Additional antitumor, pharmacologic, and toxicologic studies were performed, and the drug entered clinical trials approximately 2 years ago. Two studies were initiated, with the plan to initiate two additional clinical trials. Oral studies were initiated at Wayne State University at approximately one-third the minimum toxic dose (3 mg/m^2) in the most sensitive animal species, the beagle dog [1]. After five dose escalations, no significant toxicity was observed. At this dose, 36 mg/m^2, free carminomycin was detected in the plasma. Acute intravenous studies which were initiated at the SUNY Upstate Medical Center, Syracuse, New York are the subject of this report.

The acute intravenous studies were required by the Food and Drug Administration (FDA) to commence at a dose of 1 mg/m^2 which is one-half to one-quarter the minimum toxic dose in the beagle dog, in spite of the knowledge, based upon hundreds of patients treated in the Soviet Union, that the clinically useful dose per course would probably range between 23 and 30 mg/m^2.

After 12 patients were treated on the oral schedule and 17 patients were treated with the acute intravenous schedule, with no untoward toxicities noted, all studies in the United States were suspended by the FDA for reasons relating to technical aspects of the presentation of the chemistry section in the Investigational New Drug Application (IND).

Materials and Methods

Patients were eligible for the Phase I study if they were from 16−70 years of age, had a disease and/or stage for which no known effective therapy was available, or if they had failed therapy with appropriate, nonanthracycline-containing chemotherapeutic regimens. Informed consent was obtained from all patients. Patients were required to have normal hematopoietic, renal, and hepatic function, and no evidence for active cardiac disease. Pretreatment tests included an electrocardiogram, cardiac enzymes, complete blood count and platelet count, liver function tests, creatinine, BUN, and electrolytes. Appropriate radiologic and radionuclide studies were performed in all patients. Patients had repeat chest X rays and electrocardiograms at least every 4 weeks. Complete blood counts and platelet counts, as well as cardiac enzymes, were repeated weekly, and liver and renal function tests were repeated at least every 4 weeks. Most patients had continuous cardiac monitoring during drug administration and for 4−6 h after discontinuing the infusion. If measurable disease was present, measurements were performed at least every 4 weeks. Patients were examined weekly.

The drug was administered by rapid intravenous injection. Repeat courses were administered every 4 weeks if stable disease or a partial response occurred. Doses were not escalated within individual patients.

After extraction from 1-ml serum samples, carminomycin and carminomycinol levels were measured by high pressure liquid chromatography.

Results

A total of 17 patients were studied with doses of $1-15$ mg/m^2 prior to the suspension of the study. No consistent drug-related acute effects or myelosuppression were noted at doses below 15 mg/m^2 with or without multiple courses. The number of patients treated at each dose is presented as a percent of the expected maximally tolerated doses (MTD) based upon Soviet studies in Fig. 2. Fourteen patients received doses less than 15 mg/m^2.

All of the three patients treated at 15 mg/m^2 developed leukopenia. Two of three patients had stable disease (one metastatic renal cell carcinoma and one metastatic adenocarcinoma from an unknown primary source) for 7.5 and 8 months, respectively. Each received multiple courses of carminomycin therapy. The degree and timing of the leukocyte nadir is presented in Fig. 3. No evidence for cumulative myelosuppression was noted. In the patient who received multiple courses associated with reproducible leukopenia the WBC nadir occurred regularly at $1-2$ weeks, and recovery to $> 4\,000$ cells/mm^3 always occurred by 4 weeks. One patient developed transient thrombocytopenia after two courses of therapy (115×10^3/mm^3).

Nausea and vomiting occurred regularly in one patient directly after drug administration and lasted for $1-2$ days. No patient experienced total alopecia. Total

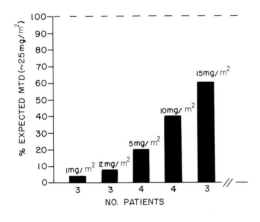

Fig. 2. Number of patients treated with carminomycin at each dose level presented as a percentage of the expected MTD based upon Russian studies

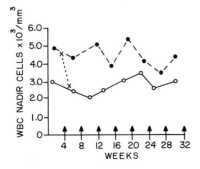

Fig. 3. Leukopenia associated with 15 mg/m^2 carminomycin. Leukocyte nadir is presented for each patient. The arrows represent the time of drug administration. All patients exhibited recovery of the white blood cell count to $\geq 4\,000$ cells/mm^3 by 4 weeks

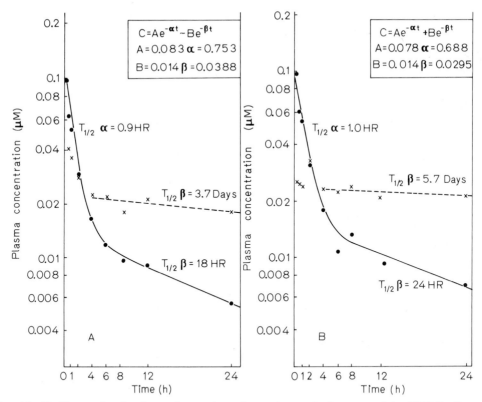

Fig. 4A, B. Plasma levels of carminomycin and carminomycinol measured by HPLC after bolus injection of 15 mg/m². PT: Q (SUNY), Carminomycin ●; Dose: 15 mg/m², Carminomycinol ×

doses of 120 and 135 mg/m² were administered to both patients treated with 15 mg/m² who had stable disease. No evidence for cardiac toxicity was apparent either from continuous cardiac monitoring during and directly after the infusion, or chronically. No hepatic or renal toxicity was noted.

Plasma carminomycin and carminomycinol levels were obtained in two patients receiving the drug at the 15 mg/m² dose (Fig. 4a, b). The carminomycin terminal phase half-life was 18 and 24 h, respectively. Carminomycinol rapidly appeared in the plasma, was persistently higher than parent compound levels, and decayed from the plasma very slowly with a half-life of 3.7 and 5.7 days, respectively.

Discussion

Large clinical trials performed in the Soviet Union have indicated that carminomycin is an active antitumor agent with acceptable acute toxicities. Most interestingly, the drug is well absorbed orally and significant cardiotoxicity has not been reported. All of these factors appropriately led to interest in the agent and the initiation of clinical trials in the United States. Unfortunately, after 26 patients had been treated with either the oral or intravenous preparation at nontoxic and almost certainly ineffective doses, further study was suspended. As a result no cancer patients are currently being treated with carminomycin in the United States.

Of the 17 cancer patients treated in our study, fourteen received doses of ≤ 10 mg/m^2. No significant drug-related toxicity — and no therapeutic effects — were noted. This pattern was predictable considering that these doses are well below the clinically effective doses employed in Russian studies. Mild, reproducible myelotoxicity occurred at doses of 15 mg/m^2 administered every 4 weeks. Although no objective responses were noted, two of three patients experienced stabilization of metastatic disease for 7.5 and 8 months, respectively. Further studies with this agent using the acute intravenous schedule are being performed in Europe.

In addition to the interest generated from the Russian clinical data, carminomycin is of increasing interest because of the recently reported data indicating that the drug may have a mechanism of action different from that of adriamycin [4] and because of our preliminary pharmacokinetic data showing the high, prolonged carminomycinol levels after bolus injection.

References

1. Baker LH, Kessel DH, Comis R, Riech SD, Defuria DM, Crooke ST (to be published) Phase I stdies of carminomycin in the United States. Cancer Treat Rep
2. Bradner WT (1977) Unpublished work
3. Crooke ST (1977) Carminomycin clinical brochure. Bristol Laboratories
4. Duvernay VH, Pachter JA, Crooke ST (1979) Carminomycin — evidence for a mechanism of action distinct from adriamycin. Proc Am Assoc Cancer Res 20: 35
5. Gause GF, Braznikova MG, Shorin VA (1974) A new antitumor antibiotic, carminomycin (NSC-180024). Cancer Chemother Rep 58: 255–256
6. Merski JA, Daskal Y, Crooke ST, Busch H (1979) Acute ultrasturctural effects of the antitumor antibiotic, carminomycin on the nucleoli of rat tissues. Cancer Res 39: 1239–1244
7. Perevodchikova NI, Gorbunova VA, Lichinister MR, Borisov VI, Alekseyev NA (1976) First phase of clinical study of the antitumor antibiotic carminomycin. Antibiotika 20: 853–856
8. Perevodchikova NI, Gorbunova VA, Lichinister MR, Moroz LV (1976) Carminomycin therapy in soft tissue sarcomas. Antibiotika 21: 657–660
9. Shorin VA, Brazhanov VS, Averbuch A, Lepeshkina GM, Grinshtein AM (1973) Antitumor activity of a new antibiotic, carminomycin. Antibiotika 18: 681–686
10. Shorin VA (1976) Unpublished work
11. Vertogradova TP, Goldberg LY, Filipposyants ST, Belova IP, Stepanova EG, Shepelevtseva NG (1974) Mechanism of the toxic effect of the antitumor antibiotic, carminomycin. Antibiotika 19: 50–57
12. Zbinden G, Brandle E (1975) Toxicologic screening of daunorubicin (NSC-32151), adriamycin (NSC-123127) and their derivatives in rats. Cancer Chemother Rep Part 1 59: 707–715

New Anthracycline Antibiotic Aclacinomycin A: Experimental Studies and Correlations with Clinical Trials

T. Oki, T. Takeuchi, S. Oka, and H. Umezawa

Central Research Laboratories, Sanraku-Ocean Co. Ltd., 4-9-1 Johnan, J − Fujisawa 251

Aclacinomycin A (ACM-A) is an anthracyclic antibiotic whose structure is represented in Fig. 1. It consists of the tetracyclic quinoid aglycone aklavinone linked to the aminosugar L-rhodosamine and to two other deoxysugars, 2-deoxy-L-fucose and L-cinerulose A [19, 20, 23, 24].

ACM-A is prepared by aerobic fermentation of *Streptomyces galilaeus* MA144-M1 and its mutants followed by solvent extraction and chromatographic purification. The antibiotic is a yellow amorphous powder of free base of is precipitated as the hydrochloride salt from chloroform and *n*-hexane. The physicochemical properties of ACM-A are summarized in Table 1. For the quantitative analysis of ACM-A, in addition to a microbiologic method using *Bacillus subtilis* as test organism, we used the spectrophotometric method based on the determination of absorbance at 433 nm and the fluorometric method using excitation and emission maxima at 440−445 nm and at 505 nm, respectively [9]. For estimation of ACM-A in mixtures with other pigments, such as in biologic fluids and extracts, we separated these other constituents by using thin-layer and high-performance liquid chromatographies.

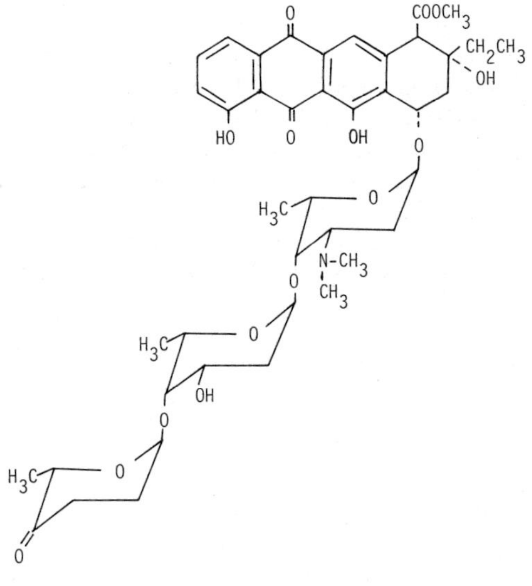

Fig. 1. Structure of aclacinomycin A

Table 1. Properties of aclacinomycin A

Empirical formula	$C_{42}H_{53}NO_{15}$
Molecular weight	811.9
pKa (50% DMF)	8.33, 9.55
Melting point (°C)	151–153
$[\alpha]_D^{22}$ (c = 1, $CHCl_3$)	−11.5°

Chromatographic Rf values on Silica gel plates:

$CHCl_3$-MeOH (20:1)	0.36
THF-DMF-H_2O (20:1:1)	0.70
$CHCl_3$-MeOH-AcOH-H_2O (15:2:0.5:0.05)	0.34

IR spectrum (KBr pellet): Major band (cm^{-1})
3450, 2980, 2945, 2820, 2760, 1735, 1620,
1600, 1010

Ultraviolet spectrum: λ_{max} (nm) ($E_{1\,cm}^{1\%}$)

90% MeOH	229.5 (550), 259 (326), 289.5 (135), 431 (161)
0.1 N HCl	229.5 (571), 258.5 (338), 290 (130), 431 (161)
0.1 N NaOH	239 (450), 287 (113), 523 (127)

In Vivo Antitumor Activity

The antitumor activity of ACM-A was tested in comparison with that of adriamycin (ADM) and daunomycin (DM) on various experimental tumors and is summarized in Table 2. An increased life span (ILS) ranging from 40%−122% was obtained at doses of 1−5 mg/kg once daily for 9 days for L1210 and P388 leukemias, but this activity was somewhat less than that of ADM [6]. ACM-A was moderately active on ascitic Lewis lung carcinoma and slightly active on B16 melanoma, and has been reported to be more effective than ADM in the treatment of various human xenograft tumors, CD mammary carcinoma, and colon 38 solid tumors [13]. The optimal dose of ACM-A was about twice that of ADM and DM. The influence of treatment schedule on the activity of ACM-A agaist IP-inoculated L1210 leukemia was studied, and ACM-A was more effective in daily and intermittent doses than in a single dose, as shown in Table 3. It was schedule-dependent for multiple dosing in this tumor system. The effect of the drug route on the ACM-A activity against IP- or IV-inoculated L1210 leukemia is summarized in Table 4. An interesting observation is that ACM-A is active on oral administration, differing from ADM and DM. This suggests that ACM-A could be well absorbed from the gastrointestinal tract. The marked inhibitory effects of oral ACM-A administration against sarcoma 180, lymphoma 6C3HED, and colon 26 solid tumors were also observed and are shown in Table 5. Combination therapy with ACM-A and vincristine, endoxan, cytosine arabinoside, natulan, or bleomycin against IP-implanted P388 leukemia and rat hepatoma AH66 was performed by Fujimoto et al. [3] and Kato et al. [8]. The most significant synergistic effect was seen in P388 leukemia system with the combination of 4 mg ACM-A/kg given every other day for 10 days, followed by endoxan at 200 mg/kg on day 7 (T/C = 460, 80-day survivors: 5 of 6), and 0.5 mg vincristine/kg given on days 1, 5, and 9, followed by ACM-A at 4 mg/kg on days 5, 9, and 13.

Table 2. Antitumor activity of aclacinomycin A

Tumor	Treatment		Opt. dosage (mg/kg/dose	%	
	Route	Day		ILS	Inh.
Ascites					
L-1210	IP	1−9	4	113	
	IP	1, 3, 5	16	80	
	PO	1−9	10	69	
P388	IP	1−9	5	108, 122[a]	
	IP	1, 5, 9	15	81[b]	
P388/ADM	IP	1. 5, 9	15	36[b]	
Ehrlich	IP	1, 5, 9	4	133	
B16	IP	1, 5, 9	3	43[a]	
Lewis lung	IP	1, 5, 9	1.6	50[a]	
Rat AH13 (IP)	IP	3−12	2	168	
Hepatoma AH44 (IV)	PO	3−12	2	200	
AH66, AH66F (IP)	IP	3−12	2	>170, 112	
AH7974 (IP)	IV	3−12	2	125	
AH41C (IV)	IV	3−12	2	200	
Solid					
Sarcoma 180	IP	1−10	6		94
	PO	1−9	10		62
Ehrlich	IP	1−10	6		74
CD mammary carcinoma	IP	1−9	6		100[a]
Colon 38	IP	5, 12, 19	12		84[a]
6C3HED/OG lymphoma	IP	0−10	1		56
Human xenograft					
Colon CX-1, IR	IP	1−10	1		91[a]
Colon CX-5, IR	IP	1−10	2		24[a]
Lung LX-1, IR	IP	1−10	2		64[a]
Breast MX-1, IR	IP	1−10	2		80[a]
Breast, SC	IP	1, 5, 9	9.4		47[a]
St-4 (Gastric adenocarcinoma, poorly diff.), SC	IP	1−10	3		64
St-15 (Gastric adenocarcinoma, poorly diff., muncinous), SC	IP	1−10	3		67
Co-3 (colon adenocarcinoma, well diff. tub.), SC	IP	1−10	3		56

Data obtained from: [a] Dr. J. D. Douros, NCI, USA
[b] Dr. F. M. Schable, Southern Research Institute
ILS (%): Increase in median life span,   Inh. (%): Inhibition of tumor growth (weight)

In Vitro Biologic Activity

ACM-A shows strong antimicrobial activity against gram-positive bacteria [21]. Mutagenicity of ACM-A was studied by means of two microbial mutation tests, the Ames' test [27] and the *rec* assay using *Bacillus subtilis* [28]. The drug was confirmed as

Table 3. Effect of treatment schedule of aclacinomycin A against L-1210 leukemia

Schedule (IP)	Optimal dosage (mg/kg/dose)	% ILS
Day 1 only	20.16[a]	62.58[a]
Day 3 only	20	46
Day 6 only	51	
Days 1, 5	15	66
Days 1, 3, 5	10	53
Days 1, 4, 7, 10	7.5	42
Days 1, 3, 5, 7, 9	5	74
Daily days 1−9	4	86 100[a]

10^5 cells, IP/CPF$_1$ mouse
[a] Data obtained from Bristol Laboratories (10^6 cells, IP/BDF$_1$ mouse)

Table 4. Influence of route of drug administration on the activity of aclacinomycin A in L-1210 leukemia inoculated intraperitoneally and intravenously

Route of tumor implantation	drug administration	Dose (mg/kg/day)	Mean survival days	ILS (%)
IP	IP	10	8.3	1.9
		5	12.3	51.2
		2.5	17.3	113.0 ($^1/_8$ cure)
		1.25	11.5	42.0
		−	8.1	
IP	PO	20	6.2	− 19.5
		10	12.3	59.7
		5	10.6	37.7
		2.5	9.1	11.8
		−	7.7	
IV	IP	10	8.2	36.7
		5	10.3	71.7
		2.5	7.8	30.0
		1.25	6.9	15.0
		−	6.0	
IV	PO	20	6.4	1.6
		10	10.3	63.5
		5	10.8	71.4
		2.5	7.4	17.5
		−	6.3	

Inoculum size: 10^5 cells/CDF$_1$ mouse (8 per group)
Drug administration: days 1−10

Table 5. Influence of route of drug administration on the activity of aclacinomycin A in solid sarcoma 180 implanted subcutaneously

Route of drug administration	Dose (mg/kg/day)	Average tumor weight (gr ± SE)	% inhibition
IP	Control	3.26 ± 0.47	0
	5	Toxic (11.9)[a]	–
	2.5	1.24 ± 0.20	62.0
	1.25	1.48 ± 0.24	54.6
	0.63	1.63 ± 0.31	50.0
PO	20	Toxic (6.9)[a]	–
	10	1.24 ± 0.13 ± 62.0	62.0
	5	1.83 ± 0.27	43.9
	2.5	1.66 ± 0.31	49.1

Incolum size: 2×10^6 cells/dd mouse
( )[a]: Mean survival (days)
Drug administration: days 1–10

Table 6. 50% Inhibition concentrations for cell growth and incorportion of ^{14}C-thymidine, ^{14}C-uridine, and ^{14}C-leucine into acid-insoluble materials

Drug	IC_{50} (μM)				
	RNA synthesis	DNA synthesis	DNA/RNA ratio	Protein synthesis	Cell growth (day 2)
Aclacinomycin A	0.12	1.5	12.5	7.8	0.041
Adriamycin	1.1	3.9	3.6	13.8	0.033
Daunomycin	0.78	1.3	1.7	19.2	0.049

Medium: RPMI 1640–20% calf serum at 37° C in a CO_2 incubator
Cell density: $5–7 \times 10^4$ cells/ml for growth test; $4–6 \times 10^5$ cells/ml for incorporation test
Pulse labeling: 60 min at 37° C in 0.05 μCi/ml precursor

having no mutagenic activity even at the 100-fold concentration of ADM, while ADM and even its aglycone adriamycinone had mutagenic activity.

We compared the inhibitory effects of ACM-A, ADM, and DM on the growth and nucleic acid biosynthesis of cultured L1210 cells. Table 6 shows 50% inhibition concentration (IC_{50} values) of the incorporation of ^{14}C-uridine, ^{14}C-thymidine, and ^{14}C-leucine into the TCA-insoluble materials and the cell growth of cultured L1210 cells on day 2 [19, 21]. The cytotoxicity of ACM-A was a little stronger than that of DM and weaker than ADM on a molar basis. ACM-A had much greater inhibitory effect on RNA synthesis than did ADM and DM. Calculating the ratio of the IC_{50} value for DNA synthesis to the IC_{59} for RNA synthesis, ACM-A inhibited RNA synthesis at about 10-fold lower concentrations than those required to inhibit DNA synthesis, while ADM and DM inhibited DNA and RNA syntheses at approximately equal concentrations. Crooke et al. [2] found that class II anthracyclines including ACM-A inhibit nucleolar RNA synthesis of Novikoff hepatoma N_1S_1 cells at a 170-fold

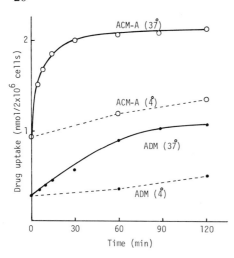

Fig. 2. Effect of time and temperature on uptake of aclacinomycin A and adriamycin by L-1210 cells. Cell: 2×10^6 cells/ml of L-1210 cells, Drug: 5 μM, Buffer: PBS (+) supplemented with 5.5 mM glucose (pH 7.0)

lower concentration than is necessary to inhibit DNA synthesis. Recently, Kajiwara et al. [7] reported that the drug blocks replication of HeLa cells by interfering with the synthesis of an RNA that is required for the chromatin maturation process.

The blockage by ACM-A of RNA polymerase reaction in *E. coli* is reversed by increasing amounts of the template DNA, but is not significantly affected by increased enzyme, suggesting that the inhibition is caused by the interaction with template DNA. Native calf thymus DNA appeared to possess one binding site per ca. six nucleotides for the drug with an apparent association constant of ca. $1.2 \times 10^6 \, M^{-1}$. Heat-denatured DNA showed much less affinity for the drug: one binding site per six nucleotides with an apparent binding constant of ca. $3.5 \times 10^4 \, M^{-1}$ [16]. The difference of association constants between double- and single-stranded DNAs suggested that ACM-A may be intercalated between base pairs of the DNA double helix. ^{14}C-ACM-A exhibited higher affinity for poly(dAdT) than for poly(dIdC).

Cellular uptake and accumulation of ACM-A and ADM by L1210 cells was examined according to the method of Bachur et al. [1]. Binding of ACM-A to the cells was faster and approximately 2- to 3-fold higher than that of ADM, as shown in Fig. 2. After 1-h incubation at 37° C, about 52% of the total ACM-A was taken up by the cells, whereas only 21% of the total ADM was accumulated in the cells.

Toxicity

The toxicity of ACM-A administered IP and IV to normal mice, rats, and dogs on various schedules of administration was studied. LD_{10}, which is the maximum tolerated dose per injection, the total LD_{10}, and total LD_{10} relative to the LD_{10} for a single treatment on only day 1 were determined and are shown in Table 7. The data indicate that the toxicity of ACM-A on successive doses is not cumulative; in other words, the maximum tolerated dose increased extensively on successive doses, while the toxicity of ADM on successive doses has been reported to be essentially additive, and consistent with the cumulative toxicity observed, even with intermittent dose schedules [5]. Therefore, ACM-A appears to be extensively metabolized in vivo in tissues.

Table 7. Maximum tolerated dose for aclacinomycin A in various dose schedules

Animal	Route	Schedule	MTD (mg/kg)		
			Per dose	Total dose	Total dose relative to
Mice (dd)	IP	1 dose	23	23	1
		qd × 9	6	54	2.3
		q4d × 3	15	45	2
Rats (Wistar)	IP	1 dose	15	15	1
		qd × 5	5	25	1.7
		qd × 30	1.5	45	3
		qd × 180	0.4	72	4.8
Dogs (beagle)	IV	1 dose	5	1	
		qd	2	14	2.8
		qd	1	75.5	15.1

The subacute toxicity test in beagle dogs given a daily intravenous dose of 0.3, 0.6, 1.0, and 1.4 mg ACM-A/kg for 3 months showed toxic signs such as weight loss, nausea, and vomiting when given 1–1.4 mg/kg. Bone marrow suppression and hepatic impairment developed and were dose-dependent to a certain degree, suggesting limiting factors for clinical trials. In fact, the phase I study of ACM-A conducted by Ogawa et al. [17], Majima et al. [14], Furue et al. [4], and Sakano et al. [25] revealed that gastrointestinal toxicity was not related to the dose and was well tolerated, but that thrombocytopenia, leukopenia, and transient and reversible hepatic dysfunction were dose dependent and limited the treatment. Concerning hematologic toxicity, the maximum tolerated dose of ACM-A in humans is considered to be 4 mg/kg. Autopsies and histologic findings on the dogs that died within 8 weeks after administration of 1.4 mg/kg showed bleeding of the gastrointestinal membranes, atrophic changes in the thymus and the spleen, and destruction of spermatocytes in the seminiferous tubules.

An ACM-A cooperative study group consisting of 35 institutions throughout Japan was organized, and the phase II trial is underway, employing the dose schedules as shown in Table 8. Tables 9 and 10 report the principal toxic manifestations related to the total dose and to the dose schedule of the drug. As described in a previous paper [18], loss of hair to complete alopecia, stomatitis, and ECG changes are extremely rare. Various degrees of nausea, vomiting, and anorexia occurred in the large majority of patients, but they were related neither to the dose schedule nor to the total dose. There is a high degree of individual patient variation. Hepatic dysfunction, including abnormal elevations of GTP, GOT, and LDH, was observed clearly after single-dose administration with a maximum tolerated dose level of 3.5–4 mg/kg. Major dose-limiting toxicity was hematologic, with moderate and severe leukopenia, thrombocytopenia, and anemia increasing in frequency with total doses of more than 6 mg/kg. In general, thrombocytopenia reached its nadir in a few days, prior to leukopenia, and both returned to prior levels within a week with prompt recovery. The median WBC and platelet nadir was related to the total dose level given and to the dose schedule. The toxic effects of ACM-A in the phase II study were predictable, usually reversible, and similar to those seen in the phase I study.

Table 8. Schedule model for the aclacinomycin phase II study

Single dose mg (mg/kg)	Schedule	Average weekly dose (mg)
20 (0.4)	Daily	140
	Daily, q2w	70
30−40	× 3/wk, day 1, 2, 3	90−120
(0.6−0.8)	× 3/wk, q2d	
40−60	× 2/wk, day 1, 2	80−120
(0.8−1.2)	× 2/wk, q3d	
80−100	× 1/wk	80−100
(1.6−2)		

MTD ≑ 4 mg/kg
Safety dose mark for weekly administration: 2 mg/kg

Table 9. Side effects related to dose schedule in the phase II study (IV)

Dose	Percentage of patients experiencing toxicity on dose schedule						
mg (mg/kg) No.	20 (0.4) daily (34)	20−40 (0.4−0.8) 3/wk (75)	40−60 (0.8−1.2) 2/wk (91)	60−100 (1.2−2) 1/wk (48)	> 100 (2) $1/_2$−3 wks (9)	Others (29)	Total (286)
Fever	6	4	2	4	11	3	4
Anorexia	47	32	52	54	56	48	46
Nausea and vomiting	32	41	47	63	78	66	49
Diarrhea	12	3	5	6	11	0	5
Lassitude	24	8	10	27	0	10	14
Phlebitis and vascular pain	3	3	4	2	0	3	3
Loss of hair	0	0	0	4	0	0	1
Stomatitis	9	3	11	0	0	7	6
Leukopenia[a]	26	27	44	38	89	7	34
Thrombocytopenia[b]	24	25	25	31	78	14	27
Anemia	21	17	19	15	44	0	17
Hemorrhage	3	1	1	4	0	3	2
Liver impairment	6	8	5	4	22	3	6
Kidney impairment	0	0	0	0	0	0	0
ECG changes	0	4	3	8	0	10	5
Others	6	5	1	0	0	3	3
No side effects	24	23	16	10	0	21	18

[a] Leukocytes, > 4000 cells/mm^3
[b] Platelets, > 100000 pl./mm^3

Cardiotoxicity

In studies designed to assess the cardiotoxicity of ACM-A in hamsters, rats, rabbits, and dogs, ACM-A displayed transient and reversible effects on cardiac function with both single and prolonged treatment at doses of more than 3−10 times those of ADM.

Table 10. Side effects related to cumulative dose in the phase II study (IV)

Total dose	% of side effects					
Per patient (mg) No. of case	< 100 (37)	101−300 (116)	301−500 (83)	501−1000 (39)	> 1001 (11)	Total (286)
Fever	3	4	5	3	0	4
Anorexia	43	41	53	51	36	46
Nausea and vomiting	57	50	40	56	64	49
Diarrhea	5	3	6	10	9	5
Lassitude	11	13	13	23	0	14
Phlebitis and vascular pain	3	3	1	8	0	3
Loss of hair	0	1	1	0	0	1
Stomatitis	5	3	7	13	0	6
Leukopenia	8	30	41	51	45	34
Thrombocytopenia	8	25	33	41	9	27
Anemia	3	14	20	28	27	17
Hemorrhage	3	3	0	3	0	2
Liver impairment	3	5	7	10	9	6
Kidney impairment	0	0	0	0	0	0
ECG changes	5	5	0	8	18	5
Others	8	3	1	3	0	3
No side effects	24	18	20	5	18	18

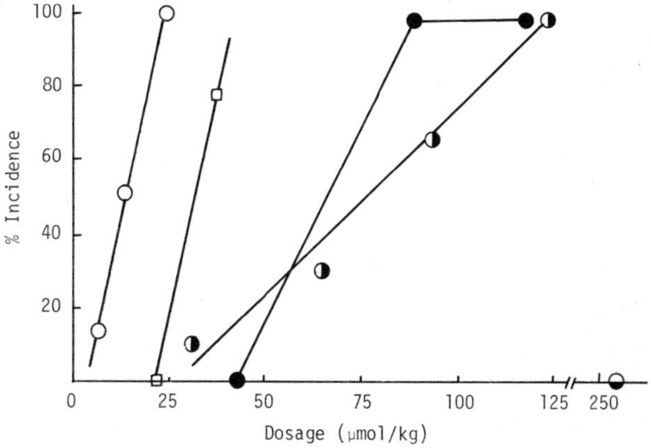

Fig. 3. Incidence of ECG alterations in hamsters by a single intravenous dose. ○, ADM; ●, ADMN; □, DM; ◑, ACM-A; ◓, AKN

Acute cardiotoxicity of ACM-A and ADM was examined in golden hamsters after a single intravenous administration. Male golden hamsters, 4−8 per group, were anesthetized intraperitoneally with sodium pentobarbital, and the test compound was injected into the femoral vein in a dose volume of 0.3 ml. Electrocardiograms were monitored by the standard lead II. The percent incidence of ECG alterations is shown in Fig. 3 on the molar basis of the molar basis of the compounds. ADM had the highest incidence on acute ECG alteration, and adriamycinone aglycone still retained the acute effect on ECG at a dose more than 4 times that of ADM. In contrast, ACM-A caused similar alterations on ECG at a dose more than tenfold that of ADM, as shown

Table 11. Acute ECG alterations of aclacinomycin A, adriamycin, and their aglycones (Single IV dose, STD lead II)

Compound	Dose (mg/kg)	ECG alteration	
Aclacinomycin A	100	Transient arrhythmia	Bradycardia (heart decrease) T wave flattening Transient extension of PR interval R wave amplitude reduction
Aklavinone	100	None	
Adriamycin	6.25	Arrhythmia S-T segment elevation Extrasystole	Bradycardia T wave flattening Transient extension of PR interval
		A-V block Bundle branch block	Transient elevation of R wave amplitude Transient reduction of S wave amplitude
Adriamycinone	36	S-T segment depression A-V block	Bradycardia

in Table 11, but aklavinone did not show any ECG alteration, even at a dose of 265 μmol/kg (100 mg/kg). Acute ECG alterations caused by ACM-A were reversible, but those caused by ADM were not.

Ultrastructural observation of cardiac myocyte in ADM-treated hamsters 10 min after receiving a single IV dose of 6.25 or 1.5 mg/kg indicated an extensive vacuolization of the sarcoplasmic reticulum, lipid deposition, formation of myelin figures, and mitochondrial damage (Fig. 4). A single IV dose of 25 mg ACM-A/kg did not produce any ultrastructural changes in the myocardia of hamsters, and an acute 100 mg/kg dose caused only scarce vacuolization, lipid deposition, and mitochondrial damages (Fig. 5).

A chronic cardiotoxicity test was conducted according to the NCI protocol in order to study the clinical and histopathologic alterations in rabbits treated with ACM-A and ADM and has just been finished. Male New Zealand white rabbits weighing 2 kg received IV ACM-A at 1, 2, 4, and 8 mg/kg and ADM at 2 mg/kg body wt. once a week for 13 weeks. As reviewed by Young [29], preliminary electron microscopic examination of the myocardium in rabbits treated with ADM revealed extensive reduction in myofibrillar bundles, myofibrillar lysis, and distortion and disruption of the Z band; mitochondria were swollen, their cristea disrupted, and they contained inclusion bodies. Glycogen granules were reduced (Fig. 6). On the contrary, the myocardial lesions in rabbits treated with ACM-A at 4 and 8 mg/kg once a week for 13 weeks were characterized by only slight swelling of mitochondria and rare myofibrillar lysis (Fig. 7), and these myocardial changes appeared to be reversible and not significant.

In the phase II study of ACM-A, there were no clinical signs of congestive heart failure which were considered to be due to the treatment, but there were acute and reversible

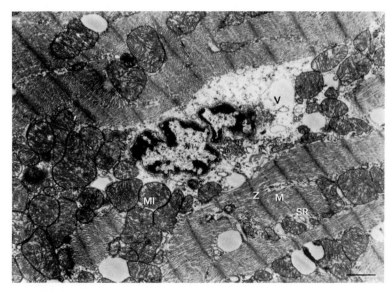

Fig. 4. Myocardium from a golden hamster 10 min after intravenous injection with 1.5 mg/kg of ADM. *Z*, z-band; *M*, M-line; *MI*, mitochondria; *SR*, sarcoplasmic reticulum; *T*, T-tube; *V*, vacuole

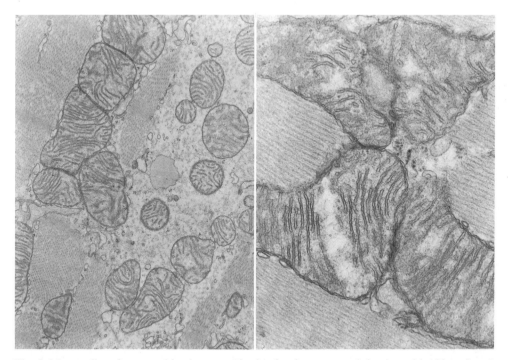

Fig. 5. Myocardium from a golden hamster 10 min after intravenous injection with 100 mg/kg of ACM-A

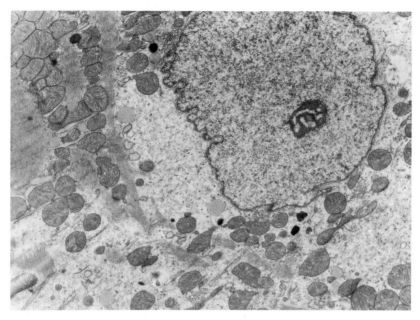

Fig. 6. Myocardium from a New Zealand white rabbit 7 days after intravenous treatment once a week for 13 weeks with 2 mg/kg ADM

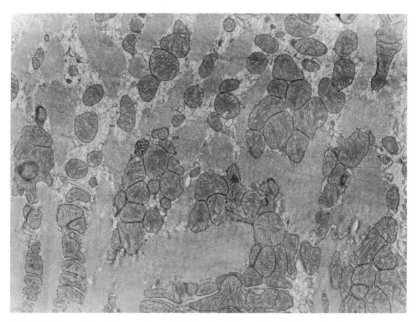

Fig. 7. Myocardium from a New Zealand white rabbit 7 days after intravenous treatment once a week for 13 weeks with 8 mg/kg ACM-A

ECG changes; flattening or inversion of T wave, ST depression, and sinus tachycardia increased in the patients who received a large dose of ACM-A − over 1 000 mg in total or over 2 mg/kg per dose.

Metabolism

Metabolic pathway and biotransformation of ACM-A was examined with rat liver homogenate [10, 12]. ACM-A was converted to the glycosidic metabolites M1 and N1 in the presence of NADPH or NADH under aerobic conditions [12]. From the structural analysis of M1 and N1, this reaction was found to be the non-degradative reduction of L-cinerulose to L-rhodinose or L-amicetose at the C-4'' keto group of ACM-A. Fractionation of rat liver cells demonstrated that three enzymes were involved in the formation of N1 and M1; first was the NADPH-dependent M1-forming enzyme, named as soluble cinerulose reductase I (mol. wt., 38 000), located in the soluble fraction. Two kinds of enzymes were involved in the formation of N1: one, in

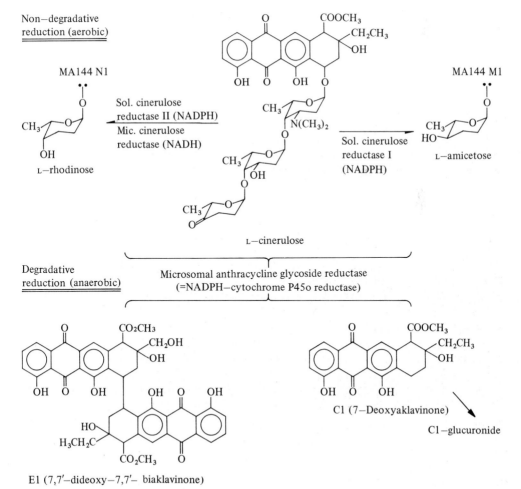

Fig. 8. Metabolism of aclacinomycin A

the soluble fraction and NADPH-dependent, was named as soluble cinerulose reductase II (mol. wt., 150 000); the other, located in the microsome fraction, was NADH-dependent microsomal cinerulose reductase [10], as shown in Fig. 8. These glycosidic metabolites retained antitumor activity in vivo and in vitro against L1210 leukemia comparable to that of ACM-A. These three enzymes could not reduce at the C-13 position of ADM and DM, and thus they might be different enzymes from the aldo-keto reductase. In contrast, under anaerobic conditions, ACM-A was degraded to the aglycone-type metabolites C1 (7-deoxyaklavinone) and E1 (7,7'-di-deoxy-7,7'-biaklavinone) by rat liver homogenate in the presence of NADPH or NADP through the reductive glycosidic cleavage at the C-7 position of anthracycline glycosides. Enzyme activity was found in the microsomal fraction, and the anthracycline glycoside reductase was extracted and purified from rat liver cells by solubilizing the microsome fraction with trypsin. Characterization of the enzyme revealed that this reductase is identical with the hepatic microsomal NADPH-cy-tochrome C reductase [11, 22]. The resulting aglycone metabolites were further resolubilized by conjugation with glucuronic acid and probably with sulfate to be excreted in the urine as shown in Fig. 8. This enzyme had the broad substrate specificity for various anthracyclic compounds to reduce not only the glycosidic bond of glycosides but also the C-7 hydroxyl group of aglycones [22]. Subcellular fractionation indicated a difference in the distribution of anthracycline glycoside reductase activity between the NADH system and the NADPH system. Although the highest activity was observed in the microsome fraction with NADPH, the result suggests that there may exist other NADH- or NADPH-dependent anthracycline glycoside reductases that possess low activity in comparison with NADPH-cytochrome P450 reductase. In fact, our preliminary experiments indicated that partially purified mitochondrial NADH dehydrogenase, soluble DT diaphorase after ammonium sulfate fractionation, and xanthine oxidase (obtained commercially) possessed the anthra-cycline glycoside reductase activity [11].

Pharmacology

The blood level and clearance of ACM-A in rabbits were examined by an IV injection of 5 mg ^{14}C-labeled ACM-A/kg in which the C-9 position and methyl groups at the C-10 position of aklavinone and at the C-3' position of rhodosamine were labeled biosynthetically by the incorporation of ^{14}C-1-propionate and methyl-^{14}C-methionine. As shown in Fig. 9, shortly after administration, the blood level of radioactivity decreased rapidly and remained nearly constant at a low level for a long period of time. A small amount reappeared with a characteristic rebound curve 6−9 h after injection. A substantial part of the drug in the blood was glycosidic metabolites M1 and N1. ACM-A was cleared for plasma with an initial half-life of about 2−5 min. The excretion pattern of ACM-A in the urine and feces following an IV injection of 5 mg ^{14}C-labeled ACM-A/kg in rabbits is shown in Fig. 10. Cumulative excretion of radioactivity into the urine of the injected radioactivity was about 50% within 72 h. However, excretion of chloroform-soluble radioactivity, corresponding to the fluorescent metabolites including aglycones and glycosidic metabolites, was only about 4%−5%. Therefore, most of the radioactivity excreted into the urine is due to water-soluble polar metabolites, including the conjugated metabolites, C1- and F-glucuronide, and sugar residues. Cumulative excretion of the radioactivity in

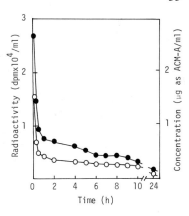

Fig. 9. Blood levels of aclacinomycin A in rabbit after intravenous injection. ^{14}C-ACM-A (10,296 dpm/μg): 5 mg/kg; whole blood: −●−; plasma: −○−

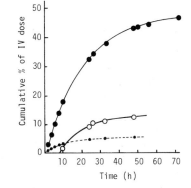

Fig. 10. Excretion of ^{14}C-aclacinomycin in rabbit after intravenous injection. ACM-A: 5 mg/kg (9.88×10^7 dpm/rabbit); Urine: −●− total, -- ● -- in CHCl$_3$; Feces: −○− in CHCl$_3$

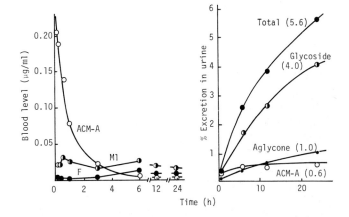

Fig. 11. Blood levels and urinary excretion of aclacinomycin A and its metabolites in humans (2 mg/kg, IV)

chloroform extract of feces was about 13% over 50 h. This radioactivity was found substantially in chloroform extract; water-soluble fraction contained little. A major metabolite in the feces was 7-deoxyaklavinone.

Blood level and urinary excretion in a cancer patient administered IV 2 mg ACM-A/kg were determined by the TLC-fluorescence method. As shown in Fig. 11, 0.2 μg ACM-A/ml was detected in whole blood 10 min after administration of the drug, and then decreased rapidly to low level. ACM-A was not detectable in plasma and blood cellular fraction 24 h after drug administration, but active metabolite M1 appeared shortly after drug administration and remained at 0.02−0.03 μg/ml for long period of time. The same trends were observed in several other patients. Total urinary excretion in this case was 5.6% within 24 h, and 4% of glycoside metabolites and 0.6% of ACM-A were recovered for 24 h. Urinary excretion in humans turned out to be highly variable concerning the duration of measurable excretion in different patients and the percentage of the dose administered.

Tissue distribution patterns of ACM-A in beagle dogs administered a dose of 15 mg/kg orally and intravenously are shown in Fig. 12. Tissue distribution was similar after both

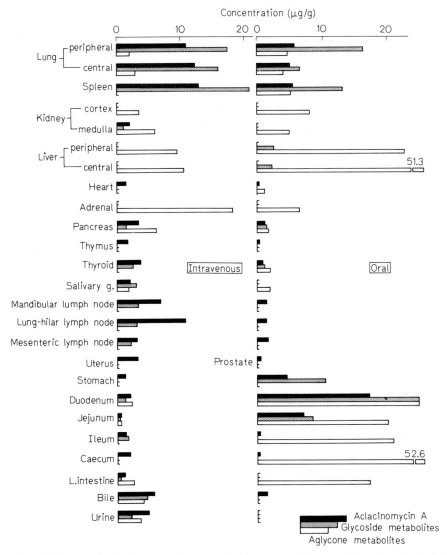

Fig. 12. Tissue distribution of aclacinomycin A in dogs 2 h after IV and oral administrations (15 mg/kg)

oral and intravenous routes, except that distribution was more extensive in the digestive tracts and the liver when ACM-A was orally administered. ACM-A and its active glycosidic metabolites were extensively distributed to the lung, spleen, lymphnodes, and bile, and also detected in the pancreas, thymus, thyroid, and salivary gland in both routes. Inactive aglycone metabolites were significantly distributed to the liver, kidney, and adrenal. In case of oral administration, the same inactive aglycone metabolites were predominant in the large intestine, cecum, and ileum as found in faces. Thus, orally administered ACM-A was well and rapidly absorbed through the digestive tracts and detected in blood and various tissues. No substantial differences were observed in absorption and excretion patterns between oral and intravenous administration of ACM-A.

Table 12. Response to malignant lymphoma to ACM-A treatment

	No. of cases	NR	PR	CR
Lymphosarcoma	9	2	6	1
Reticulum cell sarcoma	9	4	3	2
Hodgkin's disease	7	4	2	1
Total	25	10	11	4

Response rate ⩾ PR: 60%

Table 13. Therapeutic effect of ACM-A alone various recurrent and advanced cancers (IV + IA + IP)

Diagnosis	No. of cases	Karnofsky criteria			Response rate (%)
		< O-C	I-A	> I-B	> IA
Breast cancer	39	31	7	1	21
Uterine cancer	6	6			
Ovarian cancer	11	8	3		27
Lung cancer	45	40	5		11
Esophagus cancer	3	2		1	
Gastric cancer	58	52	5	1	10
Intestinal cancer	14	13	1		7
Hepatoma	3	3			
Pancreatic	6	6			
Urinary bladder cancer	11[a]	4	4	3	64
Sarcoma	7	5	1	1	
Head and neck cancer	5	4	1		
Miscellaneous	13	12		1	
Total	221	186	27	8	16

[a] 10 cases by IP instillation

Table 14. Therapeutic effect of ACM-A alone on solid tumors versus total doses

Total doses (mg)	No. of cases	Response (≥ I-A)	
		Cases	Rate (%)
101–300	79	2	3
301–500	71	9	13
500–1000	47	13	28
< 1001	14	4	29
Total	211	28	13

Clinical Effects with ACM-A Alone in the Phase II Study

Phase II clinical trials of ACM-A are underway at 35 institutions in Japan. From April 1978 to March 1979, 221 evaluable cases with various types of tumor were enlisted in this trial. Of the total number of patients treated with ACM-A alone, 207 patients received the drug IV through rapid infusion with several dose schedules as described above; 19 patients with gastric cancer were administered IA daily or intermittently with a dose of 0.4 −0.8 mg/kg through the abdominal aorta; 10 patients with metastatic peritonitis were given injections directly into the peritoneal cavity, and 11 patients with urinary bladder cancer had instilled 20−30 ml of the ACM-A solution at a concentration of 200−1 000 µg/ml into the bladder. Objective responses were observed in patients with malignant lymphoma (Table 12), breast cancer, ovarian cancer, lung cancer, gastric cancer, intestinal cancer, the urinary bladder cancer by IV and IP infusions, or bladder instillation as shown in Tables 13 and 14. Dr. K. Yamada and his co-workers recently achieved complete remission with the ACM-A treatment in two cases of acute myelogenous leukemia refractory to conventional multicombination chemotherapy, as previously reported by Mathé et al. [15].

We will continue the phase II study of ACM-A, searching for an adequate dose schedule in the treatment of mainly gastric and colon cancers, and then the combination therapy will be studied. In parallel, oral administration of ACM-A will be evaluated in the very near future.

Acknowledgments. The clinical study of ACM has been done by members of the ACM Cooperative Study Group in collaboration with the following institutions: National Sapporo Hospital, Research Institute for Tuberculosis, Leprosy and Cancer, Tohoku University Group, National Cancer Center Hospital, National Medical Center Hospital, Cancer Institute Hospital, Cancer Chemotherapy Center, Tokyo, Keio University Hospital Group, Teikyo University Hospital, Tokyo University Hospital, Chiba-Cancer Center Hospital, National Tachikawa Hospital, Shizuoka Red Cross Hospital, National Nagoya Hospital, Aichi Cancer Center Hospital, Nagoya University Hospital, Kyoto University Hospital, Research Institute for Microbial Diseases, Osaka University, The Center for Adult Diseases, Osaka, Okayama University Hospital, Research Institute for Nuclear Medicine and Biology, Hiroshima University, Kyushu University Hospital, National Kyushu Cancer Center Hospital.

We express our sincere thanks to all participants in this study for their generosity to permit this publication, and to Prof. Takashi Wakabayashi, Department of Pathology, Nagoya City University Medical Schoool, for his extensive electron microscopic observation.

References

1. Bachur NR, Steele M, Meriwether WD, Hildebrand RC (1976) Cellular pharmacodynamics of several anthracycline antibiotics. J Med Chem 19: 651−654
2. Crooke ST, Duvernay VH, Galvan L, Prestayko AW (1978) Structure-activity relationships of anthracyclines relative to effects on macromolecular syntheses. Mol Pharmacol 14: 290−298
3. Fujimoto S, Inagaki J, Horikoshi N, Ogawa M (to be published) Combination chemotherapy of a new anthracycline glycoside, aclacinomycin A, with active drugs to malignant lymphomas in P388 mouse leukemia system. Gan
4. Furue H, Komita T, Nakao I, Furukawa I, Yokoyama T, Kanko T (1978) Phase I and II study of aclacinomycin A. Int Cancer Congr (Abstr) 23: 9
5. Goldin A, Johnson RK (1975) Experimental tumor activity of adriamycin (NSC-123127). Cancer Chemother Rep 6: 137−145
6. Hori S, Shirai M, Hirano S, Oki T, Inui T, Tsukagoshi S, Ishizuka M, Takeuchi T, Umezawa H (1977) Antitumor activity of new anthracycline antibiotics, aclacinomycin-A and its analogs, and their toxicity. Gan 68: 685−690
7. Kajiwara K, Rogers AE, Mueller GC (1979) Effect of aclacinomycin A on chromatin and cell replication. AACR (Abstr), p 239
8. Kato T, Fujikawa T, Matsumoto F, Ota K (1979) Experimental study on the antitumor activity of aclacinomycin A and its combination chemotherapy. Cancer Chemother 6: 355−361
9. Kitamura I, Oki T, Inui T (1978) A sensitive analytical method for aclacinomycin A and its analogs by thin-layer chromatography and fluorescence scanning. J Antibiot (Tokyo) 31: 919−922
10. Komiyama T, Oki T, Inui T, Takeuchi T, Umezawa H (1978) NADH-dependent cinerulose reductase in rat liver microsomes. Biochem Biophys Res Commun 82: 188−195
11. Komiyama T, Oki T, Inui T, Takeuchi T, Umezawa H (to be published) Reduction of anthracycline glycoside by NADPH-cytochrome P-450 reductase. Gan
12. Komiyama T, Oki T, Inui T, Takeuchi T, Umezawa H (to be published) Reduction of cinerulose in aclacinomycin A by soluble and microsomal cinerulose reductases. Gan
13. Kubota T, Shimosato Y, Moon YH, Matsumoto S, Ishibiki K, Abe O (1978) Experimental cancer chemotherapy of human stomach and colon carcinomas serially transplanted in nude mice. IV. Anthracyclines. Cancer Chemother 5: 535−534
14. Majima H, Oguro M, Takagi T (1978) Phase I study of aclacinomycin A. Int Cancer Congr (Abstr) 23: 8
15. Mathé G, Bayssas M, Gouveia J, Dantchev D, Ribaud P, Machover D, Misset JL, Schwarzenberg L, Jasmin C, Hayat M (1978) Preliminary results of a phase II trial of aclacinomycin in acute leukemia and lymphosarcoma. Cancer Chemother Pharmacol 1: 259−262
16. Misumi M, Yamaki H, Akiyama T, Tanaka N (1979) Mechanism of action of aclacinomycin A. II. The interaction with DNA and with tubulin. J Antibiot (Tokyo) 32: 48−52
17. Ogawa M, Inagaki J, Horikoshi N, Inoue K, Chinen T, Ueoka H, Nagura E (to be published) Clinical study of aclacinomycin A. Can Treat Rep
18. Oka S (1978) A review of clinical studies on aclacinomycin A − Phase I and preliminary phase II evaluation of ACM. Sci Rep Res Inst Tohoku Univ [Med] 25: 37−49

19. Oki T, Matsuzawa Y, Yoshimoto A, Numata K, Kitamura I, Hori S, Takamatsu A, Umezawa H, Ishizuka M, Naganawa H, Suda H, Hamada M, Takeuchi T (1975) New antitumor antibiotics, aclacinomycins A and B. J Antibiot (Tokyo) 28: 830−834
20. Oki T, Shibamoto N, Matsuzawa Y, Ogasawara T, Yoshimoto A, Kitamura I, Inui T, Naganawa H, Takeuchi T, Umezawa H (1977) Production of nineteen anthracyclic compounds by *streptomyces galilaeus* MA144-M1. J Antibiot (Tokyo) 30: 683−687
21. Oki T (1977) New anthracycline antibiotics. Jpn J Antibiot 30: 70−84
22. Oki T, Komiyama T, Tone H, Inui T, Takeuchi T, Umezawa H (1977) Reductive cleavage of anthracycline glycosides by microsomal NADPH-cytochrome C reductase. J Antibiot (Tokyo) 30: 613−615
23. Oki T, Kitamura I, Yoshimoto A, Matsuzawa Y, Shibamoto N, Ogasawara T, Inui T, Takamatsu A, Takeuchi T, Masuda T, Hamada M, Suda H, Ishizuka M, Sawa T, Umezawa H (to be published) Antitumor anthracyclic antibiotics, aclacinomycin A and its analogues. I. Taxonomy, production, isolation and physicochemical properties. J Antibiot (Tokyo)
24. Oki T, Kitamura I, Matsuzawa Y, Shibamoto N, Ogasawara T, Yoshimoto A, Inui T, Naganawa H, Takeuchi T, Umezawa H (to be published) Antitumor anthracyclic antibiotics, aclacinomycin A and its analogues. II. Structural determination. J Antibiot (Tokyo)
25. Sakano T, Okazaki N, Ise T, Kitaoka K, Kimura K (1978) Phase I study of aclacinomycin A. Jpn J Clin Oncol 8: 49−53
26. Sunaga T, Fujino H, Nishiyama K, Ohmori K, Uchiyama I, Sugiyama H, Hattori M, Maezawa H (1978) Fine structure of adriamycin or aclacinomycin induced cardiomyopathy. J Electron Microsc (Tokyo) 11: 5−6
27. Umezawa K, Sawamura M, Matsushima T, Sugimura T (1978) Mutagenicity of aclacinomycin A and daunomycin derivatives. Cancer Res 38: 1782−1784
28. Yoshimoto A, Oki T, Inui T (1978) Differential antimicrobial activities of anthracycline antibiotics on rec⁻ *bacillus subtilis*. J Antibiot (Tokyo) 31: 92−94
29. Young DM (1975) Pathologic effects of adriamycin (NSC-123127) in experimental systems. Cancer Chemother Rep 6: 159−175

Current Status of PEP Bleomycin Studies in Japan

S. Ikeda, H. Miyasato, H. Nakayama, K. Tajima, and A. Sato*

Department of Dermatology, Saitama Medical School, Moroyama-cho,
J — Saitama Prefecture 350-04

Introduction

Bleomycin is an antitumor antibiotic produced by an actinomyces, *Streptomyces verticillus,* isolated from soil by Umezawa et al. [19] in 1962, and occurs as a complex of basic, water-soluble polypeptides made up of 13 bleomycins different in terminal amine, with bleomycin A_2 as the chief component. In 1965, Ichikawa et al. [4] made its clinical application, proving it to be effective in treating squamous cell carcinoma. The drug was later shown to be effective against malignant lymphoma as well. In the meantime, the characteristic adverse reactions to this drug have been revealed, indicating that the drug, unlike the other carcinostatics introduced to date, is accompanied by less adverse effects on the hematopoietic organs, while it may give rise to pulmonary fibrosis, which has recently been accepted as occurring with a frequency of 5%−10% [8, 11]. Such situations have led to a desire for the introduction of a new bleomycin (BLM) that is no less effective than the currently available bleomycin, but which is accompanied by lower incidences of adverse reactions. About 300 new derivatives of BLM, having the same basal BLM structure but different terminal amines, were screened, and pepleomycin (experimental code: NK 631), which was found in animal experiments to be close to the above-mentioned target properties, was chosen [5, 9, 12, 15, 17, 18]. Its chemical structure is shown in Fig. 1. It occurs as a single compound differing from the present BLM in the terminal amine of moiety VII.

On the basis of the phase I study made in 1977, the preliminary phase II study was started in April, 1977 at 42 medical facilities in Japan. The present paper summarizes the result of this study achieved during the period from April, 1977, through March, 1979 at the 42 institutes, including 75 cases of malignant skin tumors treated with pepleomycin.

A randomized comparison of pepleomycin with the present bleomycin has shown the former to be at least equal to or perhaps much better than the present bleomycin due

* We are greatly indebted to the assistance given by the Pepleomycin Research Project of Japan, Dermatological Section (Dr. A. Kukita, at the University of Tokyo, Tokyo; Dr. M. Tashiro, at Kagoshima University, Kagoshima; Dr. Y. Miura, at Hokkaido University, Sapporo; Dr. T. Arao, at Kumamoto University, Kumamoto; Dr. H. Urabe, at Kyushu University, Fukuoka, and Dr. M. Matsunaka, at Wakayama Medical College, Wakayama)

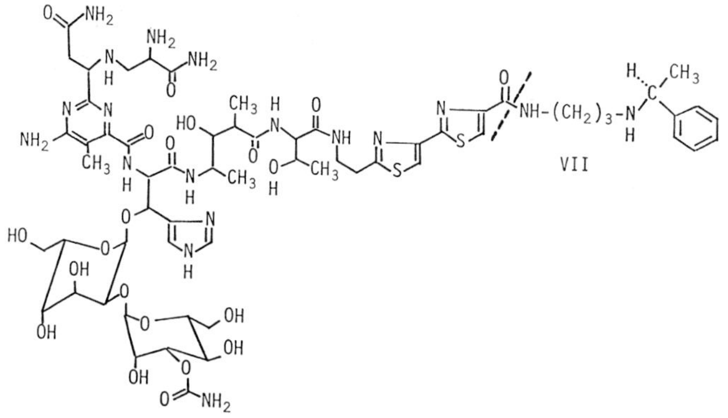

Fig. 1. Chemical structure of pepleomycin

Table 1. Responses to pepleomycin (by single use)

Malignancies	Evaluable cases	Antitumor effects			
		+++ (%)	++ (%)	+ (%)	− (%)
Head and neck (S.C.C.)	250	50 (20)	74 (30)	61 (24)	65 (26)
Skin (S.C.C.)	36	15 (42)	12 (33)	6 (17)	3 (8)
Malignant lymphoma	24	15 (63)	5 (21)	2 (8)	2 (8)
Lung (various malignancies)	34	0	3 (9)	6 (18)	25 (74)
Prostate (various malignancies)	22	0	5 (23)	5 (23)	12 (55)
Total cases	366	80	99	80	107

Table 2. Comparison between toxic effects of pepleomycin and those of bleomycin

Toxic effects	Pepleomycin		Bleomycin[a]	
	Number of cases	Incidence (%)	Number of cases	Incidence (%)
Alopecia	92	27.4	476	29.5
Anorexia	90	26.8	463	28.7
Fever	88	26.2	642	39.8
Generalized malaise	48	14.3	258	16.0
Stomatitis	45	13.4	215	13.3
Eruption	37	11.0	109	6.8
Change of nails	34	10.1	180	11.2
Pigmentation	33	9.8	297	18.4
Sclerosis	31	9.2	353	21.9
Nausea and vomiting	29	8.6	236	14.6
Pulmonary changes	20	6.0	165	10.2
Others	25	7.4		
No toxicity	138	37.7		

[a] Quoted from the Summary of Adverse Reactions to BLM submitted to the Japanese Ministry of Health and Welfare in October, 1973, covering 1613 patients treated at 92 institutions

to its possible less toxicity. In 366 cases analyzed in the Pepleomycin Research Project of Japan, an overall response rate of 86% has been achieved in the cases of squamous cell carcinoma and in cases of non-Hodgkin's lymphoma. In all the cases, the response occurred, regardless of the administration regimen employed (Table 1).

Table 2 compares the toxic effects of pepleomycin with those of bleomycin. Analysis of these toxic effects by their frequencies indicates, however, that fever and pulmonary toxicity were less frequent, but anorexia, malaise, and skin eruptions were more frequent under pepleomycin treatment.

Materials

A total of 86 cases of malignant skin tumors were treated with pepleomycin during the 23-month period from April, 1977, through March, 1979; and the effects of the treatment were evaluable in 75 of them. The data from these 75 cases are summarized in Table 3.

Dosage Schedule

Pepleomycin was mainly administered IM. In a few cases, however, it was given by drip infusion because of poor general condition. After the first or sometimes after the second administration of 5 mg of this drug, its dosage was increased to 10 mg, 3 times a week. One course of pepleomycin treatment consisted of a total dose of 200 mg. Many cases, however, responded markedly to lower doses. In such cases, no further administration of the drug was done.

In squamous cell carcinoma, we performed one course of pepleomycin treatment, and then operation, irradiation, or cryosurgery in order to attain a complete cure for the disease. In some recent cases, simultaneous combination therapy with pepleomycin and bestatin (30 mg per day, orally) was performed, and the therapy, with a total dose of 100 mg pepleomycin, proved markedly effective in half of them.

Likewise, malignant lymphoma was generally treated with pepleomycin on a similar dosage schedule to that for squamous cell carcinoma. When one course of pepleomycin treatment proved successful, the treatment was "switched over to consolidation therapy with vincristine, cyclophosphamide, 6-mercaptopurine and prednisolone (VEMP), and further to maintenance therapy with cyclophosphamide and 6-mercaptopurine (EM)".

In stage IV malignant melanoma, pepleomycin alone was not expected to be so effective. Therefore, we tried 3-drug combination chemotherapy with pepleomyin, 10 mg, IM, 5 times a course, from day 1 through day 9, to a total dose of 50 mg; Me-CCNU, 100 mg, orally, once a course, on day 1, and vincristine (VCR), 1 mg, IV, also once a course, on day 1. At 2-week intervals, this course was repeated 3−4 times, depending on its antitumor effect and side effects. This schedule is different from the protocol of De Wasch described in Table 4.

Lately, the same 3-drug combination chemotherapy has been performed even in cases of operable, stage I or II malignant melanoma in order to improve prognosis. We also make it a rule to use bestatin simultaneously in all cases of malignant melanoma, irrespective of stage.

Table 3. Clinical responses to pepleomycin (April, 1977–March, 1979)

Malignancies	Number of cases entered	Number of evaluable cases	Antitumor effects				Response rate (%)
			+++	++	+	−	
1. Squamous cell carcinoma	45	36	15	12	6	3	91.7
2. Oral florid papillomatosis	1	1	1	0	0	0	100
3. Keratocanthoma	2	2	2	0	0	0	100
4. Malignant lymphoma	16	14	6	5	2	1	92.2
5. Immunoblastic lymphadenopathy	1	1	1	0	0	0	100
6. Malignant melanoma	8	5	0	1	2	2	60
7. Bowen's disease	3	3	0	0	0	3	0
8. Actinic keratosis	2	2	0	0	0	2	0
9. Basal cell epithelioma	3	3	0	0	0	3	0
10. Mammary Paget's disease	1	1	0	0	0	1	0
11. Genital Paget's disease	1	1	0	0	0	1	0
12. Dermatofibrosarcoma protuberans	1	1	0	0	0	1	0
13. Alveolar soft part sarcoma	1	1	0	0	0	1	0
14. Angiosarcoma	1	1	0	0	0	1	0

Table 4. Triple drug combination chemotherapy for malignant melanoma (De Wasch et al. 1976)

Pepleomycin 10 mg (IM)											Pepleomycin 10 mg (IM)						
↓ ↓ ↓ ↓ ↓ ○	○	○	○	○	○	↓	↓	↓	↓	↓ ○ ○							
1 3 5 7 9 11	13	15	17	19	21	23	25	27	29	31 (days)							

1 3 5 7 9 11 · 13 · 15 · 17 · 19 · 21 · 23 · 25 · 27 · 29 · 31 (days)
↑
mCCNU, 100 mg, orally
↑
VCR, 1 mg, IV
[← 1st course →]
Pepleomycin + mCCNU + VCR, 3–4 courses

23
↑
mCCNU, 100 mg, orally
↑
VCR, 1 mg, IV
[← 2nd course →]

BLM (IV) 15 mg, 1/w, 20 times
CCNU (orally), 200 mg, 1/6 w
VCR (IV), 1.4–2 mg, 1/w, 20 times

Evaluation of Effects of Pepleomycin

The antitumor effects (primary effects) of pepleomycin were evaluated clinically by the following criteria:
(1) Marked effect (+++) – a regression of tumor by not less than 90%, (2) moderate effect (++) – a regression of tumor by not less than 50%; (3) slight effect (+) – a regression of tumor by not less than 25% but less than 50%; and (4) no effect (−) – a regression of tumor by less than 25% or "no change" or an enlargement of tumor.

Results

Squamous Cell Carcinoma

Of 36 cases of squamous cell carcinoma, 15 showed a marked response; 12, a moderate response, and six, a slight response. An effective rate of 100% was achieved in one case of oral florid papillomatosis and two of keratoacanthoma (Figs. 2–5). The interrelationship between Ts (the local extensions of primary tumors) of squamous cell carcinoma and clinical effects of pepleomycin against the malignancy was examined. In T_1 and T_2 cases, a marked response was attained, but in T_3 and T_4, the effect of the drug was not so prominent. A correlation was noted between the number of T and the average total dose of pepleomycin: in many T_1 and T_2 cases, a total dose of less than 100 mg of pepleomycin proved markedly effective, whereas in (T_3 and) T_4 cases, even as large a total dose as 270 mg of pepleomycin was only moderately effective (Table 5).
Of six cases of squamous cell carcinoma in which pepleomycin was used in combination with bestatin, three showed a marked response even to such lower doses

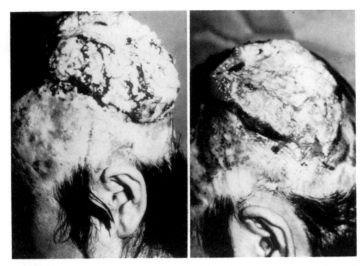

Fig. 2. *(Left)* A 44-year-old female with a huge squamous cell carcinoma on a scar $(T_4N_0M_0)$; before treatment. *(Right)* After treatment with a total dose of 210 mg pepleomycin. The tumor is promintenly diminished in size

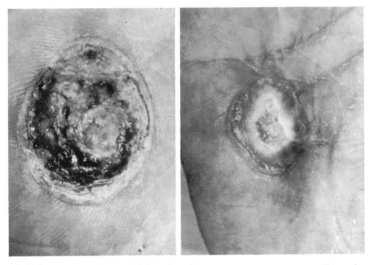

Fig. 3. *(Left)* A 40-year-old male with recurrent squamous cell carcinoma of the palm. It has been operated on at another hospital several times $(T_2N_0M_0)$; before treatment. *(Right)* After treatment with a total dose of 120 mg pepleomycin. The treatment has been markedly effective both clinically and histologically

of pepleomycin as 65–120 mg. We have an impression that the effect of pepleomycin is augmented by bestatin when the two drugs are used in combination. Lymph node metastasis responded poorly to pepleomycin. Especially, neither of two N_3 cases showed any response (Table 5).

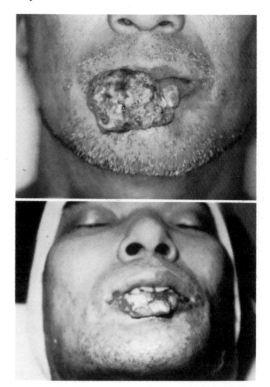

Fig. 4. *(Top)* A 47-year-old male with a huge squamous cell carcinoma of the lower lip ($T_3N_0M_0$); before treatment. *(Bottom)* After treatment with half a course of pepleomycin combined with bestatin (30 mg, orally, every day)

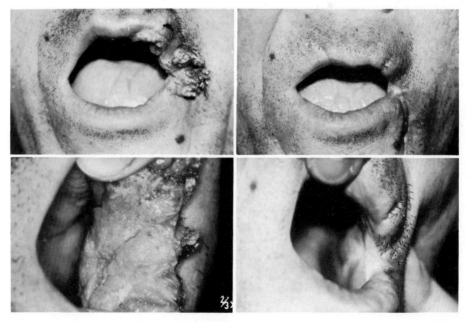

Fig. 5. *(Left)* A 64-year-old male with oral florid papillomatosis; before treatment. *(Right)* 14 months after treatment with a total dose of 200 mg pepleomycin

Table 5

	Number of cases	Clinical effects				Response rate (%)
		+++	++	+	−	
(1) Interrelationship between Ts and clinical effects						
T_1	8	6	2	0	0	100
T_2	14	7	5	2	0	100
T_3	8	2	2	2	2	75
T_4	6	0	3	2	1	83.3
	36	15 (41.7%)	12 (33.3%)	6 (16.7%)	3 (0.83%)	91.7%
(2) Interrelationship between Ns and clinical effects						
N_1	6	0	3	1	2	66.7
N_3	2	0	0	0	2	0
	8	0	3	1	4	50%

Table 6. Clinical responses of malignant lymphoma to pepleomycin

Malignancies	Number of cases	Clinical responses			Response rate (%)
		Complete remission	Partial remission	No response	
Non-Hodgkin's lymphoma					
Lymphocytic type	2	1	1	0	100
Lymphoblastic type	2	2	0	0	100
Histiocytic type	5	2	2	1	80
Mycosis fungoides	4	3	1	0	100
Reticulosis cutis	1	1	0	0	100
Total	14	9	4	1	92.9
Immunoblastic lymphadenopathy	1	1	0	0	100

Malignant Lymphoma

Pepleomycin was used in the treatment of 14 cases of non-Hodgkin's lymphoma. A complete remission was obtained in nine, and a partial remission in four, with a response rate of 92.4%.

Pepleomycin yielded a response rate of 80% in reticulum cell lymphoma, 100% in mycosis fungoides, and also in lymphocytic and lymphoblastic lymphoma (Table 6; Figs. 6 and 7).

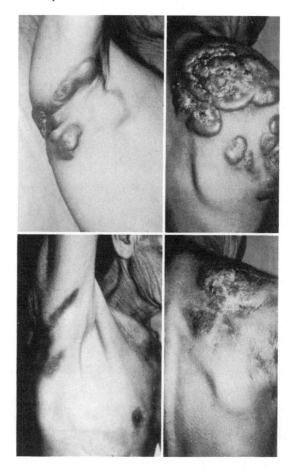

Fig. 6. *(Top)* A 67-year-old male with stage II reticulum cell lymphoma; before treatment. *(Bottom)* After treatment with a total dose of 195 mg pepleomycin. Two months later, huge tumor developed in the lungs and GI tract, and the patient died 6 months later

In a case of immunoblastic lymphadenopathy, an excellent effect was attained by one course of pepleomycin treatment, followed by a successful maintenance therapy with bestatin alone for 9 months.

Malignant Melanoma

Eight cases of malignant melanoma (2 stage I, 2 stage II, and 4 stage IV cases) were treated by three-drug combination chemotherapy. In one of the stage I cases, the primary tumor diminished in size in response to one preoperative course of the therapy. After a radical operation, we performed three additional course. Nine months later, the patient is alive with no evidence of active disease (Table 7).

The triple drug combination chemotherapy has been evaluated as slightly to moderately effective in two of the four stage IV cases. However, these two cases terminated fatally from metastases to the brain in spite of the two to four courses of this combination chemotherapy. We assume that the three-drug combination chemotherapy is in no way effective against brain metastasis (Figs. 8 and 9).

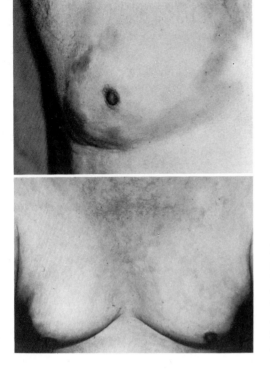

Fig. 7. *(Top)* A 67-year-old male with stage IV lymphoblastic lymphoma; before treatment. *(Bottom)* After treatment with a total dose of 55 mg pepleomycin. Three months later, huge tumors developed in bilateral epididymides and retroperitoneum, and the patient died of uremia

A maximum period of 2 years has passed since the end of the combination chemotherapy in the cases of stage I and II operable melanomas, but neither recurrence nor metastasis has been observed. At the present moment, it is difficult to evaluate the effect of the combination therapy in these cases; and it appears necessary to follow-up further their courses so as to prove whether relapse or metastasis occurs or whether the treatment exerts any life-prolonging effect or not.

Antitumor Spectrum of Pepleomycin

Since pepleomycin alone scarcely yields any effect against carcinoma in situ (e.g., two cases of actinic keratosis, and three of Bowen's disease), three cases of basal cell epithelioma, adenocarcinoma (e.g., one case of mammary Paget's disease, and one of genital Paget's disease), and soft tissue sarcoma (e.g., one case each of dermato-fibrosarcoma protuberans, alveolar soft part sarcoma and angiosarcoma), the antitumor spectrum of pepleomycin against malignant skin tumors should unfortunately by considered no broader than that of bleomycin (Table 1).

Side Effects of Pepleomycin

The sorts of side effects of pepleomycin are almost the same as those of bleomycin, that is, anorexia, fever following injection, alopecia, generalized malaise, nausea and vomiting, pigmentation of the fingers and palms, skin rashes, edema of the fingers,

Table 7. Clinical effects against malignant melanoma (March, 1979)

Case No.	Age and sex	TNM	Stage	Stage of administration	Dosage	Response	Prognosis
1	71, M	$pT_3N_0M_0$	I	Preoperative Postoperative	1 course 2 courses	+ ?	Alive for 9 months; no evidence of active disease
2	54, F	$pT_3N_0M_0$	I	Postoperative	4 courses	?	Alive for 5 months; no evidence of active disease
3	52, M	$pT_3N_1M_0$ $\rightarrow$ $T_0N_0M_0$	II	Postoperative	270 mg	?	Alive for 24 months; no evidence of active disease
4	67, M	$pT_3N_1M_0$	II	Postoperative	70 mg	?	Alive for 1 month; no evidence of active disease
5	38, M	$T_0N_0M_1$	IV		4 courses	++	The patient died of cancer in 4 months
6	16, F	$T_0N_0M_1$	IV	Preoperative Postoperative	1 course 2 courses	− ?	Alive for 26 months, with disease
7	24, M	$T_0N_0M_1$	IV		2 courses	+	The patient died of cancer in 5 months
8	64, M	$pT_3N_1M_1$	IV		1 course	−	The patient died of cancer in 2 weeks

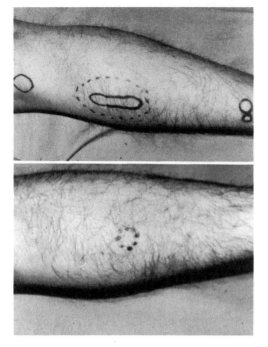

Fig. 8. *(Top)* A 38-year-old male with extensive metastases only to the skin and subcutaneous tissue of malignant melanoma ($T_0N_0M_1$, stage IV); before treatment. *(Bottom)* After three courses of three-drug combination chemotherapy with pepleomycin, mCCNU, and VCR. Several subcutaneous metastases diminished in size and decreased in number. Several months later, the patient died of brain metastasis

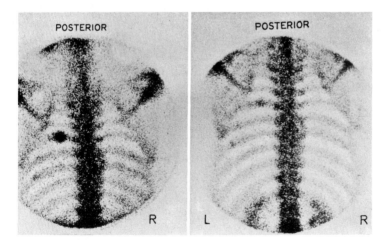

Fig. 9. *(Left)* A 24-year-old male with a metastasis to the left VI rib ($T_0N_0M_1$, stage IV); before treatment. *(Right)* After three courses of a three-drug combination chemotherapy. Markedly reduced uptake of the isotope by the same rib. Three months later, the patient died of brain metastasis

peripheral nerve symptoms, derformity of nails, hyperkeratosis in pressure areas, extremely pulmonary fibrosis and shocklike symptoms. Neither hepatic and renal toxicities or bone marrow depressions have been observed. However, we have been impressed that the fever under pepleomycin treatment is milder and less frequent than that under bleomycin treatment (Table 8). Lung toxicities were observed in two only

Table 8. Comparison between side effects of pepleomycin and those of bleomycin

Toxic effects	Pleomycin (75 cases)		Bleomycin (68 cases)	
	Number of cases	Incidence (%)	Number of cases	Incidence (%)
1. Anorexia	31	41.3	23	33.8
2. Fever	26	34.7	25	36.8
3. Alopecia	26	34.7	21	30.9
4. Generalized malaise	21	28	18	26.5
5. Pigmentation of finger and palm	15	20	15	22.1
6. Nausea and vomiting	12	16	10	14.7
7. Eruption				
1) Scratch dermatitis	6 ⎱ 12		5 ⎱ 13.2	
2) Exudative erythema	3 ⎰		4 ⎰	
8. Edema of fingers	5	6.7	8	11.8
9. Peripheral nerve symptoms	3	4	6	8.8
10. Deformities of nails	3	4	5	7.4
11. Hyperkeratosis of pressure area	3	4	3	4.4
12. Stomatitis	2	2.7	2	2.9
13. Pulmonary toxicities	2	2.7	6	8.8
14. Shock	1	1.3	1	1.5

of the 75 cases. It is quite impressive that lung toxicities occurred less frequently under pepleomycin treatment than under the treatment with the present bleomycin on the same dosage schedule. Table 2 shows the frequencies of side effects of this drug, compared with those of bleomycin.

Discussion

Squamous Cell Carcinoma

Pepleomycin has an obviously superior antitumor effect against squamous cell carcinoma to the present bleomycin, being markedly to moderately effective in many cases. Of the 36 treated cases of this malignancy, pepleomycin was evaluated as markedly effective in 15 (41.7%), moderately effective in 12 (33.3%), and slightly effective in six (16.7%), the effective rate being 91.7%. In our department, bleomycin was evaluated as markedly effective in 11 (20%), moderately effective in 10 (18%) and slightly effective in 23 (41.8%) of 55 cases of the same malignancy, giving an effective rate of 80% (Table 9).

In T_4 cases, even pepleomycin cannot be expected to be as effective (Table 5). It appears necessary to consider combination therapy with pepleomycin and other carcinostatics, radiotherapy, or cryosurgery in such cases.

Bleomycin proved hardly effective against lymph node metastasis, while pepleomycin was moderately effective in three slightly effective in one and ineffective in two of six N_1 cases. Pepleomycin was also ineffective in two N_3 cases: thus, it appears somewhat effective against lymph node metastais. But the data that either of the two N_3 cases showed no response suggests that pepleomycin as well is not as effective clinically.

Table 9. Comparison between clinical effects of pepleomycin and those of bleomycin

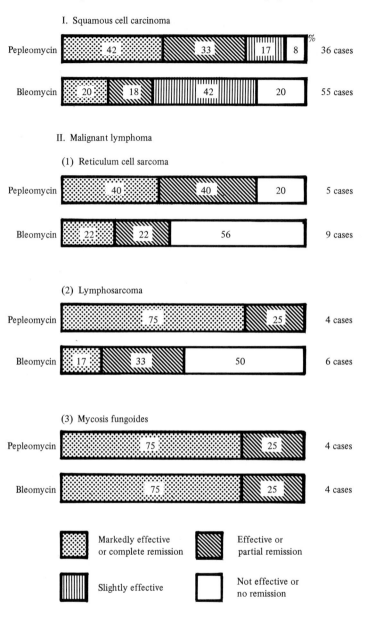

I. Squamous cell carcinoma

Pepleomycin | 42 | 33 | 17 | 8 | % | 36 cases

Bleomycin | 20 | 18 | 42 | 20 | 55 cases

II. Malignant lymphoma

(1) Reticulum cell sarcoma

Pepleomycin | 40 | 40 | 20 | 5 cases

Bleomycin | 22 | 22 | 56 | 9 cases

(2) Lymphosarcoma

Pepleomycin | 75 | 25 | 4 cases

Bleomycin | 17 | 33 | 50 | 6 cases

(3) Mycosis fungoides

Pepleomycin | 75 | 25 | 4 cases

Bleomycin | 75 | 25 | 4 cases

Markedly effective or complete remission   Effective or partial remission

Slightly effective   Not effective or no remission

Oral Florid Papillomatosis. The excellent effect of pepleomycin against oral florid papillomatosis calls for attention. In oral surgery in the United States, bleomycin is accepted as the first choice for this tumor, and it is likely that pepleomycin will take the place of bleomycin. We have encountered a case of the same disease successfully treated by cryosurgery alone. Combination therapy with pepleomycin and cryosurgery should be tried in the future. Since oral florid papillomatosis is a rare disease in Japan, it is desirable to continue further studies in a larger number of cases [16, 20].

Keratoacanthoma. Pepleomcycin treatment with a total dose of 50 mg and of 75 mg proved markedly effective in each of two cases of keratoacanthoma. The primary effect of pepleomycin against keratoacanthoma seems to evolve early and to be striking, compared with that of bleomycin [6, 7, 10]. Clinical differentiation between keratoacanthoma and squamous cell carcinoma is sometimes difficult, but when the diagnosis of this tumor is established by biopsy, it may be adequate to use pepleomycin for the purpose of accelerating the tendency to spontaneous healing.

Malignant Lymphoma

The antitumor effect of pepleomycin against non-Hodgkin's lymphoma appears to be slightly higher than that of bleomycin. In the group of 13 cases of this malignancy, a complete remission was achieved in two (40%), a partial remission in two (40%), and no remission in two (20%) of five cases of reticulum cell lymphoma; a complete remission in three (75%) and a partial remission in one (25%) of four cases of lymphosarcoma; a complete remission in three (75%) and a partial remission in one (25%) of four cases of mycosis fungoides. The results of pepleomycin treatment in 19 cases of the same malignancy reported by Kimura et al. [14] and Higuchi et al. [3] are: a complete remission in two cases (22%), a partial remission in two cases (22%), and no remission in five (56%) of nine cases of reticulum cell lymphoma; a complete remission in one (16.7%), a partial remission in two (33.3%), and no remission in three (50%) of six cases of lymphosarcoma; a complete remission in two cases (33.3.%) and a partial remission in two (50%) of four cases of mycosis fungoides. It is clear that pepleomycin is superior to bleomycin in induction therapy for non-Hodgkin's lymphoma.

Immunoblastic Lymphadenopathy. A case of immunoblastic lymphadenopathy was treated with pepleomycin, and responded markedly. This is the first case to be treated with pepleomycin and reported in Japan. An additional study is planned in which we intend to try combination therapy with pepleomycin and corticosteroid.

Malignant Melanoma

There has been no case of malignant melanoma, irrespective of stage, in which pepleomycin, used individually, was evaluated as effective. Therefore, we performed three drug combination chemotherapy with pepleomycin, mCCNU and VCR in eight cases of malignant melanoma, and the treatment was evaluated as slightly effective in a stage I case, and slightly to moderately effective in two of four stage IV cases (Figs. 8 and 9).
Three-drug combination chemotherapy with DTIC, mCCNU, and VCR is an internationally accepted regimen for malignant melanoma [1]. Six cases were treated in our department, but in no way reponded to this combination chemotherapy. We replaced DTIC with pepleomycin, and the treatment was then, as described above, evaluated as slightly to moderately effective in some of the cases. Clinical effects of this modified combination chemotherapy are now being studied in a larger number of cases. De Wasch et al. [2] reported that three-drug combination chemotherapy with bleomycin, CCNU, and VCR gave an effective rate of 48.5% against stage IV

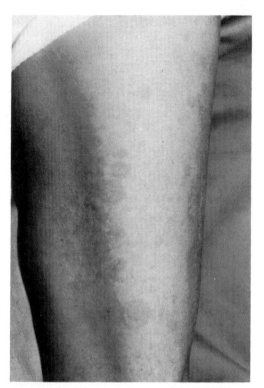

Fig. 10. A 60-year-old female with a big basal cell epithelioma in the parietal region ($T_4N_0M_0$). Exudative erythema-like eruptions appeared after pepleomycin treatment with a cumulative dose of 20 mg. The same exanthemata had formerly been observed following administration of the present bleomycin and bleomycin A_5

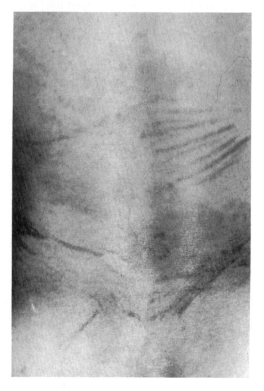

Fig. 11. A 52-year-old male with stage II malignant melanoma on the left leg. After administration of pepleomycin to a total dose of 50 mg, scratch dermatitis appeared on the trunk and extremities

malignant melanoma, but their protocol differs in dosage schedule from our regimen.

In malignant melanoma, it is preferable to combine the immunopotentiator, such as BCG, picibanil polysaccharide Kureha (PSK) and bestatin, with the chemotherapeutic agent to improve response rate and prognosis. We usually perform chemoimmunotherapy using pepleomycin, mCCNU, and VCR combined with bestatin. For an exact evaluation of the chemoimmunotherapy, however, it is necessary to administer this regimen in a larger number of cases for many years.

Side Effects of Pepleomycin

Adverse reactions to pepleomycin appear similar in sort and frequency to those to bleomycin. However, we have an impression that the fever under pepleomycin treatment is milder and less frequent than that under bleomycin treatment, while anorexia, nausea, and vomiting are more frequent under the former.

In a case of basal cell epithelioma, exudative erythema-, or urticaria-like eruptions were formerly observed following the administration of the present bleomycin and bleomycin A$_5$. It was of interest to see that pepleomycin produced the same kind of exanthemata in thise case (Figs. 10 and 11).

Pulmonary complications were found in two (2.7%) of the 75 cases, which indeed is less frequent than six (8.8%) of 68 cases treated with bleomycin. One has to be discreet in applying to man the experimental finding that in small animals and dogs pepleomycin has less pulmonary toxicity. Considering that pepleomycin is identical in basal structure to bleomycin and different only in terminal amine from the latter, and that even pepleomycin, if used in overdosage, gives rise to pulmonary complications even in animal experiments, it is desirable to monitor the lung function (vital capacity, Pao$_2$, DLco, etc.) and to check chest X ray films frequently during treatment with pepleomycin. This, we consider, will help to prevent pulmonary complications.

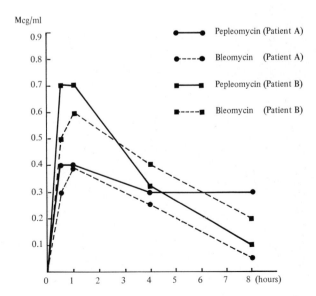

Fig. 12. Serum levels of pepleomycin and bleomycin in man (by crossover technique). Dose: 10 mg/man, IM (pepleomycin). 15 mg/man, IM (bleomycin)

Absorption and Excretion

We have been impressed that 10 mg (potency) of pepleomycin is slightly more potent both in clinical effects and adverse effects than 15 mg (potency) of bleomycin. We therefore studied the absorption and excretion in man of 10 mg (potency) of pepleomycin and those of 15 mg (potency) of bleomycin. The study was made on two

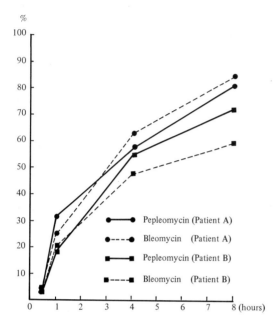

Fig. 13. Urinary recovery of pepleomycin and bleomycin in man (by crossover technique). Dose: 10 mg/man, IM (pepleomycin). 15 mg/man, IM (bleomycin)

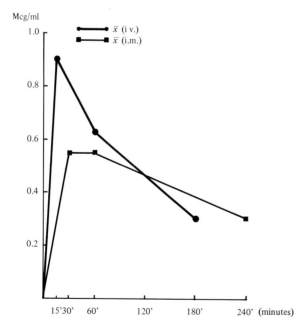

Fig. 14. Serum levels of pepleomycin in man. Dose: 10 mg/man IV or IM

cancer patients by the IM route and by the crossover technique. Blood levels and urinary outputs of the drugs during the 8 h after their IM injections were determined. The blood levels of pepleomycin after the injections of 10 mg (potency) of this drug were similar to those of bleomycin after the injection of its 15 mg (potency) dose in each of the two patients. The peak blood level of pepleomycin occurred slightly earlier (at 30 min). The blood levels vary from patient to patient (Fig. 12).

There was virtually no difference between the urinary outputs of the two drugs in each patient, with 60%−80% of the injected dose of each drug recovered in 8 h (Fig. 13).

The blood levels of pepleomycin by IV and IM routes were compared. The blood level by the IV route remained higher during the first hour, but that by the IM route was higher at 3 h (Fig. 14).

Summary

1. The therapeutic effects of pepleomycin seem superior to those achieved with bleomycin against squamous cell carcinoma and malignant lymphoma.
2. In basal cell epithelioma, carcinoma in situ (e.g., actinic keratosis, Bowen's disease), adenocarcinoma (e.g., mammary and genital Paget's disease), and adult soft tissue sarcoma, pepleomycin as well as bleomycin was clinically ineffective.
3. Of the two cases of stage IV malignant melanoma, pepleomycin combined with MeCCNU and VCR exerted a moderate effect against multiple disseminated skin metastases in one, and a slight effect against a VI rib metastasis in the other.
4. The sorts of side effects of pepleomycin were almost the same as those of bleomycin. Lung toxicities were less frequent under pepleomycin treatment than those under bleomycin treatment.

References

1. Comis RL (1976) DTIC (NSC-45388) in malignant melanoma; a perspective. Cancer Treat Rep 60: 165−173
2. De Wasch G, Bernheim J, Michel J, Lejeune F, Kenis Y (1976) Combination chemotherapy with three marginally effective agents, CCNU, vincristine, and bleomycin, in the treatment of stage III melanoma. Cancer Treat Rep 60: 1273−1276
3. Higuchi K, Goto M, Kurita R (1969) Studies of bleomycin in dermatology (Clinical study). Jpn J Dermatol Ser A 79: 593−609
4. Ichikawa T (1968) Introduction of bleomycin (BLM). Jpn J Cancer Clin 14: 296
5. Ichikawa T (1978) Basic and clinical studies of antitumor spectra of anticancer agents (4) with particular reference to bleomycin. Chemotherapy 26: 91−96
6. Ikeda S, Miyasato H, Imai K, Seki M, Nakayama H, Mori Y, Mizutani H (1975) Local chemotherapy of skin tumors (I) with particular reference to clinical application of bleomycin ointment. Jpn J Clin Dermatol 29: 734−478
7. Ikeda S, Kawamura T, Miyasato H, Imai K, Nakayama H, Ishihara K, Mizutani H (1975) Local chemotherapy of skin tumors (II) basic study of bleomycin ointment. Jpn J Clin Dermatol 29: 827−839
8. Ikeda S, Hamamatsu T, Ishihara K (1976) Effects of bleomycin on skin cancer. Gann 19: 235−250

 9. Ikeda S, Hamamatsu T, Tazima K, Miyasato H, Imai K, Nakayama H, Mizutani H (1976) Clinical trial of NK5033 in dermatology. Med Treat 9: 981−999
10. Ikeda S, Nakayama H, Hamamatsu T, Miyasato H, Imai K, Seki M (1976) Local oil BLM therapy in dermatology. Med Treat 9: 1237−1254
11. Ikeda S, Hamamatsu T, Miyasato H, Imai K, Nakayama H (1977) Skin cancer, a new therapy. J Ther 59: 903−920
12. Ikeda S, Miyasato H, Nakayama H, Kobayashi Y (1979) Clinical trial of pepleomycin in dermatology. J Jpn Soc Cancer Ther 14: 384
13. Imamura Y (1978) Immunoblastic lymphadenopathyconcept of disease and study of cases reported in Japan. Intern Med 41: 436−442
14. Kimura K, Sakai Y, Konda C, Kashiwada N, Kitahara T, Inagaki H, Itano T, Fujita H, Izuka N, Mikuni N (1969) Chemotherapy of malignant lymphoma, with particular reference to bleomycin. Jpn J Clin Med 27: 1593−1601
15. Matsuda A, Yoshioka O, Yamashita T, Ebihara K, Umezawa H, Murata T, Katayama K, Yokoyama M, Nagai S (1978) Fundamental and clinical studies on new bleomycin analogs. Recent Results Cancer Res 63: 191−210
16. Miyasato H (1978) Two cases of oral florid papillomatosis treated by cryosurgery. J Cryosurg Res Group 4: 29−30
17. Takita T (1977) Development of new drugs; chemical and biological modifications of bleomycin. Chem Ind 28: 1271−1277
18. Tanaka W (1977) Development of new bleomycins with potential clinical utility. Jpn J Antibiot (Tokyo) [suppl] 30: 41−48
19. Umezawa H (1965) Bleomycin and other antitumor antibiotics of high molecular weight. Antimicrob Agents Chemother 1965: 1079−1085
20. Wolff K, Toppeiner J (1976) Oral florid papillomatosis. In: Andrade R, Gumport SL, Popkin GL, Rees TD (eds) Cancer of the skin; vol 1. Saunders, W. Washington Square, pp 797−813

Phase I and II Study of a New Bleomycin Analog (Pepleomycin)

T. Miura, K. Katayama, and T. Wada

Second Department of Surgery, University of Tokyo Faculty of Medicine, Hongo 7, Bunkyo-ku, J – Tokyo 113

Introduction

It is well known that bleomycin, developed by Umezawa et al. in 1965, is now widely used not only in Japan but also in other countries as an anticancer drug, specifically effective against squamous cell carcinoma and malignant lymphoma, giving excellent clinical effects. It is, however, accompanied by the occurrence of pulmonary fibrosis as one of its adverse effects, creating problems as to the measures to counteract it.

As its chemical structure was later elucidated, about 300 bleomycin analogs were semisynthesized, and some analogs screened out of them have been tested to find an anticancer agent with less adverse effects but with a more potent anticancer effect.

Pepleomycin (experimental code: NK631), a new bleomycin derivative, was recently developed, and its fundamental studies have shown that the agent has an antitumor effect mostly comparable to or slightly more potent than that of its parent compound, bleomycin. It is distributed into tissues at high concentrations, especially, into the stomach at a high concentration with a statistical significance, and has proved effective even against experimental rat stomach cancer. Studies of its toxicology have also revealed that pepleomycin has a slightly higher systemic toxicity than bleomycin, but is accompanied by only about one-third the incidence of pulmonary fibrosis in mice with the latter [1].

With reference to these findings in the fundamental studies, we made the phase I and II study of pepleomycin in 23 cases of various advanced cancers during the period from October, 1976, through September, 1978; and the results are presented in this paper.

Subjects

In the phase II study, which attempted to find a wider range of indications for it, pepleomycin was, as shown in Tables 1 and 2, administered in the cases of various adenocarcinomas in addition to the cases of squamous cell carcinoma and of malignant lymphoma.

Of the cases entered in the study, nine cases, i.e., two cases of malignant lymphoma, one of tongue cancer, five of primary lung cancer, and one of lung metastasis of

Table 1. Cases treated with pepleomycin

Case No.	Patient, age and sex	Clinical diagnosis (histologic diagnosis)	TNM stage	Location (metastasizing site)	Past history	Compli-cation	Previous treatment
1	K. K. 52, ♂	Malignant lymphoma (reticulosarcoma)	Stage IV	Left cervical region	None	None	5-FU, MMC; radiotherapy
2	M. K. 31, ♂	Malignant lymphoma (reticulosarcoma)	Stage IV	Colon	None	None	Operation; 5-FU, MMC FT-207
3	Y. S. 53, ♂	Hepatic cancer	Stage IV	Liver	None	Liver cirrhosis	Operation (exploratory laparotomy)
4	O. O. 27, ♂	Malignant chorio-epithelioma	Stage IV	Colon, retroperi-toneum (lung)	None	None	Operation
5	H. H. 65, ♂	Prostatic cancer	Stage IV	Prostate (lung)	None	None	Operation; stilbesterol
6	T. H. 65, ♂	Cervical metastasis of tongue cancer (squa-mous cell carcinoma)	Stage IV	(cervical region)	None	None	Operation; radiotherapy
7	F. K. 63, ♀	Lung cancer (squa-mous cell carcinoma)	Stage IV	(Pleurae)	None	None	None
8	G. O. 56, ♂	Prostatic cancer	Stage IV	Prostate (bone)	None	None	Stilbesterol
9	K. Y. 41, ♀	Lung cancer (squa-mous cell carcinoma)	Stage IV	Lung	None	None	Radiotherapy, MMC, 5-FU
10	C. T. 74, ♂	Lung cancer (squa-mous cell carcinoma)	Stage IV	Lung	None	None	None
11	K. K. 60, ♂	Lung cancer (squa-mous cell carcinoma)	Stage IV	Lung	None	None	None
12	S. T. 69, ♂	Lung cancer (squa-mous cell carinoma)	Stage IV	Lung (supraclavic-ular lymph nodes)	None	None	MMC, 5-FU
13	S. O. 69, ♀	Stomach cancer	Stage IV	Stomach (liver)	None	None	Operation

[a] I.Pl: intrapleurally

Dosage schedule				Primary effect antitumor effect and/or Karnofsky classification	After therapy	Adverse effect (kind and severity)	Prognosis (months) survival or death	Remarks
Route	Dose at time × freq./week	Period (days)	Total dose (mg)					
IV IA	5−10 mg × 7/wk. 5 mg × 3/wk. fr. 17. Jan. '77 to 12. Feb. '77	27	170 65 Total: 235	I-B	Chemo-therapy	Stomatitis	3.5 mos.; death	
IV IA	5−10 mg × 7/wk. 5−10 mg × 3/wk. fr. 8. Nov. '76 to 8. Feb. '77	91	295 140 Total: 435	I-C	Chemo-therapy	Nausea	20 mos., surivival	
IV IA	10 mg × 2 10 mg × 7/wk. fr. 21. Oct. '76 to 25. Nov. '76	34	20 140 Total: 160	0-C			1 mo.; death	
IV IA	5−10 mg × 7/wk. 5−10 mg × 2/wk. fr. 5. Oct. '76 to 6. Nov. '76	30	125 25 Total: 150	0-B		Alopecia	1 mo.; death	
IA	5−10 mg × 2−4/wk. fr. 18. Nov. '76 to 14. Dec. '76	27	110	0-C			1 mo.; death	
IV	5−10 mg × 7/wk. fr. 25. Dec. '76 to 1. Mar. '77	95	365	I-B		Change of skin, stomatitis, fever	12 mos.; death	
IV IA I.Pl.[a]	5 mg × 3/wk. 20 mg × 2	76	305 40 Total: 345	I-C	Chemo-therapy	Dermatitis	24 mos.; survival	
IV IA	5−10 mg × 7/wk. 5−10 mg fr. 19. Jan. '77 to 5. Feb. '77.	20	75 45 Total: 120	0-C		Stomatitis, dermatitis	20 days; death	
IV IA	5−10 mg × 2/wk. 5 mg × 5 fr. 22. Nov. '76 to 3. Mar. '77	101	140 25 Total: 165	0-A			Death	
IV IA	5−10 mg × 3/wk. 5−10 mg 3/wk. fr. 19. Oct. '76 to 14. Dec. '76	62	50 220 Total: 270	0-A		Dermatitis	Death	
IV	5−10 mg × 7/wk. fr. 3. Nov. '76 to 30. Nov. '76	28	205	0-A	Chemo-therapy		Survival	
IV IA	5−10 mg × 7/wk. 5−10 mg × 2/wk. fr. 8. Dec. '76 to 27. Dec. '76	20	155 50 Total: 205	0-A			Death	
IA	10 mg × 2−12/wk. fr. 9. Oct. '76 to 29. Oct. '76	21	120	0-0		Stomatitis	Death	

Table 1 (continued)

Case No.	Patient, age and sex	Clinical diagnosis (histologic diagnosis)	TNM stage	Location (metastasizing site)	Past history	Compli- cation	Previous treatment
14	I. M. 45, ♂	Stomach cancer	Stage IV	Stomach (rectum)	None	None	MMC, 5-FU
15	M. S. 55, ♂	Renal cancer (clear cell carcinoma)	Stage IV	Kidneys (perito- neum, stomach, Virchow's nodes)	None	None	None
16	H. S. 57, ♂	Leiomyosarcoma originating in the retroperitoneum	Stage IV	Retroperitoneum (inguinal lymph nodes)	None	None	5-FU
17	E. A. 63, ♀	Stomach cancer (un- differentiated carci- noma)	Stage IV	Stomach (pancreas, retroperitoneum, spleen, liver)	None	None	None
18	G. S. 68, ♂	Thyroid cancer (un- differentiated carci- noma)	Stage IV	Thyroid	None	None	None
19	A. U. 50, ♂	Lung metastasis of parotid cancer (adenocarcinoma)	Stage IV	(lung)	None	None	Operation
20	S. F. 37, ♂	Hepatic metastasis of colonic cancer	Stage IV	(liver)	None	None	Operation; 5-FU, MMC
21	S. O. 72, ♂	Lung metastasis of laryngeal cancer (squamous cell carci- noma)	Stage IV	(lung)	None	None	Operation
22	Y. K. 54, ♂	Hepatic cancer	Stage IV	Liver	None	None	None
23	K. M. 58, ♀	Hepatic metastasis of duodenal cancer (leiomyosarcoma)	Stage IV	(liver)	None	None	Operation

pharyngeal cancer, were what had been accepted as indications for bleomycin. The other 14 cases, made up of one case of lung metastasis of parotid cancer, three of stomach cancer, two of primary hepatic cancer, one of hepatic metastasis of colonic cancer, one of hepatic metastasis of leiomyosarcoma, one of thyroid cancer, one of kidney cancer, two of prostatic cancer, one of leiomyosarcoma, and one of malignant chorioepithelioma had not been considered to be the indications for bleomycin; however, in an attempt to expand the range of indications for pepleomycin, these cases were entered in this study so as to find their responses to local A administration of large doses.

Dosage schedule				Primary effect antitumor effect and/or Karnofsky classification	After therapy	Adverse effect (kind and severity)	Prognosis (months) survival or death	Remarks
Route	Dose at time × freq./week	Period (days)	Total dose (mg)					
IV IA	5−10 mg × 7/wk. 5 mg × 7 fr. 11. Dec. '76 to 10. Jan. '77	30	165 35 Total: 200	0-0			Death	
IV IA	5−10 mg × 7/wk. 5−10 mg × 13 fr. 27. Nov. '76 to 11. Jan. '77	44	225 75 Total: 300	0-0			Death	
IA	10 mg × 2/wk. fr. 10. Nov. '76 to 11. Dec. '76.	32	100	0-A		Fever	Death	
IA	10 mg × 2/wk. fr. 14. Dec. '76 to 6. Jan. '77	23	60	0-0			Death	
IA	10 mg × 2 fr. Oct. '76	2	20	0-0			Death	
IV IA	5−10 mg × 7/wk. 20 mg × 2 fr. 8. Nov. '77 to 28. Nov. '77	21	160 40 Total: 200	0-0			4.5 mos.; death	
IV IA	5 mg × 6/wk. 5 mg × 3/wk. fr. 16. Feb. '78 to 5. Mar. '78	18	30 45 Total: 75	0-C		Stomatitis	2.5 mos.; death	GOT ↘ GPT ↘ LDH ↘ Al-P ↗
IV IA	5 mg × 7/wk. 5−10 mg × 2/wk. fr. 30. Mai '78 to 20. Oct. '78	141	135 100 Total: 235	0-A			5 mos.; survival	Blood sedimen-tation rate ↘
IV IA	5 mg × 7/wk. 5 mg × 3/wk. fr. 18. Feb '77 to 5. Mar. '77	16	40 30 Total: 70	0-B		Stomatitis	1 mo.; death	GPT, Al-P, LDH and α-feto-protein, slight ↘
IA	5 mg × 3/wk. fr. 7. Nov. '77 to 14. Dec. '77	37	105	I-A			4 mos.; death	

The effects of pepleomycin treatment were evaluated according to the Karnofsky classification [2].

Dosage Schedule

For the purpose of proving its clinical effects as early as possible, it was decided to administer pepleomycin locally at as high a concentration as possible; and the IA infusion [3−5] was employed as a rule. With reference to the findings in the

Table 2. Routes of administration of pepleomycin

Disease	Route of administration			Total
	Selective intra-arterial administration	Subselective intra-arterial administration	Intravenous administration	
	Cases	Cases	Cases	Cases
Malignant lymphoma	1	1		2
Tongue cancer			1	1
Primary lung cancer		4	1	5
Metastatic lung cancer		2		2
Stomach cancer		3		3
Primary hepatic cancer	2			2
Metastatic hepatic cancer	1	1		2
Thyroid cancer	1			1
Renal cancer		1		1
Prostatic cancer	2			2
Leiomyosarcoma		1		1
Malignant chorio-epithelioma		1		1
Total	7	14	2	23

fundamental studies, its dose at a time was decided to be 5−10 mg, which was administered 2−7 times a week, depending on the response of the patient, until any objective adverse reaction appeared.

Results

IA infusion or IV injection of pepleomycin was performed on a dosage schedule of 5−10 mg at a time, 2−3 times a week or every day. Intrapleural injection of the drug was made on a dosage schedule of 20 mg at a time. Of the 23 cases, the drug was administered chiefly by IA infusion in 21: selectively into the local artery in seven, and subselectively into the aorta in 14; and IV injection also was employed in them. It was in only two cases that the drug was administered IV as a systemic route.

Table 3 summarizes the clinical effects of pepleomycin treatment in these 23 cases. Of the nine cases of malignant lymphoma and squamous cell carcinoma, it was in four that the treatment gave a I−B or better effect by the Karnofsky classification. Of the 14 cases of adenocarcinomas, the treatment gave a 0−C or I−A effect in five cases. Thus, the treatment proved less effective in these cases than in the former, but the local IA infusion of large doses of this drug gave a 0−A or better effect with a regression of tumor in seven of the cases of adenocarcinomas.

The typical cases are presented here. The patient in *case 1* was a 52-year-old male with malignant lymphoma (Fig. 1.). His cervical lymph nodes became swollen 6 years before, when the disorder was diagnosed as malignant lymphoma. At that time, a

Table 3. Results of pepleomycin treatment

Karnofsky classification	Group of malignant lymphoma and squamous cell carcinoma		Group of adenocarcinoma	
0-0			Stomach cancer	3 cases
			Renal cancer	1 case
			Thyroid cancer	1 case
			Lung metastasis of parotid cancer	1 case
		5/9		9/14
0-A	Lung cancer	4 cases	Retroperitoneal leiomyosarcoma	1 case
	Lung metastasis of laryngeal cancer	1 case		
0-B			Hepatic cancer	1 case
			Malignant chorio-epithelioma	1 case
0-C			Prostatic cancer	2 cases
			Hepatic cancer	1 case
			Hepatic metastasis of colonic cancer	1 case
I-A			Hepatic metastasis of duodenal leio-myosarcoma	1 case
		4/9		5/14
I-B	Malignant lymphoma	1 case		
	Cervical metastasis of tongue cancer	1 case		
I-C	Malignant lymphoma	1 case		
	Lung cancer	1 case		
Total	9		14	

complete remission was achieved by the combination of infusion of 5-fluorouracil (5-FU) and mitomycin C (MMC) into the left subclavian artery and ^{60}C radiation.

He was admitted this time for swelling of the right cervical lymph nodes and of the right inguinal lymph nodes; and the histopathologic examination gave the diagnosis of recurrent malignant lymphoma (reticulosarcoma). Indwelling catheterization was provide on the right subclavian artery and right common iliac artery, and a cumulative dose of 65 mg of pepleomycin was infused IA, and a total of 170 mg was systemically administered by IV injection during a period of 4 weeks.

The treatment was withdrawn for stomatitis at the stage when a total dose of 235 mg had been administered; however, the cervical and inguinal lymph nodes were not palpable at all at the stage when a cumulative dose of 185 mg (50 mg by IA infusion and 135 mg by IV injection) had been administered. Fever that had persisted before the treatment was also completely controlled to normal, and the general condition was markedly improved. The evaluation by the Karnofsky classification was I−B.

The patient in *case 2* was a 31-year-old-male with malignant lymphoma (Fig. 2). The patient was admitted for intestinal obstruction ileus due to malignant lymphoma (reticulosarcoma) the size of a hen egg located at the terminal ileum incarcerating into the cecum and the ascending colon. A 25-cm-long portion of the terminal ileum and a 15-cm-long portion of the cecum and ascending colon were resected, and the regional lymph nodes enlarged to the size of the thumb top, dissected as far as possible; however, numerous lymph nodes enlarged to the size of the little fingertip remained in the root of the mesentery, and were undissectable; hence, the operation ended in noncurative resection.

After the operation, MMC and 5-FU were subselectively infused via the indwelling catheter provided on the abdominal aorta, and, at the same time, IV drip infusion of 5-FU and oral administration of 1-(2-tetrahydrofuryl)-5-fluorouracil were performed for prevention of recurrence. The lymph nodes at the root of the mesentery, however, markedly enlarged 7 months later, and a large recurrent metastatic focus the size of a fist was palpable as an upper abdominal mass.

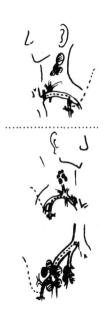

1971: Malignant lymphoma of the left neck.

MMC
5FU } Selective infusion into the subclavian artery.

^{60}Co radiation in combination.

A complete remission of the tumor was achieved.

1977: Recurrence in the right neck.
       Recurrence in the right inguinal region.

Pepleomycin: selective infusion into the subclavian artery
              selective infusion into the common iliac artery.

Fig. 1. Case 1

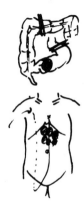

Reticulosarcoma of the terminal ileum.

April, 1976: ileus.
              resection of the right colon.
              MMC } Infusion into the abdominal aorta, and
              5FU } IV drip infusion
              FT-207 orally.

              A remission was achieved, and lasted 7 months;
              however, the malignancy recurred in the root of
              mesentery.

Fig. 2. Case 2

After readmission, the patient immediately received IV drip infusion of 5–10 mg of pepleomycin, every day, and also subselective IA infusion of 5–10 mg into the abdominal aorta every other day.

As a result, at the stage when a total dose of 280 mg had been administered (185 mg by IV infusion and 95 by IA infusion), the recurrent metastatic focus the size of a fist in the upper abdomen completely disappeared, accompanied by a marked improvement in general condition.

Even after discharge, the patient continued to receive IA and IV infusion of pepleomycin once a week on an ambulatory basis. However, he began to complain of nausea when a cumulative dose of 420 mg had been administered and the treatment was withdrawn at the stage when a total dose of 435 mg had been administered (295 mg by IV infusion and 140 mg by IA infusion).

The patient has since been treated with 5-FU, MMC, and 1-(2-tetrahydrofuryl)-5-fluorouracil, and is now healthy 2 years since the start of the pepleomycin treatment, and the treatment was evaluated as I–C by the Karnofsky classification.

The patient in *case 3* was a male aged 53 with cirrhosis of the liver and hepatoma (Fig. 3). Palpation revealed that the liver was enlarged six fingerbreadths, and this was a case of hepatoma associated with severe cirrhosis of the liver. Laboratory studies showed that total protein was 7.8 mg/dl; albumin, 2.4 mg/dl; A/G ratio, 0.7; SGOT, 80 units; SGPT, 18 units; LDH, 3033 units; TTT, 7.0 units; ZTT, 27.5 units, and α-fetoprotein, positive.

Laparotomy disclosed the retention of about 500 ml of ascites, associated with portal hypertension, and ended in an exploratory laparotomy. The IV injection of 100 mg of pepleomycin was performed twice immediately; indwelling catheterization was then performed on the hepatic artery, and 10 mg of pepleomycin was administered by one-shot IA injection every day through the catheter. The primary lesion began to regress at the stage when a cumulative dose of 50 mg had been administered (20 mg by IV injection, and 30 mg by IA injection), and was hardly palpable at the stage when a cumulative dose of 100 mg had been administered. At this stage, the primary lesion also was greatly regressed even on the liver scintigram. On the other hand, ascites began to be retained about 2 weeks after the start of pepleomycin treatment (by which time a cumulative dose of 70 mg had been administered), and became striking at the stage when a cumulative dose of 160 mg had been administered.

The left hepatic lobe, enlarged 6 fingerbreadths.
Febrile type.

Oct. 23, 1976: Catheterization on the hepatic artery.

Pepleomycin: 140 mg, IA
                20 mg, IV

The liver function was improved, and the liver markedly regressed; however, ascites was retained markedly from 2 weeks of treatment.
The patient died of hemorrhage from gastric ulcer at 38 days of treatment.

Fig. 3. Case 3

Laboratory studies revealed that AFP was improved; LDH rapidly decreased at 1 week of pepleomycin treatment but was increased at 3 weeks again; and SGOT increased transiently at 1 week of the treatment, but then decreased, and again tended to increase slightly from 3 weeks of pepleomycin treatment.

In this case, signs and symptoms were transiently improved by the IA injection of pepleomycin, but the patient died of bleeding from gastric ulcer at 38 days of the treatment.

The patient in *case 4* was a 27-year-old male with colonic and retroperitoneal malignant chorioepithelioma. About 1 month after colectomy and resection of a tumor located in the retroperitoneum, a large tumor relapsed in the retroperitoneum, associated with lung metastasis. The patient immediately received 5−10 mg of pepleomycin at a time by IV drip infusion every day. Furthermore, an indwelling catheter was provided on the abdominal aorta [3] at 14 days of this treatment in order to administer 5−10 mg of pepleomycin at a time by IA one-shot injection, twice a week. The tumor began to regress at 7 days of this treatment (from the broken line circle to the solid line circle in Fig. 4), and the abdominal tumor completely disappeared with a total dose of 150 mg (125 mg IV and 25 mg IA). At this stage, however, massive melena occurred, requiring blood transfusion. On the other hand, the lung metastases were aggravated (Fig. 5). The patient was later transferred to another hospital, and died of brain metastasis. The pepleomycin was evaluated as having given a 0−B effect by the Karnofsky classification.

The patient in *case 5* was a 65-year-old male with prostatic cancer. He underwent orchiectomy for prostatic cancer, and was then treated orally by endocrinologic therapy with 300 mg stilbesterol daily for 6 months; however, the treatment did not prove markedly effective, and, dysuria persisting, he was hospitalized.

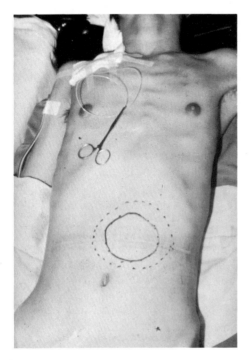

Fig. 4. Case 4, a 27-year-old male patient with colonic and retroperitoneal malignant chorioepithelioma

Because this was a case of inoperable advanced cancer, it was decided to perform IA chemotherapy, and an indwelling catheter was provided on each of the bilateral internal iliac arteries. Following the method [4] the author employs for operation on patients with unresectable rectal cancer and uterine cancer, the patient was placed in a prone position; the superior gluteal artery was exposed deep in the gluteus maximus muscle and at the greater sciatic foramen on the superior margin of the piriform muscle, where a Teflon catheter 1 mm in external diameter was inserted toward the internal iliac artery and fixed there.

The IA injection of 5−10 mg of pepleomycin was repeated at a rate of 2−3 times a week, with a cumulative dose of 110 mg administered during the first 4 weeks. The hard, enlarged prostatic cancer lesion softened and regressed markedly, and dysuria was markedly improved due to disappearance of narrowing of the urinary passage.

The left half section of Fig. 6 shows the pyeloureterogram before the treatment: the pelvis of the kidney on either side is enlarged, and the ureter on either side is also dilated, indicative of the presence of dysuria. The right half section of the figure illustrates the pyeloureterogram after IA infusion of 90 mg of pepleomycin: it is clear that the pelvis of the kidney and the ureter on either side are no longer enlarged or dilated, indicating the disappearance of the dysuria.

In this case, a metastatic focus 2 cm in diameter was found in the right upper lung lobe. Probably because the pepleomycin, which had been injected into the internal iliac artery, returned to the heart to act on the focus, this metastatic focus also responded to the treatment, considerably regressing already at the stage when a cumulative dose of 40 mg had been administered (Fig. 7).

No adverse reactions to the treatment were observed until the stage when a cumulative dose of 110 mg had been administered, and the patient ran a favorable course. However, he died of heart failure at 28 days of the treatment. The treatment was evaluated as 0−C by the Karnofsky classification.

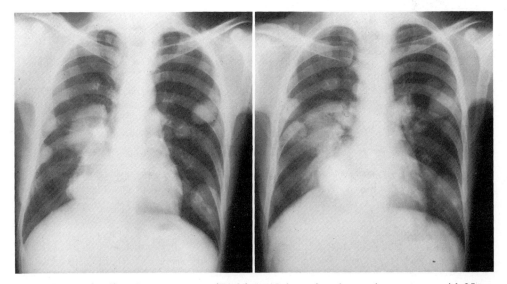

Fig. 5. Case 4. (*Left*) Before treatment. (*Right*) At 18 days of pepleomycin treatment with 25 mg IA and 115 mg IV in total

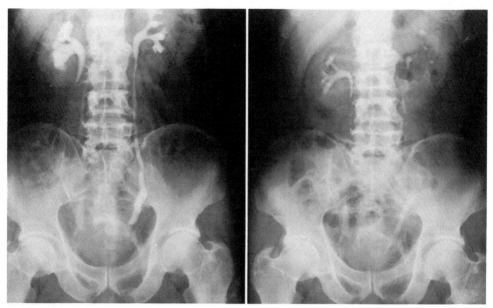

Fig. 6. Case 5, a 65-year-old male patient; pyeloureterogram of prostatic cancer. (*Left*) Before treatment. (*Right*) After pepleomycin treatment with 90 mg IA in total

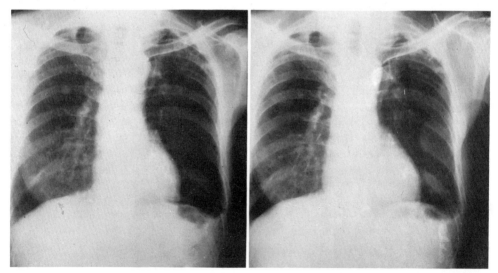

Fig. 7. Case 5, a 65-year-old male patient with a metastatic focus 2 cm in diameter in the right upper lung lobe. (*Left*) Before treatment. (*Right*) After pepleomycin treatment with 40 mg IA in total

The patient in *case 6* was a 65-year-old male with metastasis of tongue cancer to the neck. Using an electric surgical knife, he was operated on in March, 1976 for resection of tongue cancer the size of a thumb top that had developed in the tongue margin. The patient appeared to be following a favorable course after the operation. Metastases to the right cervical lymph nodes developed 3 months later, which rapidly enlarged to form a giant ulcer the size of the palm. He was admitted for severe pain, secretions with a offensive odor, and persistent hemorrhage, but on the condition that he should be treated with only narcotics and daily blood transfusion as a forlorn patient. Because one of the authors, Miura, could not stand looking at this patient treated only that way, he administered pepleomycin, which, to his surprise, exerted a marked antitumor effect resulting in a drastic improvement in signs and symptoms.

Figure 8 shows a clinical photo of the condition at 10 days of pepleomycin treatment, with 10 mg daily by IV drip infusion, when the hemorrhage has stopped and the lesion has begun to regress. Figure 9 shows a clinical photo at 3 months of the treatment with a cumulative dose of 260 mg administered: the giant cancerous ulcer has markedly regressed and been cleaned, covered with a clean crust; the secretions with an offensive odor have disappeared; and the hemorrhage has stopped, showing a marked curing tendency. Along with palliation of the pain, the oral food intake increased, the general condition was markedly improved, and the patient could return to the routine work (Fig. 10).

The pepleomycin treatment was started by administering 10 mg daily for the first 14 days, and then 5−10 mg every other day. However, the treatment was withdrawn for dermatitis as the stage when a cumulative dose of 230 mg had been administered. After a 10-day withdrawal, it was resumed with 10 mg at a time by IV drip infusion; however, it was finally withdrawn, because of such adverse reactions as dermatitis, stomatitis, and fever, at 95 days of the treatment counted from its very beginning, with a total dose of 365 mg administered.

This was a once given-up case of recurrent terminal cancer, but pepleomycin treatment exerted a marked effect, which was evaluated as I−B by the Karnofsky classification. Local recurrence was seen again about 9 months after the start of the treatment, and the patient died 12 months after the start of the treatment.

The patient in *case 7* was a female aged 63 with squamous cell carcinoma of the lung. The lesion was located in the left lower lung field; a large amount of effusion was retained in the pleural cavity; and the patient was admitted for complaints of dyspnea and chest pain. The patient coughed frequently, expectorated a large amount of sputum, had anorexia, and was severely weakened; and the malignancy, being an advanced cancer, was diagnosed as not indicating surgery. Puncture of the thoracic cavity was performed to remove pleural exudate and to infuse 20 mg of pepleomycin into the pleural cavity; and 5 mg of pepleomycin was administered by IV drip infusion 3 times a week. As the pleural effusion was retained again, the thoracic cavity was again punctured to infuse 20 mg of the drug into the pleural cavity at 23 days. The cytologic diagnosis of the effusion drained each time was squamous cell carcinoma.

This was a case where the combined intrapleural infusion and IV infusion of pepleomycin proved markedly effective (Fig. 11): the treatment completely eradicated the pleural effusion, eliminated the cough, sputum and chest pain, restored appetite, and markedly improved the general condition. The treatment, however, was withdrawn for dermatitis at 76 days of the treatment, by which stage a total dose of 345 mg had been administered, 305 mg by IV infusion, and 40 mg by intrapleural infusion.

The treatment was then switched to combination chemotherapy with MMC and 5FU; remission was achieved by chemotherapy alone without resorting to radiotherapy, and the patient is healthy today, 2 years after the start of pepleomycin treatment. The treatment was evaluated as I−C by the Karnofsky classification.

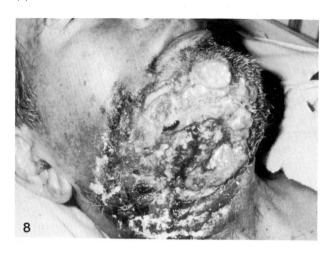

Fig. 8. Case 6, a 65-year-old male patient with metastasis of tongue cancer to the neck; at 10 days of pepleomycin treatment with 90 mg IV in total

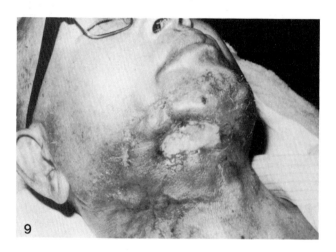

Fig. 9. Case 6; at 3 months of pepleomycin treatment with 260 mg IV in total

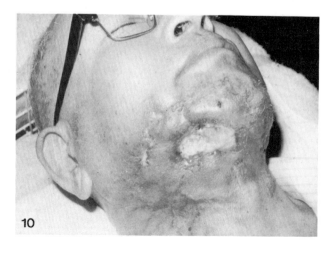

Fig. 10. Case 6; at the end of pepleomycin treatment with 365 mg IV in total

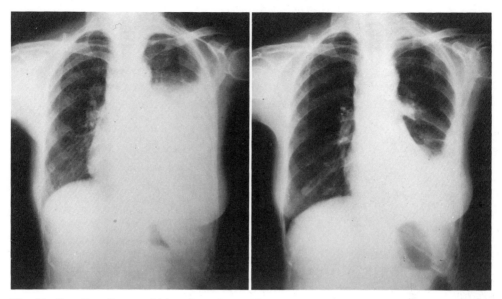

Fig. 11. Case 7, a 63-year-old female patient with squamous cell carcinoma of the lung. (*Left*) Before treatment. (*Right*) At 1 month of pepleomycin treatment with 40 mg intrapleurally and 150 mg IV, which proved markedly effective

Laboratory Findings

Various laboratory parameters were sequentially studied in these cases during the pepleomycin treatment. Changes in the parameters are shown in Figs. 12–26.

Changes in RBC, WBC, Hematocrit Value, and Hemoglobin Level

Figures 12–15 show changes in hematologic parameters during the treatment with pepleomycin. Changes in RBC with different total doses of pepleomycin are given in Fig. 12: RBC did not virtually change even with a increase in the total dose of pepleomycin. This also held true of hematocrit value and hemoglobin level (Figs. 14 and 15).

Figure 13 shows the relation of WBC to the total doses of pepleomycin: WBC in no way tended to decrease even with an increase in the total dose of the drug.

From these findings, pepleomycin, like bleomycin, was considered to have no severe myelodepressive effect.

Changes in Total Protein

The total protein, as shown in Fig. 18, did not tend to decrease with an increase in the total dose of pepleomycin.

T. Miura et al.

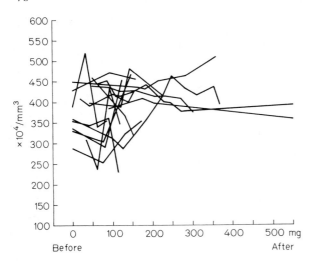

Fig. 12. Changes in RBC

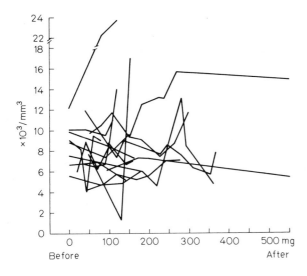

Fig. 13. Changes in WBC

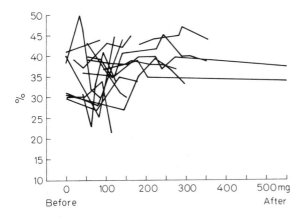

Fig. 14. Changes in hematocrit

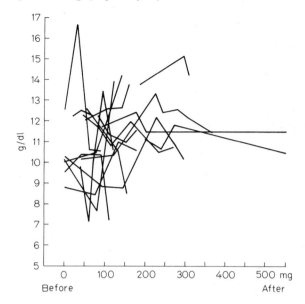

Fig. 15. Changes in hemoglobin

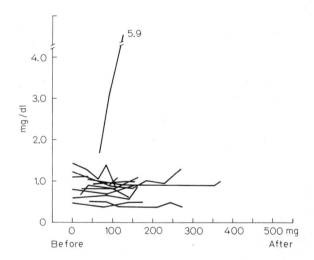

Fig. 16. Changes in creatinine

Changes in Cholesterol

As shown in Fig. 17, there was no given correlation between the total doses of pepleomycin and changes in cholesterol level.

Changes in BUN and Creatinine (Figs. 16 and 19)

BUN was found to be increased in two cases, and creatinine was found to be increased in one. These increases occurred in the cases of recurrent stomach cancer with hepatic metastasis and of terminal prostatic cancer with bone metastasis where renal disorders

T. Miura et al.

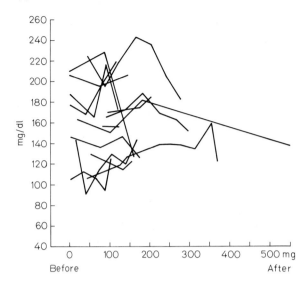

Fig. 17. Changes in cholesterol

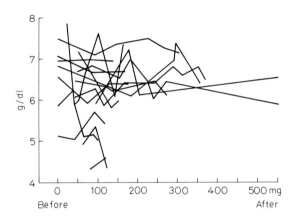

Fig. 18. Changes in total protein

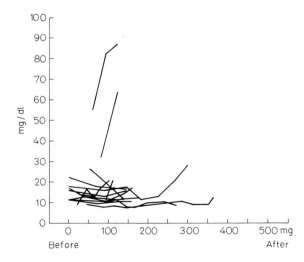

Fig. 19. Changes in BUN

had already existed prior to the pepleomycin treatment; hence, the increases in BUN may be considered to have resulted from aggravation of the malignancies but not from the toxicity of pepleomycin.

Changes in GOT, GPT, and LDH (Figs. 20–22)

GOT, GPT, and LDH were abnormally elevated in three of the cases. These were one case of hepatic cancer, one of malignant chorioepithelioma and one of recurrent stomach cancer with hepatic metastasis, and the elevations of these parameters resulted from aggravation of the malignancies while there occured no marked changes in potassium, chlorine, calcium and sodium levels as illustrated in Figs. 23a–d. Hence, it could not be judged whether the elevations were directly related to be pepleomycin treatment itself.

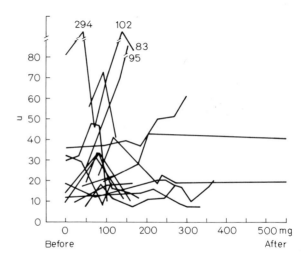

Fig. 20. Changes in GOT

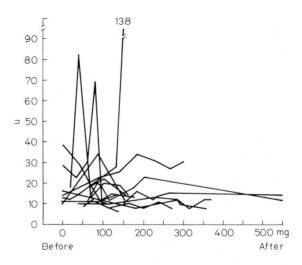

Fig. 21. Changes in GPT

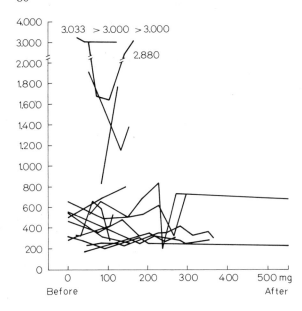

Fig. 22. Changes in LDH

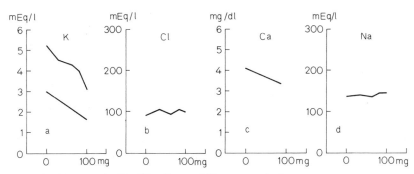

Fig. 23. Changes in K, CL, Ca, and Na respectively

Table 4. Adverse effects of pepleomycin

Without adverse effects	12/23
With adverse effects	11/23
Stomatitis	6
Dermatitis	4
Fever	2
Alopecia	1
Nausea	1
Bone marrow depression	0
Diarrhea	0
Live disorders	0
Renal disorders	0
Pulmonary fibrosis	0

Adverse Effects

As shown in Table 4, some adverse effects or the other were observed in 11 of the 23 cases, i.e., stomatitis in six (26%), dermatitis in four (17.4%), fever in two (8.7%), alopecia in one (4.3%), and nausea also in one case (4.3%). Myelodepression occurred in none of the cases, and pulmonary fibrosis, which was observed in bleomycin treatment, was not encountered in any of the cases. Pulmonary function was measured in some of the cases, but no striking changes were found.

Discussion

In view of the fact that pepleomycin, a bleomycin derivative, proved effective against rat stomach cancer and that the study of its pulmonary toxicity in mice showed it to be accompanied by only about one-third the incidence of pulmonary fibrosis with bleomycin, it was clinically anticipated that it would have a wider anticancer spectrum and that the incidence of pulmonary fibrosis with it would be lower.

We did not carry out the phase I and II study of pepleomycin rigidly, but with reference to the findings administered 5−10 mg at a time IA or IV, 2−3 times a week, or every day, while placing the patient under careful observation. We also administered 20 mg at a time intrapleurally.

Adverse effects appeared without so intimate a relation to the total doses of pepleomycin administered. The adverse effects evolved even in some cases treated with a total dose of less than 50 mg, while no adverse effects appeared in the other cases treated with even 300 mg or more.

These adverse effects, like those of bleomycin, were frequent stomatitis, fever, and changes of the skin, while myelodepression and pulmonary fibrosis were encountered in none of the cases.

The relation of the total doses of pepleomycin to its effects was such that the treatment, as shown in Fig. 24, gave a I−B or better effect in four of the cases of malignant lymphoma and of squamous cell carcinoma; and in three of the four cases, not less than 300 mg pepleomycin was administered. However, it is not true to say that the treatment was so effective in these cases because such a large dose could be administered, rather that the antitumor effect evolved relatively early in them, and such a large total dose was the result of a lack of adverse effects.

In one case of lung cancer treated with a total dose of 345 mg and one case of malignant lymphoma treated with a total dose of 435 mg, the patients have been healthy for 2 years.

The pepleomycin treatment, on the other hand, was not so effective against adenocarcinomas as against malignant lymphoma and squamous cell carcinoma. Even in the cases of adenocarcinomas, pepleomycin, when administered IA locally, gave a I−A effect (in one case of lung metastasis of duodenal cancer) and a 0−C (in two cases of prostatic cancer, one of hepatic cancer, and one of hepatic metastasis of colonic cancer). In one of the two cases of prostatic cancer, the local IA administration of pepleomycin not only caused a local improvement but was effective against the lung metastases. Subselective IA administration of pepleomycin was performed in three cases of stomach cancer, but was effective in none of them.

As described above, it was greatly anticipated that pepleomycin would find a wider range of indications than bleomycin; however, although the drug, when administered

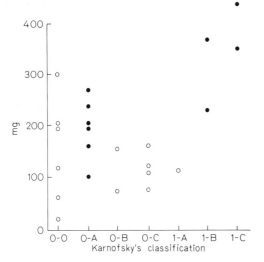

Fig. 24. Correlations between total doses and effects

locally, gave some antitumor effect in adenocarcinomas, it was considered difficult to find a wider range of indications for it by systemic administration only.

Conclusion

The phase I and II study of pepleomycin was made in 23 cases of various advanced cancers. Although pepleomyin failed to give a marked antitumor effect against adenocarcinomas, except for the effects against hepatic cancer and prostatic cancer (I−A and 0−C effects), it was accompanied by low incidences of adverse effects, especially, by a low incidence of pulmonary fibrosis. Hence, this drug may be considered to take the place of bleomycin.

References

1. Brochure of preclinical studies of NK631. Institute of Microbial Chemistry (1976) Brochure of preclinical studies of NK631. Nippon Kayaku, Tokyo
2. Karnofsky DA (1961) Meaningful clinical classification of therapeutic response to anticancer drugs. Clin Pharmacol Ther 2: 709−712
3. Miura T, Ishida M (1974) Effects of triple agent chemotherapy with mitomycin C, 5-FU and cylocide in 31 cases of various tumors; i.a. therapy using uronase. Jpn J Cancer Clin 20: 255−263
4. Miura T, Wada T, Katayama K, Miyahara T, Hashimoto D, Konishi T, Haida K, Haida S (1977) Surgical chemotherapy of colonic cancer. Cancer Chemother 4: 971−982
5. Miura T, Wada T (1978) Evaluation of chemotherapy of hepatic carcinoma, with particular reference to chemotherapy by selective infusion into the hepatic artery. Surg Diagn Treat 20: 144−154

Tallysomycin, A Third Generation Bleomycin Analog

S. T. Crooke, J. E. Strong, W. T. Bradner, J. Schurig,
A. Schlein, and A. W. Prestayko*

Bristol Laboratories, Thompson Road, USA – Syracuse, NY 13201

Introduction

The bleomycins, discovered in 1966 by Umezawa and colleagues [12], have been the focus of intense interest for a number of years. Unique molecular pharmacologic, clinical pharmacologic, and toxicologic characteristics, and substantial clinical activities have resulted in significant analog development efforts. At present more than 300 analogs of bleomycin have been reported, and these analogs can be divided into three generations. First generation analogs can be thought of as the initial 13 bleomycins isolated. Second generation analogs are those that differ from the initial bleomycins only by changes in the terminal amine structure, or by very minor modifications in the bleomycinic acid portion of the molecule. Third generation analogs can be thought of as those differing significantly from the bleomycins in the bleomycinic acid portion of the molecule. The tallysomycins are third generation bleomycin analogs.

The goals of the development of bleomycin analogs, to which various programs have been directed, include the reduction in toxicities, particularly pulmonary toxicities, mucocutaneous toxicities, and hyperpyrexia. An expanded spectrum of activity which would include activity against adenocarcinomas and compounds which have different pharmacokinetic characteristics have also been targets of analog programs.

Chemistry

Figure 1 shows the structure of tallysomycin A, compared to the structures of a number of other bleomycin analogs [5–7]. Inasmuch as the structural proof for tallysomycin was based on the structure of bleomycin, the recently reported alteration of the structure of bleomycin is reflected in the proposed structure of tallysomycin. In a manner analogous to the development of bleomycin analogs, a number of tallysomycin analogs have been prepared which differ in the terminal amine structure.

* The authors thank Ms. Julie Durantini for excellent typographical assistance, and Dr. Harris Busch for his continuing guidance and support

Molecular Pharmacology

The molecular pharmacologic characteristics of tallysomycin are similar to those of the bleomycins. Tallysomycin A interacts with transition metals in a manner similar to the bleomycins. At a 1 : 1 tallysomycin : metal ion concentration, tallysomycin has been shown to bind Cu (II), Zn (II), and Fe (II) at a site equivalent to the bleomycin site. At higher metal ion to bleomycin ratios, a second Cu (II) or Zn (II) ion can be bound. This site employs the amino group of the L-talose moiety, and amino groups in the β-lysine and spermidine portion of the molecule. This site is significantly less thermodynamically stable than the primary site, and does not bind to Fe (II) [3]. After binding to Fe (II) in the primary binding site, tallysomycin has been shown to facilitate rapidly the oxidation of Fe (II) to Fe (III) [4].

Tallysomycin binds to DNA in a manner similar to bleomycin [10]. Employing fluorescence quenching techniques, tallysomycin has been shown to bind to DNA with greater affinity than bleomycin (Km for salmon sperm DNA : $8.47 \pm 1.06 \times 10^5 \ M^{-1}$

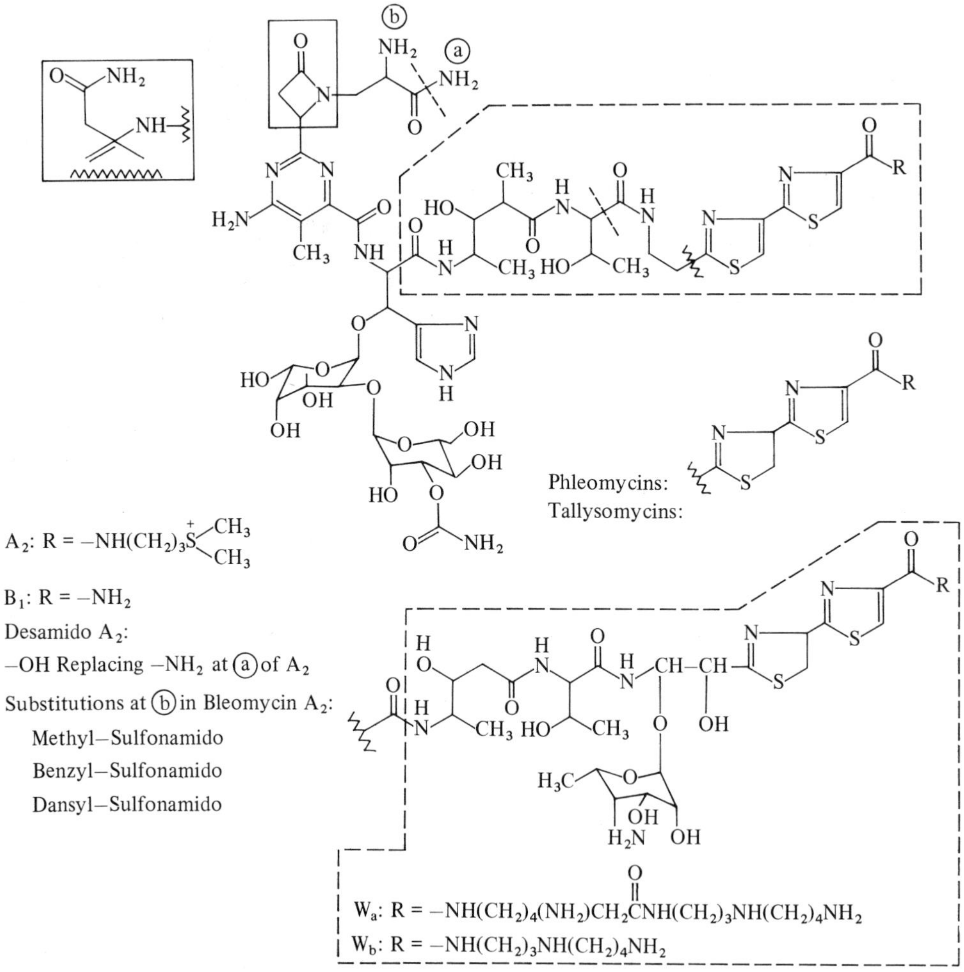

A_2: R = $-NH(CH_2)_3\overset{+}{S}\overset{CH_3}{\underset{CH_3}{<}}$

B_1: R = $-NH_2$

Desamido A_2:

$-OH$ Replacing $-NH_2$ at (a) of A_2

Substitutions at (b) in Bleomycin A_2:

   Methyl–Sulfonamido

   Benzyl–Sulfonamido

   Dansyl–Sulfonamido

Phleomycins:

Tallysomycins:

W_a: R = $-NH(CH_2)_4(NH_2)CH_2\overset{O}{\overset{\|}{C}}NH(CH_2)_3NH(CH_2)_4NH_2$

W_b: R = $-NH(CH_2)_3NH(CH_2)_4NH_2$

Fig. 1. Structures of bleomycin analogs

versus $3.41 \pm 0.42 \times 10^4\ M^{-1}$). However the number of nucleotides per molecule of tallysomycin were equivalent to the number of nucleotides per bleomycin A_2 molecule (4.04 ± 0.13 versus 3.39 nucleotides per molecule). Binding of tallysomycin to DNA is inhibited by higher ionic strength buffers and by EDTA and Cu (II) and Zn (II) [4].

Tallysomycin has been shown to induce DNA breakage in a manner similar to bleomycin A_2. The pH optima, ionic strength optima, metal ion effects, the effects of reducing agents, and the temperature optima were equivalent for tallysomycin and bleomycin A_2 [9]. Moreover, tallysomycin and bleomycin were both shown to induce single- and double-strand breaks in PM-2 DNA [10]. However, although tallysomycin has greater affinity for DNA, it was shown to be a less potent DNA degradative agent than bleomycin. This is probably due to acquiring a greater energy of activation for DNA degradation [9].

Treatment of Novikoff hepatoma cells and HeLa cells in vitro has been shown to inhibit DNA synthesis and to result in degradation of intracellular DNA [9]. Preliminary studies have demonstrated that tallysomycin has effects on the cell cycle similar to those of bleomycin A_2.

Biologic Activities

Tallysomycin A is a highly potent antibacterial agent. It has minimal inhibitory concentrations against gram-positive and gram-negative organisms including *Pseudomonas* and *Proteus* species under 2 µg/ml. It is more than 20-fold more potent than bleomycin against most organisms studied. It is also a highly potent antifungal agent with minimal inhibitory concentrations of $0.8-12.5$ µg/ml against *cryptococcus neoformans*, *aspergillus niger*, and *candida albicans*. It is more than 20-fold more potent than bleomycin against most fungi tested [1].

In general, the spectrum of activity against rodent tumors in vivo of tallysomycin A is similar to that of bleomycin. However, in all tumors tested, tallysomycin has proved to be more potent. Table 1 shows a comparison of the potencies of tallysomycin A and bleomycin against various tumors. The potency ratios for tallysomycin A to bleomycin

Table 1. Comparison of in vivo antitumor potencies of tallysomycin A and bleomycin

Tumor	Maximum MST		Potency radio[a] TLM : BLM
	BLM	TLM A	
L-1210 Leukemia	Inactive	Inactive	
P388-J Leukemia	131	150	8−12
Lewis lung	200	165	1
B16 Melanoma (S.C.)	163	183	10
B16 Melanoma (IP)	Inactive	138	
B16 Melanoma (solid)	136	151	2
Walker 256	> 489	> 489	4
Sarcoma 180	193	> 293	10
Colon 38	Inactive	Active	

[a] Potency ratios determined by comparing doses required to give maximum mean survival time. Potencies are compared at the dose that induced the maximum survival increase

against all tumors studied has ranged from 3–20, demonstrating clearly that tallysomycin A is a more potent antitumor agent than bleomycin [1, 5]. However, against some tumors, tallysomycin has not resulted in as significant a maximal increase in survival time as bleomycin, e.g., B16 melanoma, and Lewis lung carcinoma. Neither drug is active against L1210 leukemia, and neither drug demonstrated oral activity against a bleomycin sensitive line of P-388 leukemia.

Pharmacokinetics

A radioimmunoassay for tallysomycin A has been developed [2]. The maximum sensitivity of the assay is approximately 2.5 ng/ml as shown in Fig. 2. The radioimmunoassay does not cross-react with other antibiotics, antineoplastic agents, or the closely related bleomycins (Table 2). Tallysomycin B and its fragment Wb (see Fig. 1) cross-react only to the extent of 5%. However, when complexed with copper,

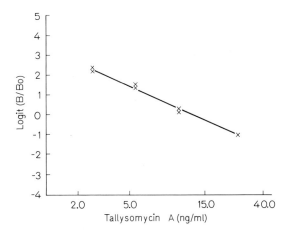

Fig. 2. Sensitivity of tallysomycin RIA

Table 2. Cross-reactivity of Tallysomycin antisera

Drug	%Cross-reactivity[a]	Drug	%Cross reactivity
Tallysomycin A	100	Bleomycin	< 0.1
Vincristine	< 0.1	Desamidobleomycin	< 0.1
Peptichemio	< 0.1	Phleomycin	< 0.1
Neocarzinostatin	< 0.1	Tallysomycin A with copper	100
Methotrexate	< 0.1	Peptide Wa	62
Adriamycin	< 0.1	Tallysomycin B with copper	33
Carminomycin	0.1	Tallysomycin B	5.0
		Tallysomycin E_{1a} with copper	5.0
		Tallysomycin S_2 B with copper	< 1.0
		Peptide Wb	5.0

[a] Cross-reactivity was defined as the molar concentration of drug required to produce 50% inhibition of the iodine-125 tallysomycin bound by antiserum relative to unlabeled tallysomycin A

tallysomycin B showed 33% cross-reactivity. The peptide fragment Wa cross-reacted extensively, but compounds with modified terminal amines cross-reacted minimally.

Employing the tallysomycin A radioimmunoassay, the pharmacokinetics of tallysomycin have been compared to bleomycin in the beagle dog and the monkey [11]. Both compounds exhibited biphasic plasma elimination characteristics, and were extensively absorbed after intramuscular administration. The elimination half-lives of tallysomycin in the dog were 2.03 ± 0.50 h and 2.04 ± 0.41 h after intravenous or intramuscular administration respectively. These values were significantly longer than the comparable intravenous (1.1 ± 0.14 h) and intramuscular (1.31 ± 0.17) elimination half-lives for bleomycin. Figure 3 shows the serum elimination curves in a dog that was administered bleomycin and tallysomycin A simultaneously. More pronounced differences were observed in the rhesus monkey. The elimination half-lives of tallysomycin was approximately 5 h and bleomycin < 0.6 h after intravenous administration.

The total apparent volumes of distribution and the total peripheral compartment volume of distribution were larger for tallysomycin than bleomycin in the dog and monkey. This may reflect greater tissue binding of tallysomycin as it has a higher affinity for its principal intracellular target, DNA, than does bleomycin. Moreover, these pharmacokinetic differences may account for the greater in vivo antitumor activity of tallysomycin than bleomycin in the absence of greater in vitro activity. The data in dogs and monkeys also suggest that the clearance of tallysomycin from the body may differ from bleomycin since the 24 h urinary recovery rate for tallysomycin was 20% as compared to 80% for bleomycin.

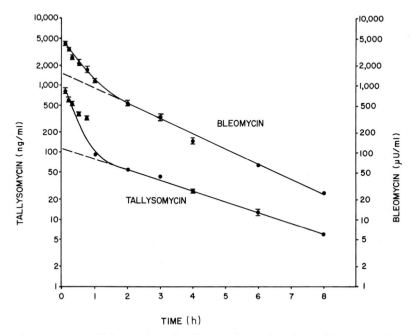

Fig. 3. The plasma decay curves of bleomycin and tallysomycin A administered intravenously simultaneously to the beagle dog. When not indicated, standard errors were smaller than the symbol employed

Toxicologic Characteristics

General. The acute and subacute toxicities of tallysomycin A and bleomycin have been compared in the mouse, rat, dog, and monkey. Again, tallysomycin A was shown consistently to be more potent than bleomycin in all species studied, and with all dose schedules employed.

Pulmonary Toxicities. The relative pulmonary toxicities of tallysomycin and bleomycin have been compared in the mouse, dog, and monkey. In the mouse, studies employing histopathologic examinations of mice treated twice weekly for 6 weeks with several doses of each drug demonstrated that tallysomycin A was less pulmonary toxic if a 4 : 1 potency ratio was assumed for tallysomycin A [1]. For example, tallysomycin A at a daily dose of 4 mg/kg induced subpleural fibrosis in three of nine animals. At a daily dose of 4 mg/kg bleomycin induced subpleural fibrosis in six of ten mice treated, and at 16 mg/kg per day (the daily dose of bleomycin comparable to 4 mg/kg tallysomycin A), bleomycin induced subpleural fibrosis in six of seven animals.
More recently, total lung hydroxyproline levels in mice have been employed to provide a quantitative, albeit indirect, estimate of the relative pulmonary toxicities of bleomycin and tallysomycin A [8]. Figure 4 shows the dose-hydroxyproline response curves obtained for tallysomycin A and bleomycin. As can be seen, tallysomycin A and

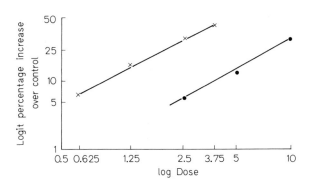

Fig. 4. Dose response curves for tallysomycin ($-\times-$) and bleomycin ($-\bigcirc-$) effects on hydroxyproline in mice after 11 weeks of treatment

Table 3. Multiple dose pulmonary toxicity in the monkey

Drug	Dose (mg/kg)	Total histopathologic score[a]		
		Alveolitis	Parenchymal fibrosis	Interstital pneumonitis
Tallysomycin A	0.752[b]	0	0	1
	0.188	0	0	5
	0.094	0	0	4
Bleomycin	4.0	12	10	10
	1.0	3	3	6
Control		0	0	3

[a] Four animals in each group were scored 0–4 for increasing severity. Maximum score: 16
[b] Drugs were administered at indicated dose intravenously every 4 days for 6 weeks

bleomycin were approximately equipulmonary toxic if a 4 : 1 potency ratio is assumed. Whether this difference in results represents strain differences or limitations of the indirect hydroxyproline assay is not yet defined.

In the monkey, tallysomycin A has been clearly demonstrated to be less pulmonary toxic than bleomycin. In this study bleomycin and tallysomycin A were administered twice intravenously to monkeys at three dose levels for 6 weeks. One half the treated animals were necropsied one week after completion of dosing. The other half was observed for 120 days after dosing was discontinued, the necropsied. Pulmonary toxicities were evaluated histopathologically.

The results of the monkey toxicologic study are shown in Table 3. At no tallysomycin dose employed was there significant evidence of pulmonary toxicity observed. However at both doses of bleomycin, evidence of pulmonary toxicity was present.

Nephrotoxicity. Although bleomycin and tallysomycin A produced qualitatively equivalent nephrotoxicity in animals, tallysomycin A has been shown to be a more potent nephrotoxin than bleomycin in all species studied. At high doses in all species studied, both drugs induced progressive, apparently irreversible renal tubular intoxication that manifested itself in increases in BUN and serum creatinine levels, and urine abnormalities.

Multiple dose studies in the dog and monkey suggest that in each species tallysomycin A is 12.5 (dog) and 5 times (monkey) as potent a nephrotoxin as bleomycin. Single dose studies in the rat, dog, and monkey suggest that tallysomycin A is 10, 24, and 12 times as potent in each species as bleomycin. If a potency ratio of 4 : 1 is assumed (in most in vivo tumor systems, tallysomycin A has proved more than four times as potent), the ratios of nephrotoxicity would be 3 and 1.25 for dogs and monkeys respectively that were treated subacutely and 2.5, 6, and 3 for rats, dogs and monkeys respectively that were treated with single doses. The state of hydration was not monitored in these studies, nor have any studies been performed to determine if hydration or diureses reduces the nephrotoxicity of either drug.

Discussion

The tallysomycins represent the first third generation analogs of bleomycin. Tallysomycin A has been shown to be very similar to bleomycin molecular pharmacologically, but to be significantly more potent as an antibacterial, antifungal, and in vivo antitumor agent. The enhanced in vivo potency may relate to a longer serum elimination half-life and greater distribution in the peripheral compartment.

Histopathologic studies suggest that tallysomycin A is significantly less pulmonary toxic than bleomycin in the mouse and the monkey. However, hydroxyproline assays suggest that tallysomycin A and bleomycin are approximately equipulmonary toxic in the mouse. Tallysomycin A is a more potent nephrotoxin than bleomycin in all species but both agents produce qualitatively equivalent toxicities.

Tallysomycin A is an analog that merits clinical investigation for the following reasons:

1) In direct histopathologic comparisons in two species, tallysomycin has been shown to induce less pulmonary toxicity than bleomycin.

2) Tallysomycin A is a potent antitumor agent with a spectrum of activity slightly broader than bleomycin.
3) Although of concern, the nephrotoxicity of tallysomycin A is not a major inhibitory factor because (a) the nephrotoxicity of tallysomycin A is qualitatively equivalent to bleomycin, an agent that does not induce clinically significant nephrotoxicity; (b) nephrotoxicity is a much simpler toxicity to evaluate, and thus to avoid, clinically than is pulmonary toxicity; and (c) recent experience with cis platinum suggests that nephrotoxicity of severely nephrotoxic agents may be ameliorated by careful hydration and diuresis.
4) Tallysomycin A differs pharmacokinetically from bleomycin.
5) Tallysomycin A is a single component.
6) Tallysomycin A may prove to be less expensive than bleomycin.

References

1. Bradner WT (1978) BU-2231, A third-generation bleomycin: Preclinical studies. In: Carter SK, Crooke ST, Umezawa H (eds) Bleomycin: current status and new developments. Academic Press, New York, pp 333–342
2. Broughton A, Strong JE, Crooke ST, Prestayko AW (to be published) A radioimmunoassay for tallysomycin. Cancer Treat Rep
3. Greenaway FT, Dabrowiak JC, van Husen M, Grulich R, Crooke ST (1978) The transition metal binding properties of a 3rd generation bleomycin analogue, tallysomycin. Biochem Biophys Res Commun 85: 1407–1414
4. Huang CH, Galvan L, Crooke ST (to be published) Quenching of flourescence of bleomycin by ferrour ion and its correlation with DNA-breakage activity. J Biochem
5. Imanishi H, Ohbayashi M, Nishiyama Y, Kawaguchi H (1978) Tallysomycin, a new antitumor antibiotic complex related to bleomycin. III. Antitumor activity of tallysomycins A and B. Antibiot (Tokyo) 31: 667–674
6. Kawaguchi H, Tsukiura H, Tomita K, Konishi M, Saito K, Kobaru S, Numata K, Fujisawa K, Miyaki T, Hatori M, Koshiyama H (1977) Tallysomycin, a new antitumor antibiotic complex related to bleomycin. I. Production, isolation and properties. J Antibiot (Tokyo) 30: 779–788
7. Konishi M, Saito K, Numata K, Tsuno T, Asama K, Tsukiura H, Takayuki N, Kawaguchi H (1977) Tallysomycin, a new antitumor antibiotic complex related to bleomycin. II. Structure determination of tallysomycin A and B. J Antibiot (Tokyo) 30: 789–805
8. Sikic BI, Mimnaugh EG, Gram TE (1978) Development of quantifiable parameters of bleomycin toxicity in the mouse lung. In: Carter SK, Crooke ST, Umezawa H (eds) Bleomycin: current status and new developments. Academic Press, New York, pp 293–297
9. Strong JE, Crooke ST (1978) Mechanism of action of tallysomycin, a third generation bleomycin. In: Carter SK, Crooke ST, Umezawa H (eds) Bleomycin: current status and new developments. Academic Press, New York, pp 343–355
10. Strong JE, Crooke ST (1978) DNA breakage of tallysomycin. Cancer Res 38: 3322–3326
11. Strong JE, Schurig J, Issell BF, Tavel A, Florczyk AP, Crooke ST (to be published) Pharmacokinetics of tallysomycin and bleomycin in the beagle dog. Cancer Treat Rep
12. Umezawa H, Maeda K, Takeuchi T, Okami Y (1966) New antibiotics, bleomycin A and B. Antibiot Ser A (Tokyo) 19: 200–209

Studies of Analogs of Fluorinated Pyrimidine in Japan

Y. Sakurai

Cancer Chemotherapy Center, Japanese Foundation for Cancer Research, Kami-Ikebukuro 1-37-1, Toshima-ku, J – Tokyo 170

Ftorafur

Ftorafur, 1-(2-tetrahydrofuryl)-5-fluorouracil, is a cancer drug very widely used in treatment of cancer in Japan; in particular, it is administered orally for treatment of tumors of the gastrointestinal tract. Recently a new preparation with an enteric coating became available for oral administration. Ftorafur itself is absorbed mainly from the jejunum and ileum, and slightly from the duodenum, but not from the stomach. This new preparation was designed to release ftorafur only in the intestine, and in experiments with beagle dogs it was shown to be absorbed more easily than the earlier preparation. With the same dose, approximately 20% greater total absorption into the blood was estimated with the new preparation. In clinical trials, side effects of the new preparation, especially to the upper digestive organs, were less evident than those of the previous one, which released nearly 100% ftorafur into the stomach within 10 min after the oral administration. The new preparation was tolerated by patients at daily doses of approximately 1 000 mg/m^2 for continuous treatment.

The merit of ftorafur in practical use promoted various attempts to find new masked-type analogs of 5-fluorouracil (5-FU), and two analogs at present have come to clinical trial in Japan. Ones is FD-1, 1,3-bis(tetrahydro-2-furyl)-5-fluoro-2,4-pyrimidindione, which was prepared by Taiho Pharmaceutical Company, and was first proved to have some effect on certain human solid cancers. However its clinical trial was recently discontinued, on account of substantial manifestation of untoward toxicity to the central nervous system.

1-Hexylcarbamoyl-5-fluorouracil

The second analog is 1-hexylcarbamoyl-5-fluorouracil (HCFU), which was first supplied by Mitsui Pharmaceuticals, Inc., in 1975 [11]. This compound was selected as the most promising analog among many derivatives of 1-alkylcarbamoyl-5-fluorouracil in respect to its balance of antitumor effect and toxicity on a series of mouse tumor models as shown by Iigo et al. [4] in 1978. They evaluated 16 analogs with six tumor models: ascitic sarcoma 180, ascitic Ehrlich carcinoma, C1498 leukemia, L1210 leukemia, adenocarcinoma 755, and Fukuoka-Nakahara sarcoma. Of these, 1-methyl- and 1-ethyl-derivatives showed marked antitumor activity, followed by 1-hexyl- and

1-octyl-derivatives. However, the former two compounds exhibited untoward side effects in mice, though they were not lethal. Abnormal behavior accompanied by tremor or paralysis of the hind legs was observed among the mice treated with these compounds. 1-Hexylcarbamoyl-5-fluorouracil (HCFU) was thus selected as an agent for clinical trial because of its better chemotherapeutic index. HCFU is a white crystalline powder that decomposes at 110° C and tastes bitter. It is easily soluble in chloroform and acetone, sparingly soluble in benzene and ethanol, and nearly insoluble in water (0.006 w/v%). Its molecular weight is about twice that of 5-FU. The effect of 5-FU derivatives on L1210 was briefly indicated in Table 1 [3].

The effect of HCFU on B16 melanoma and Lewis lung carcinoma was tested by Iigo et al. [5]. The mice bearing B16 were given the drugs orally on days 1, 3, 5, 8, 10, and 12, and the result was checked by prolongation of life span (median). Maximum increase in life span (ILS max) with HCFU was 38% at daily dose of 300 mg/kg, while ILS max with ftorafur and 5-FU were 26% at daily dose of 200 mg/kg and 9% at daily dose of 50 mg/kg. HCFU was also effective on Lewis lung carcinoma, showing ILS max of 100% at daily dose of 200 mg/kg, while ftorafur exhibited 70% ILS max at the same daily

Table 1. Effect of HCFU and its related compounds on L1210

Compounds	Dose, per os[d]		Effect	
	ILS_{30} mg/kg/day	ILS max. mg/kg/day	Max. ILS %	T.I.[a]
HCFU[b]	44	200	53	4.5
FH[c]	98	100	31	1.0
5-FU	26	50	56	1.9

[a] Therapeutic index (ILS max/ILS_{30})
[b] 1-Hexylcarbamoyl-5-fluorouracil
[c] Ftorafur
[d] Drug was given on day 1 to 5

Table 2. Effect of HCFU and 5-FU on mouse colon tumor 26

Dose (mg/kg)	ILS[a] (%)	Time to 750 mg[b] (day)	T−C[c] (day)	Tumor free survivor
HCFU 300	200	43	25	1/7
200	86	21.5	3.5	0/7
100	6	17	0	0/7
5-FU 50	58	30	12	0/7
30	86	22	4	0/7
20	1	18	0	0/7

[a] Median survival days of control were 18 days
[b] Days until the tumors of the treated mice reach 750 mg
[c] (Time to 750 mg of control mice) − (Time to 750 mg of treated mice). Time to 750 mg of the control was 18 days
The tumor was inoculated subcutaneously in the axillary region of CDF_1 mice with 3×10^5 cells. The drugs were given orally from day 1 to 28 with 3 day interval

dose. The antitumor effect of HCFU on mouse transplantable colon carcinomas was examined by Tsuruo [13]. The result with colon 26 is shown in Table 2; experiments with other colon tumors are now in progress.

The acute toxicities of HCFU and its related compounds are shown in Table 3. Tolerance of long-term oral administration was guessed from the data for dogs with repeated administration, which are shown in Table 4. Even with oral administration of HCFU for 6 months with daily doses of 5 mg/kg, all dogs of both sexes survived.

Distribution of this compound was also studied by Iigo et al. [6]. The level of concentration of HCFU and 5-FU released from the parent compound, in the serum of rats given orally 50 mg/kg of HCFU, is demonstrated in Fig. 1. In a similar experiment with rats given orally 50 mg/kg of HCFU, the cumulative excretion in the urine in the forms of HCFU and 5-FU was as indicated in Fig. 2. As for distribution of HCFU into the tissues, the highest concentration − nearly 270 μg/g tissue − was attained in the stomach from 1−2 h after administration, followed by the concentration in the small intestine and kidney (approximately 17−19 μg/g). The transition of level of HCFU and 5-FU in the serum of dogs orally given 10 mg/kg HCFU was shown in Fig. 3. Metabolites of HCFU were first pursued in male Sprague-Dawley rats with HCFU-6-^{14}C by Kobari et al. [9]. The final active metabolite is, of course, 5-FU, but

Table 3. LD$_{50}$ and LD$_{10}$ of HCFU and related compounds (oral administration, 2 weeks, mg/kg)

	Mouse		Dog	
	♂	♀	♂	♀
LD$_{50}$ HCFU	1260	1350	65	97
Ftorafur	1510	1620	48	
5-FU	390		22	
LD$_{10}$ HCFU		210		
Ftorafur		240		
5-FU		68		

Table 4. Mortality of beagle dogs orally administered HCFU and its related compounds (13 weeks)

Compounds	Daily dose mg/kg	Mortality	
		Male	Female
HCFU	1	0/3	0/3
	5	0/3	0/3
	10	2/5	1/5
	15	0/3	2/3
Ftorafur	15	3/3	3/3
5-FU	5	2/3	2/3

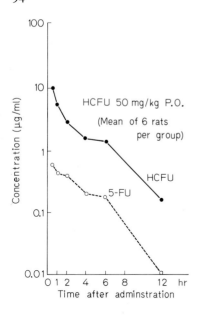

Fig. 1. Concentration of HCFU and 5-FU in the serum of rats orally given 50 mg/kg HCFU

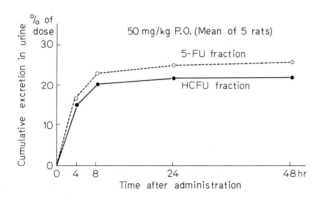

Fig. 2. Cumulative excretion in urine after oral administration of HCFU to rats (50 mg/kg)

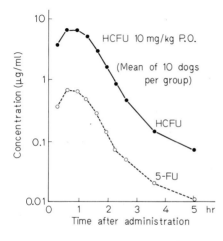

Fig. 3. Concentration of HCFU and 5-FU in the serum of dogs after oral administration of 10 mg/kg HCFU

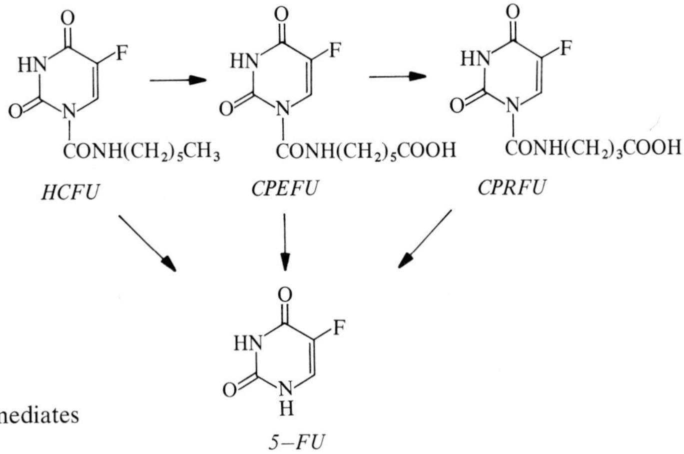

Fig. 4. Structure of intermediates of HCFU

two intermediates have been found so far: one is CPEFU (1-ω-carboxypentyl-carbamoyl-5-fluorouracil) and the other CPRFU (1-ω-carboxypropyl-carbamoyl-5-fluorouracil); these were later detected also in the urine and serum either of beagle dogs or of the patients treated in phase 1 study (Fig. 4). It must be noted that HCFU induced a rhythmic contraction of the bladder of rabbit or cat, and this movement was stronger and longer-lasting in the case of an intermediate, CPEFU, than for the parent compound.

HCFU was brought into phase I study in 1977 in Japan because of its promising efficacy with less toxicity than ftorafur or 5-FU, if it was given orally. Eleven hospitals joined in performing phase I study, and the number of patients entered were 111, which consisted of 40 cases of stomach, 22 of colorectal, 18 of breast, 10 of liver, and eight of lung cancers, and 13 of other miscellaneous malignancies. A report was issued in the name of Yoshiyuki Koyama and the HCFU clinical group [10]. The side effects were more frequent with increased dosage. Of the total of 58 trials, side effects occurred in 15 patients (25.9%), and the total number of side effects was 38. The most characteristic symptoms were pollakisuria and sensations of heat, which appeared seven and 11 times, respectively. Most cases of pollakisuria occurred 15–60 min after the oral administration and lasted from 30 min to 4 h.

These two side effects in the phase I study, heat sensation and pollakisuria, are regarded as peculiar ones, because we have not experienced the same phenomen with either 5-FU of ftorafur. Most of the patients who received HCFU complained at the moment of unpleasant feelings accompanied by these side effects. However, it may be possible in the future to find medications which alleviate these untoward side effects.

In animal experiments, the rhythmic contraction of the bladder caused by HCFU was blocked by intravenous injection of atropine or hexamethonium, but not by diphenhydramine. The contraction did not appear in the spinal cut canimals (C_1-C_2), suggesting that the action of the drug was mediated by CNS.

Maximum tolerable dose (MTD) at a single oral administration was estimated as approximately 20 mg/kg. The optimal daily dose for continuous treatment was supposed to be 9 mg/kg and 18 mg/kg with divided administration. Among 31 cases that were treated continuously for 60 days, no serious adverse reactions, such as hematologic, hepatic, renal, and CNS toxicities, were observed. Koyama stated that among 31 patients who received HCFU for more than 60 days, improvement in clinical findings was seen in seven patients, two with measurable lesions and five with evaluable lesions. The compound is now moving into phase II study.

Enhancement of Effect of Ftorafur by Simultaneous Administration of Uracil

In 1971, Garattini [2] reported that six repeated intraperitoneal injections of 20 mg/kg of 5-FU to rats induced a marked enhancement of the microsomal enzyme activity of the liver, which metabolizes the drug, while after a single shot of the same drug the activity of the liver enzyme was impaired. On the other hand, Jato et al. [7, 8] reported in 1975 that the antitumor effect of 5-FU was increased by a simultaneous administration of deoxyuridine, but no improvement in the chemotherapeutic index resulted because of accompanied increase of toxicity to the host. Many papers have recently been published which discuss positive or negative influence of pyrimidines on the antitumor effect of 5-FU. In 1979 Vogel et al. [14] published a paper on the clinical trial of 5-FU plus thymidine on patients having colorectal carcinoma. The conclusion of the paper was that the addition of thymidine to 5-FU infusion enhanced 5-FU toxicity and changed the pattern of dose-limiting side effects. The patients who received thymidine plus 5-FU at doses of one-fourth to one-half the usual 5-FU dose for infusion all suffered from myelosuppression, and fatal granulocytopenia was also seen in four of 12 patients. Gastrointestinal toxicities, including stomatitis, were only rarely observed.

It is noticeable that these doses of 5-FU would not be expected to manifest such bone marrow toxicity when infused alone, and it is well known too that the ordinary dose-limiting toxicity of 5-FU infusion is not hematologic but gastrointestinal. The action of noncytotoxic pyrimidines, which are given along with 5-FU, seemed to be involved. Pyrimidines, including 5-FU, might enhance catabolic enzyme activity of the host liver, or noncytotoxic pyrimidines might compete with 5-FU on the catabolic enzyme, resulting in protection of 5-FU from catabolic degradation in vivo.

In 1977 Toide et al. [12] compared the metabolism of 5-FU and ftorafur in animals and in vitro. According to their results, 5-FU was rapidly metabolized into fluoro-β-alanine, while ftorafur as such did not inhibit DNA synthesis, but 70% ftorafur, intravenously given to rats or mice, was slowly metabolized to 5-FU, which successively decomposed into fluoro-β-alanine. In vitro degradation of ftorafur into 5-FU took place predominantly by the microsomal fraction of the liver of both animals in the presence of NADPH, which suggested that microsomal electron transport system was concerned with this reaction.

Since it was known that uracil, cytosine, or thymine did not reverse the growth inhibition of the mammalian cells affected by 5-FU, Fujii et al. [1] anticipated that, if ftorafur was administered with uracil, the latter would prevent degradation in vivo of 5-FU, which was released from ftorafur, and thus increased the antitumor efficacy of the former. They tried in 1978 to examine the influence of uracil on the effect of ftorafur on Sarcoma 180 and a transplantable rat ascites hepatoma, AH 130. The effect on sarcoma 180 is indicated in Table 5.

It was suggested that the addition of uracil enhanced remarkably the antitumor effect of ftorafur and 5-FU, but, judging from the body weight change, increase of toxicity of ftorafur by addition of uracil was less than that of 5-FU. A similar result was obtained with rat ascites hepatoma AH 130. In this experiment, Donryu strain rats were inoculated subcutaneously with the 10^7 ascitic tumor cells. The result, shown in Table 6, seemed to indicate that an increase in the molar ratio of uracil enhanced the antitumor effect of ftorafur, with an accompanying increase in toxicity. However, there seemed to be a possibility that an optimal dose of uracil might improve the chemotherapeutic index of ftorafur. As seen in Table 6, the treatment with 60 mg/kg of ftorafur plus 68 mg/kg of uracil (molar ratio: 2) exhibited a far stronger antitumor effect than 90 mg/kg ftorafur alone, without showing a marked difference in body weight change in either treatment.

The results of a comparative determination of the level of 5-FU in the serum and tissues of rats bearing hepatoma AH 130, which were administered orally ftorafur alone or ftorafur plus uracil, are shown in Table 7. It is worth noticing that the 5-FU level in the tumor tissue rose remarkably and lasted long if uracil was added to ftorafur, while an increased concentration of 5-FU in the blood was not observed. A

Table 5. Effect of coadministration of ftorafur and uracil on sarcoma 180

	FT^a (mg/kg)	Molar ratio (U/FT)	Tumor wt. (g ± SD)	T/C (%)	Body wt. change (g)
Control	0	–	1.01 ± 0.18	–	+ 7
U^b + FT	40	2	0.23 ± 0.24	23	+ 4
U + FT	40	5	0.13 ± 0.10	13	0
FT alone	40	0	0.64 ± 0.25	64	+ 4
U + 5-FU	20	5	0.18 ± 0.04	18	– 7
U alone	0	224 mg/kg U	0.89 ± 0.30	89	+ 8

[a] Ftorafur
[b] Uracil

The tumor cells (2×10^7) were inoculated into the subepidermal tissue of ICR mice on day 0. The drugs were given orally on day 1 to 7. On day 10, tumor was removed and weighed

Table 6. Effect on AH130 of ftorafur plus uracil

FT^a (mg/kg)	Molar Ratio U^b/FT	T/C (%)	Body wt. change (g)
Control	0	–	+ 46
90	0	71	+ 38
60	2	12	+ 31
45	2	38	+ 34
30	2	52	+ 48
45	5	18	– 4
30	5	33	– 7
30	10	22	+ 8

[a] Ftorafur
[b] Uracil

The drugs were given orally once daily on day 11 to 7, and on day 10, the tumor was removed and weighed

Table 7. Level of 5-FU after administration of ftorafur plus uracil, and ftorafur alone (mcg/ml or g)

H. after administration	1		4		8	
	FT[a]	FT + U[b]	FT	FT + U	FT	FT + U
Blood	0.164	0.147	0.205	0.011	0.102	0.022
Tumor	0.222	0.871	0.329	1.334	0.325	0.594
Spleen	0.285	0.375	0.134	0.400	0.183	0.166
Bone marrow	0.189	0.174	0.214	0.126	0.034	0.040

[a] Ftorafur
[b] Uracil
A single dose of ^{3}H-ftorafur (90 mg/kg) alone, or ^{3}H-ftorafur (30 mg/kg) plus uracil (34 mg/kg) was orally administered

higher level of 5-FU than that in the blood was only detected in the spleen to a lesser degree; in other tissues, including the bone marrow, a significant rise in 5-FU level did not occur with simultaneous administration of uracil.

A reasonable explanation for this phenomenon has not yet been elucidated, but a preliminary clinical trial has begun recently in Japan using a mixture of ftorafur and uracil in a molar ratio of 1 : 4. In particular, determination of the level of 5-FU and ftorafur in human serum and tumor tissues surgically excised from patients after medication with this mixture is now in progress.

References

1. Fujii S, Ikenaka K, Fukushima M, Shirasaka T (1978) Effect of uracil and its derivatives on antitumor activity of 5-fluorouracil and 1-(2-tetrahydrofuryl)-5-fluorouracil. Gann 69 : 763−772
2. Garattini S (1971) Tumours and drug metabolism (General remarks). Proceeding of a seminar in clinical oncology. Padova, Sept 1971, pp 1−6
3. Hoshi A, Iigo M, Nakamura A, Yoshida M, Kuretani K (1976) Antitumor activity of 1-hexylcarbamoyl-5-fluorouracil in a variety of experimental tumors. Gann 67 : 725−731
4. Iigo M, Hoshi A, Nakamura A, Kuretani K (1978) Antitumor activity of 1-alkylcarbamoyl derivatives of 5-fluorouracil in a variety of mouse tumors. Cancer Chemother Pharmacol 1 : 203−208
5. Iigo M, Hoshi A, Nakamura A, Kuretani K (1978) Antitumor activity of 1-hexylcarbam-oyl-5-fluorouracil in Lewis lung carcinoma and B16 melanoma. J Pharm Dyn 1 : 49−54
6. Iigo M, Nakamura A, Kuretani K, Hoshi A (1979) Distribution 1-hexylcarbamoyl-5-fluo-rouracil and 5-fluorouracil by oral administration in mice. J Pharm Dyn 2 : 5−11
7. Jato JG, Lake LM, Grunden EE, Johnson BM (1975) Effect of deoxyuridine coadministration on toxicity and antitumor activity of fluorouracil and floxuridine. J Pharm Sci 64 : 943−946
8. Jato J, Windheuser JJ (1973) 5-Fluorouracil and derivatives in cancer chemotherapy. III: In vivo enhancement of antitumor activity of 5-fluorouracil and 5-fluoro-2′-deoxyuridine. J Pharm Sci 62 : 1975−1978

 9. Kobari T, Tan K, Kumakura M, Watanabe S, Shirakawa I, Kobayashi H, Ujiie A, Miyama Y, Namekawa H, Yamamoto H (1978) Metabolic fate of 1-hexylcarbamoyl-5-fluorouracil in rats. Xenobiotica 9: 547−556
10. Koyama Y, Hufu Clinical Group (to be published) Phase I study of a new drug, 1-hexylcarbamoyl-5-fluorouracil (HCFU) by oral administration. Cancer Treat Rep
11. Ozaki S, Mizuno H, Ishikawa K, Mori H (1977) 5-Fluorouracil derivatives. I. The synthesis of 1-carbamoyl-5-fluorouracils. Bull Chem Soc Jpn 50: 2406−2412
12. Toide H, Akiyoshi H, Minato Y, Okuda H, Fujii S (1977) Comparative studies on the metabolism of 2-(tetrahydrofuryl)-5-fluorouracil and 5-fluorouracil. Gann 68: 553−560
13. Tsuruo T (unpublished work) Antitumor effect of 1-hexylcarbamoyl-5-fluorouracil on mouse colon tumors
14. Vogel SJ, Presant CA, Ratkin GA, Klahr C (1979) Phase I study of thymidine plus 5-fluorouracil infusions in advanced colorectal carcinoma. Cancer Treat Rep 63: 1−5

The Pharmacology of Ftorafur
(R, S-1-(Tetrahydro-2-Furanyl)-5-Fluorouracil)*

J. L. Au and W. Sadée

School of Pharmacy and Department of Pharmaceutical Chemistry,
University of California San Francisco, USA – San Francisco, CA 94143

Introduction

Ftorafur (FT) was synthesized in the Soviet Union in 1966, as part of a program searching for fluorinated pyrimidines with an improved therapeutic index over that of 5-fluorouracil (FU) [29]. It bears structural resemblance to FU and 5-fluorodeoxy-uridine (FUdR), the two fluorinated pyrimidine antimetabolites in clinical use. It has been proposed that FT is metabolically activated in vivo and represents a chemical depot form of FU [12, 20, 21, 25, 34, 46, 47, 54, 56]. Clinically, FT has shown activity similar to that of FU, but it is less toxic to the bone marrow [27, 35, 58]. The reduced myelosuppression of FT has prompted clinical trials, first in the Soviet Union and Japan, and more recently in the United States [28]. However, the high neurotoxicity of FT may limit its widespread clinical use in the future [35, 58].

FU undergoes a series of metabolic conversions to its active nucleotides. Due to the complex scheme of activation, the tissue selectivity of FU may depend on a number of biochemical determinants (reviewed by Myers et al. [48] and Sadée and Wong [52] as well as its delivery to the target tissues. For example, when given as a prolonged infusion instead of a bolus injection, FU is less myelosuppressive [48, 52]. The plasma clearance of FU ranges from $0.4-2$ l/kg/h after a bolus injection to $3-60$ l/kg/h after an 8 h infusion [10, 16, 17, 39]. The reason for this drastic difference in FU pharmacokinetics is still obscure. When FU is administered in a form of metabolic prodrug, the kinetics of its release may be related to its bone marrow toxicity; moreover, the tissue selectivity is further complicated by the distribution characteristics, rate, and mechanism of activation of the FU prodrug, such as FT.

Although the clinical trials of FT were started in 1967, its pharmacology has not been fully elucidated. This chapter will review several aspects of its pharmacology, with particular emphasis on the kinetics and mechanism of metabolic activation of FT to FU.

Chemical Classification and Synthesis

FT represents a new class of heterocyclic compounds named furanidyl pyrimidines. The structure of FT is shown in Fig. 1 and is compared to those of FU and FUdR. FT is

* This work is supported by Public Health Research Grants GM-16496 from NIGMS, the Earl C. Anthony Fund from UCSF, and Training Grant GM 00728-15 from NIH

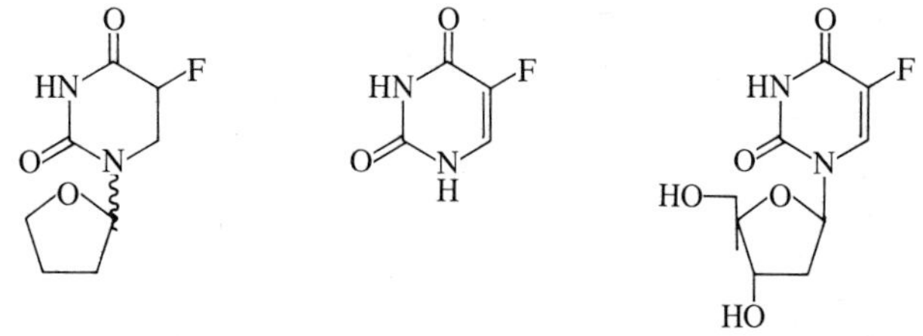

Fig. 1. Structures of ftorafur
(FT), 5-fluorouracil (FU), and
5-fluorodeoxyuridine (FUdR)

FT	FU	FUdR
pKa 7.8; MW 2oo	pKa 8.02; MW 130	pKa 7.8; MW 246

chemically unstable, and rapidly converts to FU at pH 1 or at temperatures above 80° C [28].

Numerous chemical schemes have been employed to synthesize FT. The commonly used methods include direct fluorination of tetrahydrofuranyluracil [15], and the condensation of substituted FU with tetrahydrofuranyl analogs [29, 30]. Both these methods yield the racemic mixture of R,S-FT, whereas the decarboxylation of the corresponding 2'-deoxynucleoside uronic acid anomers allows a stereospecific synthesis [32]. Resolution of the racemic FT into R-(+)- and S-(−)-FT has been achieved by fractional crystallization [64]. FT is available for clinical use as a racemic mixture.

Absorption

Pharmacokinetic studies in patients receiving an oral dose of 1g FT revealed nearly complete absorption with a peak plasma concentration of 25 µg/ml at 2 h following administration [13]. Similar results were found in rabbits [27]. In recent clinical trials in Japan with rectal administration of 1 g FT per day, peak plasma concentrations of 20 µg/ml occurred at 1−4 h postadministration [28]. In contrast to the erratic absorption of FU [16], FT is well absorbed through the gastrointestinal tract [28] with minimal degradation in the gastric juice [13].

Distribution

Following IV, oral, or rectal administration of [14]C- and ^{3}H-labeled FT to rats and mice, the administered radioactivity was recovered in the liver, small intestine, stomach, lung, spleen, kidney, tumors, and brain [12, 22, 23]. The highest concentrations of FU and FT were found in the liver [12], implicating the liver as the primary site of metabolic activation of FT to FU. FT is more lipid soluble than FU and, therefore, may cross the blood-brain barrier more rapidly [48]. Cohen [12] found that within 1 h after IV administration, the levels of FT in rat brain tissue were similar to those in liver, spleen, kidney, and small intestine. Fujita et al. [24] reported that rat brain levels of FT following an IV dose of 90 mg FT/kg were 200−300 times higher than those of FU following a similar dose of 30 mg FU/kg. However, the brain levels of FU at 1 h resulting from FT administration were slightly lower than those found after FU administration [24].

Antitumor Activities

Animal Studies

The antitumor activities of FT and FU on several transplanted tumors in rats and mice were compared. Both drugs produced comparable growth inhibition of L1210 leukemia, Sarcoma 180, Sarcoma AK, Walker's carcinosarcoma, Carcinoma HK, and Harding-Passey's melanoma, but neither drug had any activity against Sarcoma 45. FU was more effective against B16 melanoma, Gardener 6C3HED lymphosarcoma, and P388 leukemia [28]. In combination chemotherapy of L1210 leukemia, FU plus FT was no more effective than FU alone, and neither of the congeners was synergistic with either adriamycin or actinomycin D [25]. When used in combination with methotrexate, synergism was observed with FU but not with FT [25]. Sublines of L1210 leukemia were cross-resistant between FT and FU [25].

The similarity of their antineoplastic activities in animals and cross-resistance of cell lines to both drugs support the contention that FT exerts its antitumor effects primarily by activation to FU.

Horwitz et al. [32] compared the in vitro growth inhibitory effect on cultured human fibroblasts by the R-(+), S-(−) isomers and the racemic mixture of FT, and found no significant difference among these isomers. Similarly, no difference was observed in the inhibitory effects of these isomers on tumor growth in rats bearing AH-130 carcinoma and Yoshida Sarcoma [64].

Clinical Studies

Initial clinical trials with FT were performed in the Soviet Union in 1967 for treatment of various adenocarcinomas in humans. Daily IV dose of 30 mg FT/kg to a total of 30−40 g produced 50% reduction in tumor size in patients with stomach, colon, and breast cancer [35]. The activity of FT against rectal and brain tumors was considered to be superior to that of FU [9]. During the clinical trials in Japan, FT was given either orally, rectally, or intravenously to patients. The oral and rectal routes of administration were as effective as the IV administration with minimal gastrointestinal toxicity [38, 60]. The only comprehensive clinical evaluatiion of FT in the United States was completed in 1976. Valdivieso et al. [58] reported that daily doses of 2 g FT/m^2 for 5 days, repeated every 3 weeks, produced therapeutic activities comparable to those obtained with 5-day continuous IV infusion of FU against colon, stomach, and lung tumors in patients. Phase I clinical studies of FT given orally by multiple daily dosing regimen at 1−2 g/day are now on-going in the United States. Preliminary results indicate that this dosage is well tolerated with minimal gastrointestinal toxicity [1, 13, 49, 61].

Clinical Toxicities

FT is toxic to the epithelium of the gastrointestinal tract, the central nervous system, and the bone marrow. These side effects appear to be dose-related and occur at doses greater than 2 g/m^2 per day. The gastrointestinal and neurologic disturbances are the most common and dose-limiting toxicities of FT [58, 61]. Incidence of hematologic toxicity is less frequent, and a number of clinical trials indicated that FT is as effective against solid tumors, but less myelosuppressive than FU when the latter is given by bolus injection [35]. The pattern of clinical toxicities of FT, i.e., mild myelosuppression and significant gastrointestinal toxicity, is very similar to that of prolonged infusion of FU and FUdR [48].

Fujita et al. [24] compared the FU concentrations in rat brain after a dose of 90 mg FT/kg or 30 mg FU/kg. They found higher levels of FU, fluoroureido proprionic acid (FUPA), and fluoro-β-alanine (FBAL) one hour after the administration of the FU dose, during which time the neurologic toxicity of FT becomes significantly higher than that of FU. This indicates that the active component of FT contributing to its neurotoxicity is unrelated to FU, FBAL, or FUPA. The neurologic toxicities of FT, including ataxia, dizziness, and, less frequently, lethargy and headache, are shared by its structural analog, N-1,3-bis-(tetrahydrofuran-2-yl)-5-fluorouracil (FD-1) [44]. FD-1 was synthesized in Japan in 1977 and presumably also acts as a FU prodrug [36]. The dose-limiting toxicity of FD-1 observed during its clinical trials in Japan is its neurotoxicity, which represents the major factor prohibiting its further use [11, 44]. One of the major metabolites of FD-1 in rat plasma and brain tissue is γ-butyrolactone (in equilibrium with γ-hydroxybutyrate) derived from the tetrahydrofuran portion of the molecule [36]. γ-Butyrolactone is a CNS depressant and is used clinically as a general anesthetic agent [60]. The possibility of γ-butyrolactone as the FT metabolite responsible for its CNS toxicity is now being investigated in our laboratory.

Pharmacokinetics

The assays used to analyze FT in biologic fluids include ^{14}C radioactivity analysis after metabolite separation with thin layer chromatography [18], gas-liquid chromatography (GLC) following chemical derivatization [31, 62], and high-pressure liquid chromatography (HPLC) [3, 7, 63]. FT is heat-labile and decomposes to FU when exposed to the high temperature used in GLC [31, 62] which complicates the application of GLC to the simultaneous assay of FT and FU. Plasma concentrations of FT and FU and four additional FT metabolites were measured by an HPLC assay using a reverse phase C18 column, with a sensitivity range between 20 ng FU/ml and 100 ng FT/ml [3]. With some modification, the same assay could be applied to the analysis of urine samples [5]. More recently an HPLC assay using a normal phase column was also described [13]. The pharmacokinetics and metabolism of FT in experimental animals and cancer patients have been investigated using above-mentioned assays.

Following daily IV administration of 2−5 g FT/m^2 the disposition of FT in man displayed two compartment kinetics with a β-elimination half-life ranging from 6−17 h and an average plasma clearance of 0.05 l/kg-h [3, 8, 31]. FT has an average volume of distribution (Vd) during the elimination phase of 0.5 l/kg (range 0.4−0.8 l/kg) [3, 8, 31], which approximates the volume of total body water. The Vd of FT is similar to that of FU, despite their different plasma protein-binding. FU does not bind to plasma proteins, whereas FT is bound to the extent of 30%−50% at a concentration range of 6−100 μg/ml [8, 26]. We have recently studied the pharmacokinetics of FT in patients receiving 2 g FT/m^2 per day as a single chemotherapeutic agent during the first day of therapy and again together with either methyl-CCNU, adriamycin, or mitomycin C on the second day [5]. Plasma concentration-time profiles of FT from individual patients were similar after the first and second dose. This rules out significant accumulation of

FT in these patients during the two-day therapy, and also argues against major changes of FT disposition because of repeated dosing or coadministration of the antineoplastic agents used in combination.

There is some species variation in the disposition of FT; half-lives varying from 40 min to 2 h; 5 h and 10 h were reported for mice [40], rabbits [4, 62, 63], rats [11, 62, 63], and both beagle dogs and rhesus monkey [18], respectively. Wu et al. [63] reported capacity-limited metabolism in some rabbits given a high dose of 125 mg FT/kg intravenously. This nonlinearity of FT disposition was not observed in patients receiving daily doses of up to 5 g/m^2 [8].

Mechanism of Action

FT is neither a substrate nor an inhibitior of the pyrimidine nucleoside phosphorylases [49]. It has very little in vitro cytotoxicity in microbiologic systems and is a weak inhibitor of DNA and RNA synthesis in several mouse tumor cell lines [49]. FU at a concentration of $1 \times 10^{-5} M$ inhibited DNA synthesis by 90%−100%, measured by ^{14}C-formate incorporation in HeLa cells, whereas the inhibition by FT at $1 \times 10^{-4} M$ was only 15% [19, 49, 50]. In tumor-bearing animals, both FU and FT markedly inhibited the incorporation of labeled precursors into nucleic acids and proteins in Ehrlich ascites cells; however, such effect was absent when the tumor cells were incubated with FT in vitro [21]. The growth inhibition by FT of cultured Chinese hamster cells [46] and E. coli B3 [57] was accounted for by its slow conversion to FU. The growth inhibition of FU and FT on E. coli B3, a thymidine-requiring strain, was reversed by uracil, suggesting a similar mode of action for these two agents that is independent of thymidylate synthetase inhibition [57]. The enhancement of FT activity by 18-h preincubation was probably due to its spontaneous hydrolysis to FU in the culture medium [57]. Likewise, Fujita et al. [23] reported increased antibacterial activity of FT upon incubation with various organ homogenates; the highest activity was seen after incubation with liver homogenates. In addition, sublines of L1210 leukemic cells [35] and strains of E. coli B3 [57] were cross-resistant to FU and FT.

These results lead to the conclusion that FT is a chemical depot form of FU. It has insignificant cytotoxicity in vitro and exerts its in vivo activity by metabolic activation to FU. The liver has been proposed as the primary site of FT activation to FU, and the hepatic microsomal cytochrome P-450 enzyme system may be responsible for such activation [23, 51]. However, nonenzymatic hydrolysis may also occur in the acidic conditions of the gastric juice, particularly when FT is administered orally [48].

The mechanism of pharmacologic activity of FT is summarized as follows. FT is metabolized to FU, which is subsequently anabolized to 5-fluorodeoxyuridylate (FdUMP) and 5-fluorouridine triphosphate (FUTP), along with other anabolic products. FdUMP is a potent inhibitor of thymidylate synthetase which catalyzes the methylation of deoxyuridylate to thymidylate, and thus inhibits the de novo thymidylate and consequently DNA synthesis [48, 52]. Alterations of RNA metabolism by FU may also mediate cell toxicity, which involves inhibition of RNA formation or incorporation of FUTP into RNA [52]. The DNA effect of FU is usually considered as its major mode of action [48], although recent data indicate that the antitumor effects of FU may be mediated by RNA related mechanism (e.g. [55]).

Metabolism

FT undergoes extensive metabolism in vivo [8, 12, 18]. Eighty percent of a 100 mg/kg dose of 2-^{14}C-FT administered to rats was eliminated in 24 h, of which 55% was expired CO_2, 15% excreted in the urine as unchanged FT, and 10% as FU and FU-containing nucleosides and nucleotides [12]. The major routes of excretion of ^{14}C-FT in beagle dogs (30 mg/kg) and rhesus monkeys (60 mg/kg) were found to be pulmonary (35% in 24 h) and renal (30% in 24 h). FUPA was the major urinary metabolite in monkeys, but only a minor one in dogs [18]. Tumor-bearing mice eliminated FT at a faster rate. One hundred percent of the administered radiooactive FT dose (150 mg/kg) was recovered within 48 h via the renal (51%), pulmonary (38%), and fecal (1%) routes of excretion [40]. These studies show that, in spite of some species variation, FT is mainly eliminated by metabolism to FU and FU-related metabolites.

It is assumed that the metabolism of FT to active species proceeds solely via FU. This assumption is based on the following observations.

1) The antitumor activity and tissue (gastrointestinal and bone marrow) toxicity of FT are similar to those of FU [58].
2) FU is the major product of the in vitro metabolism of FT by mouse or rat liver microsomal enzyme preparations [8, 64].
3) FT lacks the structural requirements for the pyrimidine phosphokinases [6, 46] and therefore cannot undergo direct activation.

FT is administered to patients as a racemic mixture of R-(+) and S-(−) enantiomers. FT recovered from combined urine of nine patients showed no optical activity, indicating no enzymatic preference on the degradation of either isomer [31]. When these enantiomers were incubated separately with mouse liver microsomal enzmyes, each released the same amount of FU determined by its antibacterial activity against *Staphylococcus aureus* 209P [64].

It has been suggested that the liver is the primary site of metabolism and the hepatic microsomal cytochrome P-450 may be the responsible enzymes [12, 23, 46]. This is supported by the following observations during in vitro metabolism studies and in vivo studies in animals. Antibacterial activity of FT increased when incubated with human tissue homogenates, and the highest activity was seen with liver homogenates [23]. Ohira et al. [51] reported that FT produced a type II binding spectrum with rat cytochrome P-450, whereas a type I binding spectrum was seen by Meiren et al. [46]. In vitro activation of FT by liver microsomes requires NADPH [20, 46]; higher rates of FT decomposition were observed with liver microsomes harvested from mice pretreated with phenobarbital and glutathione [23]. Pretreatment of tumor-bearing mice with phenobarbital increased the survival time of the animals when treated with FT [51]. On the contrary, the elimination of FT and formation of FU were retarded in mice with hepatic lesions induced by chloroform [23]. The significance of the liver as the major organ activating FT to FU has not been established in humans. Patients with severe liver malfuntion eliminated FT at the same rate as patients without liver damage [3, 43]. Majima and Taguchi [44] pretreated patients with phenobarbital prior to FT administration and found no difference in response rate when compared to the control group.

Mechanism of Metabolic Activation

We have identified two FT metabolites in rats and rabbits given IV doses of 100–125 mg/kg of ^{14}C-labeled FT [63]. Physicochemical analysis suggests their structures to be 3' and 4'-OH-FT. These same metabolites were present in patient plasma and urine samples [3, 8, 53]. In addition, two other metabolites, i.e., dehydro-FT and MH-3, were recovered from human urine [3]. Dehydro-FT, which is chemically more labile than FT, was also observed in the plasma and urine of rats and rabbits [63], and patients given a daily oral dose of 1 g FT [14]. The fourth metabolite, MH-3, has been observed in human, but not rat or rabbit, plasma and urine; one possible structure consistent with its proton nuclear magnetic resonance and gas chromatograph mass spectral (GC-MS) data is $FU-CH_2-CO-CH_2-CH_2OH$. The structures of the other three metabolites are listed in Fig. 2.

The plasma concentration-time curves of FT and its metabolites following IV administration of FT at 2 g/m^2 to a patient are shown in Fig. 3 [3]. The relative ratios of

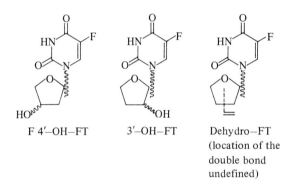

F 4'–OH–FT   3'–OH–FT   Dehydro–FT
                                      (location of the
                                      double bond   **Fig. 2.** Structures of the FT
                                      undefined)   metabolites

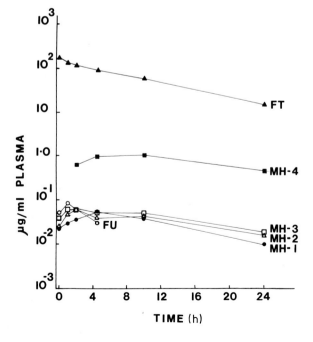

Fig. 3. Plasma concentration-time curves of FT and its metabolites, i.e., FU, MH-1(4'–OH–FT), MH-2(3'–OH–FT), MH-3, and MH-4 (dehydro-FT), in one patient given 2 g FT/m^2 by IV infusion over 30 min. Zero time refers to the end of infusion. FU concentrations were corrected for nonmetabolically generated FU as described in the text. (From Au et al. [3], generated FU as described in the text.) (From Au et al. [3], courtesy of Cancer Treat Rep)

metabolite concentrations were variable among patients, with dehydro-FT being the major circulating metabolite. The total amount of these metabolites recovered in 24 h urine from one patient represents less than 1% of the administered FT dose, indicating low renal clearances or a small extent of metabolite formation.

The hydroxylated FT metabolites are structurally similar to endogenous nucleosides and may, therefore, undergo enzymatic cleavage to FU by pyrimidine phosphorylases [6]. $4'-OH-FT$, but not $3'-OH-FT$, isolated from rabbit urine, was partially (20%) converted to FU by thymidine phosphorylase in vitro, suggesting a fraction of the $4'-OH-FT$ may be present in the β,D configuration [66]. The rather low conversion (5%) of $4'-OH-FT$ from human urine may have been caused by a more rapid metabolism of the β,D enantiomer prior to excretion in cancer patients when compared to rabbits [3, 56]. Benvenuto et al. [8] subsequently found that a mixture of these two hydroxylated FT metabolites was partially converted to FU when incubated with plasma and to a lesser extent with aqueous buffer. In order to study the activity of the hydroxylated FT metabolites, Lin et al. [45] synthesized enantiomers of $3'-OH-FT$ and $4'-OH-FT$. However, the major products were the α,D and α,L isomers of $4'-OH-FT$ and the β,D and β,L isomers of $3'-OH-FT$. These compounds showed no activity against L1210 at 100 mg/kg doses [45], possibly because thymidine phosphorylase is specific for pyrimidine deoxyribosides in the β,D configuration [6].

We have studied the stereochemistry of the hydroxylation of FT in rats using separate doses of R-(+)-FT and S-(−)-FT. The amounts of and $4'-OH-FT$ excreted in 24-h urine samples after an IP dose of S-(−)-FT at 50−100 mg/kg were significantly higher than those excreted after similar doses of R-(+)-FT [5]. This suggests that the hydroxylated products of the R-(+)-FT would have the natural β configuration, and thus might be preferentially metabolized prior to urinary excretion. This observation is in agreement with the previous findings [3, 63] that only small fraction of the $4'-OH-FT$ isolated from rabbit and human urine was present in the β,D configuration. The alternate hypothesis that S-(−)-FT is stereoselectively hydroxylated cannot be ruled out.

Benvenuto et al. [8] recovered a component with the same chromatographic behavior as the hydroxylated FT metabolites upon incubating 2-^{14}C-FT with rat and mouse liver microsomal enzyme system, suggesting the hydroxylation may be mediated by the microsomal cytochrome P-450 enzymes. The enzymes responsible for the formation of dehydro-FT and MH-3 are unknown at present.

Another potential pathway of activation currently under investigation in our laboratory is the enzymatic oxidation at the C-2′ position. The products of this reaction would be FU and γ-hydroxybutyrate (in equilibrium with γ-butyrolactone in plasma). We have modified the assay of Vree and Van der Kleijn [59] and are able to quantitate γ-butyrolactone at 200 ng/ml plasma. Preliminary results indicate that γ-butyrolactone is present at significant concentrations in patient and rabbit plasma after administration of 2 g FT/m^2 [4]. Therefore, C-2′ oxidation of FT followed by spontaneous cleavage to γ-butyrolactone and FU may represent a major activation pathway.

In summary, we have demonstrated several potential pathways of FT activation to FU:

1) Hydroxylation of FT at the C-4′ position followed by stereospecific enzymatic phosphorolysis to FU. However, the low extent of enzymatic FU formation together with the presence of rather low plasma concentrations of $4'-OH-FT$ suggest that this may be only a minor activation pathway of FT in man.

2) Dehydrogenation of FT to dehydro-FT results in a more lipophilic and chemically more labile metabolite which could undergo nonenzymatic conversion to FU in vivo. Contribution of this metabolite to FU formation and the neurotoxicity associated with FT remains to be determined.

3) Further activation pathways may exist, for example, enzymatic C-2'-oxidation followed by formation of FU and β-butyrolactone.

Kinetics of FU Formation

FU has been detected in plasma of experimental animals and cancer patients [3, 8, 24, 31, 62, 63]. However, there are large discrepancies between the reported FU plasma concentrations resulting from FT administration.

Earlier studies in animals reported significant plasma concentrations of FU detected by biologic assays [24]. Wu et al. [63] analyzed FT by a GLC method with on-column flash methylation and FU by a column chromatographic GC-MS method and found that unchanged FT accounted for most of the ^{14}C radioactivity in plasma, while FU concentrations were below 0.15% and 0.4% relative to FT concentrations in rabbits and rats, respectively.

Hills et al. [31] studied the pharmacokinetics of FT and FU formation in patients given a dose of 2.25 g FT/m^2 over 30 min by a GLC assay. In one patient, FU plasma concentrations peaked at 0.5–1 h after the dose at above 1 µg/ml and slowly declined over 24 h; FU concentrations were reported to be about 1% of FT concentrations. Hall et al. [27] and Benvenuto et al. [8] reported that FU plasma concentration peaked at 5 µg/ml which were maintained at 1.7 µg/ml for up to 96 h in patients given a rapid IV infusion of FT at a dose of 4–5 g/m^2, or a total dose of 7–8 g. The theoretical dose of an FU infusion needed to achieve such concentrations in a 70 kg man is 24 g (or the equimolar amount of 37 g FT) over 96 h, assuming a plasma clearance of 2.1 l/kg-h for FU [16]. The rapid exponential fall of initial FU levels [3, 8] excludes inhibition of FU metabolism in the presence of FT as a possible cause of the observed high FU plasma concentration.

We have investigated the kinetics of FU formation in patients receiving IV infusions of FT at 2 g/m^2 over 30 min, using storage and HPLC assay procedures that minimize in vitro conversion of FT and its metabolites to FU [3]. This assay represents a minor modification of our previous HPLC assay [63]. This assay represents a minor modification of our previous HPLC assay [63], which has been independently varified with a column chromatographic GC-MS assay confirming the very low FU plasma concentrations after FT administration to rats and rabbits [62]. Plasma concentration-time profiles of FU and FT in five patients are shown in Fig. 4. FU concentrations are corrected for the FT dose contaminated by FU (0.15%) and a 0.03% FT decomposition to FU during analysis. The plasma concentration ratios of FU to FT in all patients are below 0.2%, which is lower than those observed by Hills et al. [31] (1%), but in marked contrast to the data of Benvenuto et al. [8] and Hall et al. [27] (initially 5%, steadily increasing with time). Comparable results of low FU concentrations were observed by Diasio et al. [13]; in nine patients given an oral dose of 1 g FT/day, FU plasma concentrations assayed by a normal phase HPLC method reached a maximum of 50 ng/ml.

The high FU plasma concentrations reported by other groups can be caused by several factors; FT is chemically labile and slowly decomposes to FU upon storage and

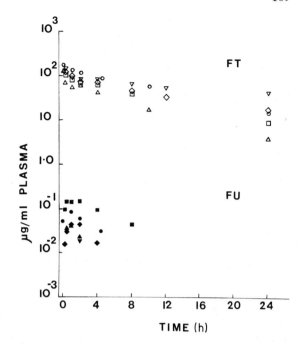

Fig. 4. Plasma concentration-time profiles of FT and FU in five patients given 2 g FT/m² by IV infusion over 30 min. Zero time refers to the end of infusion. FU concentrations were corrected for nonmetabolically generated FU as described in the text. (From Au et al. [3], courtesy of Cancer Treat Rep)

possibly during extractions using high salt concentration [31]. While such decomposition is quite small, it may be significant due to very large FT : FU concentration ratio (1 000 : 1) in the biologic samples. The hydroxylated metabolites also rapidly converted to FU in plasma at 37° C. In addition, the dehydrogenated metabolite is chemically more labile than FT itself and decomposes to FU during storage. Extraction under acidic conditions employed by Fujita and Kimura [24], and Freudenthal and Emmerling [18], would cause hydrolysis of dehydro-FT to FU, and therefore, introduce an error in FU quantitation. Our study showed that the plasma concentrations of dehydro-FT is the highest among all FT metabolites, reaching a plateau at 4 h after the FT dose and remaining essentially constant for up to 24 h. This kinetic behavior of dehydro-FT is similar to that of the FU concentrations observed by Benvenuto et al. [18]. Our data suggest that previously reported FU plasma concentrations after FT administration are caused by partial or complete in vitro decomposition of the labile dehydro-FT and possibly also the hydroxylated FT metabolites in the plasma.

Extent of FU Formation

There is no good estimate of the amount of FU formed following an FT dose. If one assumes the metabolism of FT is solely via FU, then a large fraction of the FT dose is converted to FU since 60%−80% of 2-^{14}C-FT dose administered to animals was recovered as FU metabolites. One pharmacokinetic approach to determining the extent of prodrug conversion is to compare the plasma clearance and the area under the plasma concentration-time curves of the parent drug and its active metabolite, as shown in equation 1.

$$F = \frac{CL_{FU}}{CL_{FT}} \times \frac{AUC_{FU}}{AUC_{FT}}$$

where F is the fraction of the FT dose converting to FU; CL_{FU} and CL_{FT} represent the plasma clearance of FU and FT, respectively; AUC_{FU} and AUC_{FT} are the area under the plasma molar concentration-time curves of FU and FT following an FT dose. We have used population estimates of CL_{FU} taken from the literature and, therefore, assume little intersubject or intrasubject variability. The intersubject variability of FU kinetics is indeed small provided that the rate of administration is the same among individuals [10, 16, 45]. However, there is a drastic difference in the CL_{FU} in humans when FU is administered at different rates. A 60-fold higher plasma clearance was observed in the same subject receiving FU by slow IV infusion rather than by bolus injection [10]. When FU is given in a form of slow-release metabolic prodrug, the input of FU follows a first order rate process which is different from a pulse (bolus) injection or a zero order infusion, and therefore obscures the estimation of CL_{FU}. Another assumption underlying this conventional pharmacokinetic approach is that the distribution of the drug to and from its metabolizing sites is faster than its metabolism. It is of interest to note that the plasma clearance of FU (ranges from $0.4-60$ l/kg-h depending on the rate of administration; calculated from [10, 16, 45]) exceeds the blood volume of cardiac output (6 l/kg-h); Jacquez [33] reported a diffusion constant of 1.1×10^{-5} cm/min for FU in Ehrlich ascites cells at $25°$ C, and an equilibrium between intracellular and extracellular concentrations was obtained in 1 min. It is, therefore, conceivable that the absolute rate of metabolism of FU may surpass its diffusion rate across the cell, and that FU generated from FT is localized at metabolic sites, where it is further metabolized without redistributing back into the systemic circulation. A similar "sequentila first-pass" effect of phenacetin and its metabolite, acetophen-acetin, in an isolated perfused-liver model was noted by Pang and Gillette [50]. In summary, it is presently not possible to calculate the conversion rate and extent of FT to FU based on the plasma concentrations of FU. Furthermore, FU plasma concentrations may not correspond to the extent of exposure of the various target tissues to intracellular FU generated from FT.

Other FU Prodrugs

FD-1. A structural analog of FT, FD-1 (*N*-1,3-bis-(tetrahydrofuran-2-yl)-5-fluoro-uracil), was synthesized in Japan in 1977. It is chemically more labile than FT and decomposes to FU via two intermediates, FT and *N*-3-(tetrahydrofuran-2-yl)-5-fluoro-uracil [36]. While higher FU plasma concentrations were observed with oral FD-1 administration [36], the incidence and severity of neurotoxicity are also higher than those of FT and limit the general use of FD-1 [11, 44].

HCFU. 1-Hexylcarbamoyl-5-fluorouracil (HCFU), another orally effective agent synthesized in Japan in 1976, is reported to have a broader spectrum of antitumor activity and reduced gastrointestinal toxicity than FU and FT. The central nervous system toxicity of FU, FT, and FD-1 is not seen with HCFU; instead hot sensation and pollakisuria are the dose-related toxic effects of HCFU [39].

5'-dFUR. 5'-Deoxy-5-fluorouridine was recently synthesized in the United States as an orally applicable form of FU [2, 41], 5'-dFUR is a substrate for nucleoside phosphorylase, and was found to enter the Ehrlich Ascites cells, followed first by expansion of the FU pool and, subsequently, by the FU ribosyl nucleotide pool [2].

β,D$-4'-OH-FT$. $4'-OH-FT$ was isolated uring our FT metabolism studies [3, 63]. Subsequent observations of partial phosphorolysis to FU by thymidine phosphorylase [3, 63] and of the stereochemistry of hydroxylation of the R-(+) and S-(−)-FT enantiomers [5] suggest that a fraction of the urinary $4'-OH-FT$ is present in the β,D configuration. Susceptibility of β,D$-4'-OH-FT$ to phosphorolysis, its decreased lipophilicity caused by addition of the hydroxyl function, and the low levels of thymidine phosphorylase in the brain allow us to propose β,D$-4'-OH-FT$ as a potential FU prodrug that may be devoid of the CNS toxicity of FT. β,D$-4'-OH-FT$ is presently being synthesized by Levinson and Meyer at the University of California, San Francisco.

Conclusions

The reduced myelotoxicity of FT has been attributed to its property of releasing FU slowly in vivo, and represents a significant advantage over FU. Unfortunately, the clinical use of FT is associated with a high dose-limiting neurotoxicity, and the clinical trials in the United States have not proved FT to be a superior agent when given intravenously. At present, the oral applicability of FT is the remaining advantage and phase I clinical trials of oral FT have been initiated. Preliminary results indicate that the drug is completely bioavailable and is well tolerated, with gastrointestinal toxicity being the major toxicity.

It is still debatable if an appreciable fraction of the FT dose is indeed metabolized to FU. Pharmacokinetic studies of FT disposition and FU formation have been inconclusive, largely due to the rapid metabolism of FU. After being formed intracellularly from FT, FU may be further metabolized without redistributing into the circulation, which results in relatively low FU serum concentrations in spite of extensive conversion of FT to FU. In this case, the tissue selectivity of a FU prodrug may be determined by its distribution, rate, and mechanism of activation to FU. These factors should be considered when designing further FU prodrugs. The alternative hypothesis that FT may be activated to and metabolized via other metabolites independent of FU cannot be ruled out.

References

1. Ansfield FJ, Kallas G, Singson J, Uy B (1979) Phase I-II clinical studies with iv and oral ftorafur, a preliminary report. Proc Am Assoc Cancer Res 20: 349
2. Armstrong RD, Diasio RB (1979) 5′-Deoxy-5-fluorouridine: Cellular metabolism of a new fluoropyrimidine with antioneoplastic activity. Proc Am Assoc Cancer Res 20: 260
3. Au JL, Wu AT, Friedman MA, Sadée W (1979) Pharmacokinetics and metabolism of ftorafur in man. Cancer Treat Rep 63: 343−350
4. Au JL, Sadée W (1979) Activation of ftorafur (R,S-1(tetrahydro-2-furanyl)-5-fluorouracil) to 5-fluorouracil and γ-butyrolactone. Cancer Res (submitted)
5. Au JL, Sadée W (1979) Studies on the mechanism of activation of Ftorafur (R,S-1-(tetrahydro-2-furanyl)-5-fluorouracil). Am Pharm Assoc Acad Pharm Sci (Abstr) 9: 108

6. Baker RB (1968) Specific mode of binding to enzmyes: II. Pyrimidine area. In design of active-site-directed irreversible enzyme inhibitors. Wiley, New York, p 121

7. Benvenuto JA, Lu K, Loo TL (1977) High pressure liquid chromatographic analysis of ftorafur and its metabolites in biological fluids. J Chromatogr 134: 219−222

8. Benvenuto JA, Lu K, Hall SW, Benjamin RS, Loo TL (1978) Disposition and metabolism of 1-(tetrahydro-2-furanyl)-5-fluorouracil (ftorafur) in humans. Cancer Res 38: 3867−3870

9. Blokhina NG, Vozny EK, Garin AM (1972) Results of treatment of malignant tumors with ftorafur. Cancer 30: 390−392

10. Cano JP, Rigault JP, Aubert C, Carcassionne Y, Seitz JF (1979) Determination of 5-fluorouracil in plasma by GC/MS using an internal standard application to pharmaco-kinetics. Bull Cancer 66: 66−74

11. Carter S (1979) Personal communication

12. Cohen AM (1975) The disposition of ftorafur in rats after intravenous administration. Drug Metab Dispos 3: 303−308

13. Diasio RB, Hunter HL, Labudde JA, Mayol RF (1979) Pharmacologic study of oral ftorafur: Potential for improved oral delivery of 5-fluorouracil. Proc Am Assoc Cancer Res 20: 401

14. Diasio RB (1979) Personal communication

15. Earl RA, Townsend LB (1972) The synthesis of 1-(tetrahydro-2-furanyl)-5-fluorouracil (ftorafur) via direct fluorination. J Heterocyc Chem 9: 1141−1143

16. Finn C, Sadée W (1975) Determination of 5-fluorouracil (NSC-19893) plasma levels in rats and man by isotope dilution-mass fragmentography. Cancer Chemother Rep 59: 279−285

17. Finn C, Schwandt H-J, Sadée W (1975) Application of ion-counting selected ion monitoring-mass spectrometry in pharmacokinetics. Argonne Natl Lab 129−137

18. Freudenthal RI, Emmerling DC (1977) The metabolism of ftorafur in the beagle dog and rhesus monkey. Xenobiotica 7: 757−764

19. Fujii S, Okuda H (1973) Antitumor activity of N-1-(2′-tetrahydrofuryl)-5-fluorouracil (FT-207). In: Daikos GK (ed) Prog. Chemother. (antibacterial, antiviral, antineoplast.) vol 3. Proc. VIII Int. Congr. Chemother Hell. Soc. Chemother. Athens, pp 669−679

20. Fujii S, Okuda H, Akazawa A, Yasuda U, Kawaguchi Y, Fukunaga Y, Nishikawa H (1975) Studies on the fate of 1-(2′-tetrahydrofuryl)-5-fluorouracil (FT-207), a carcinostatic agent III. Absorption, distribution, excretion and metabolism after rectal administration of FT-207. J Pharm Soc (Jpn) 95: 732−740

21. Fujimoto S, Akao T, Itoh B, Koshizuka I, Koyano K, Kitsukawa Y, Takahashi M, Minami T, Ishigami H, Nomura Y, Itoh K (1976) Effect of N-1-(tetrahydrofuryl)-5-fluorouracil and 5-fluorouracil on nucleic acid and protein biosynthesis in Ehrlich ascites cells. Cancer Res 36: 33−36

22. Fujita H, Ogawa K, Sawabe T, Kimura K (1972) In vivo distribution of N-1-(2′-tetra-hydrofuryl)-5-fluorouracil (FT-207). Jpn J Cancer Clin 18: 911−916

23. Fujita H, Kimura K (1973) In vivo distribution and metabolism of N-1-(tetrahydrofu-ran-2-yl)-5-fluorouracil (FT-207). Prog. Chemother, (antibacterial, antiviral, antineoplast), vol 3. Proc. VIII Int. Congr. Chemother. Hell. Soc. Chemother. Athens, pp 159−164

24. Fujita H, Kimura K (1977) In vivo distribution and metabolism of N-1-(tetrahydrofu-ran-2-yl)-5-fluorouracil (FT-207). Presented at the Japan. Congr. Chemother. Gifer City, Japan

25. Garibjanian BT, Johnson RK, Kline I, Valdimudi S, Gang M, Venditti JM, Goldin A (1976) Comparison of 5-fluorouracil and ftorafur. II. Therapeutic response and development of resistance in murine tumors. Cancer Treat Rep 60: 1347−1361

26. Gilev AP, Meirina DV, Khagi KhB (1974) Isuchemie farmakokinetiki 5-ftoruratsila-2-C14. Biull Eksp Biol Med 78: 59−61

27. Hall SW, Benjamin RS, Griffin AC, Loo TL (1976) Pharmacokinetics and metabolism of ftorafur (FT) in man. Proc Am Assoc Cancer Res 17:128
28. Handelsman H, Slavik M (1974) Ftorafur (FT-207), NSC 148959. Clinical brochure, div. cancer treatment. National Cancer Institute
29. Hiller SA, Zhuk RA, Lidak MY (1967) Analogs of pyrimidine nucleosides. I. N-(α-furanidyl) derivatives of natural pyrimidine bases and their antimetabolites. Dokl Akad Nauk SSSR 176:332−335
30. Hiller S, Lazdins A, Veinbergs AK, Sidorov AB (1977) N-1-(tetrahydrofuran-2-yl)-5-substituted uracils. US Patent No. 4039546
31. Hills EB, Godefroi VG, O'Leary IA, Burke M, Amdrezejewski D, Brukwinski W, Horwitz JP (1977) GLC determination for ftorafur in biological fluids. J Pharm Sci 66:1497−1499
32. Horwitz JP, McCormick JJ, Phillips KD, Maher VM, Otto JR, Kessels D, Zemlicka J (1975) In vitro biological evaluation of the R and S isomers of 1-(tetrahydrofuran-2-yl)-5-fluorouracil. Cancer Res 35:1301−1304
33. Jacquez JA (1962) Permeability of Ehrlich cells to uracil, thymine and fluorouracil. Proc Soc Exp Biol Med 109:132−135
34. Johnson RK, Garibjanian BT, Houchens DP, Kline I, Gaston MR, Syrkin AB, Goldin A (1976) Comparison of 5-fluorouracil and ftorafur. I. Quantitative and qualitative differences in toxicity to mice. Cancer Treat Rep 60:1335−1345
35. Karev NI, Blokhina NG, Vozny EK, Pershin MP (1972) Experience with ftorafur treatment in breast cancer. Neosplasma 19:347−350
36. Kawaguchi Y, Nakamura Y, Sato T, Takeda S, Marunaka T, Fujii S (1978) Studies on the fate of 5-fluoro-1,3-bis-(tetrahydro-2-furanyl)-2,4-pyrimidinedione (FD-1), a new antitumor agent. I. Absorption, distribution, excretion and metabolism of FD-1 administered orally to rats. Yakugaku Zasshi 98:525−536
37. Kawai M, Rosenfeld J, McCulloch P, Hillcoat BL (1976) Blood levels of 5-fluorouracil during intravenous infusion. Br J Cancer 33:346−347
38. Konda C, Mitani H, Sokurai N, Suzuki A, Sakai A, Sakano T, Shimoyama T, Kitahara T, Kumaokai S, Kimura K (1973) Chemotherapy of cancer with oral administration of N-1-(2'-furanidyl)-5-fluorouracil (FT-207). Jpn J Cancer Clin 19:495−499
39. Koyama Y, CHFU Clinical Group (1979) Phase I. Study of a new antitumor drug, 1-hexycarbomyl-5-fluorouracil (HCFU) by oral administration. Unpublished work
40. Kozhukhov AN, Mejrens D, Gilev AP (1977) Pharmacokinetics of ftorafur-2-^{14}C in rats with Walker-carcinosarcoma. Byull Eksp Biol Med 83:734−736
41. Kramer MJ, Trown PW, Cleeland R, Cook AF, Grunberg E (1979) 5'-Deoxy-5-fluorouridine − A new orally active antitumor agent. Comparative activity with 5-fluorouracil, 2'-deoxy-5-fluorouridine and ftorafur against transplantabel tumors in mice and rats. Proc Am Assoc Cancer Res 20:20
42. Lin AJ, Benjamin RS, Rao PN, Loo TL (1979) Synthesis and biological activities of ftorafur metabolites: 3'- and 4'-hydroxyftorafur. J Med Chem 22:1096−1100
43. Lu K, Loo TL, Benvenuto JA, Benjamin RS, Valdivieso M, Freireich EJ (1975) Pharmacologic disposition and metabolism of ftorafur. Pharmacologist 17:202
44. Majima H, Taguchi T (1978) Personal communication
45. Macmillan WE, Wolberg WH, Welling P (1978) Pharmacokinetics of fluorouracil in humans. Cancer Res 38:3479−3482
46. Meiren DV, Belousova AK (1972) Mechanism of action of ftorafur, a new antitumor agent. Vopr Med Khim 18:288−293
47. Meiren Z (1974) Comparison of the effect of fluorafur and 5-fluorouracil on the biosynthesis of DNA thymine. Opukolei 2:206−208
48. Myers CE, Diasio RB, Eliott HM, Chabner BA (1976) Pharmacokinetics of fluoropyrimidines: Implications for their clinical use. Cancer Treat Rev 3:175−183
49. Morgan LR, Browder H, Carter RD (1979) Oral ftorafur: A feasibility study. Proc Am Assoc Cancer Res 20:397

50. Pang KS, Gillette JR (to be published) Sequential first-pass elimination of the metabolite derived from its precusor. J Pharmacokin Biopharm

51. Ohira S, Maeqawa S, Watanabe K, Kitada K, Saito T (1976) Experimental approach to increase the effect of cancer chemotherapy in tumor-bearing rats pretreated with an inducer on microsomal drugmetabolizing enzyme (cytochrome P-450). In: Hellman K, Connors TA (eds) Cancer chemotherapy II. (Proceedings of the 9th Int. Congr. Chemother. London, 1975). Plenum Press, New York, pp 197−202

52. Sadée W, Wong CG (1977) Pharmacokinetics of 5-fluorouracil: Interrelationship with biochemical kinetics in monitoring therapy. Clin Pharmacokin Biopharm 2: 437−450

53. Sadée W, Au JL, Wu AT, Friedman MA (1978) Metabolic activation of 1-(tetrahydro-furan-2-yl)-5-fluorouracil (ftorafur). Proc Am Assoc Cancer Res 19: 92

54. Saunders PP, Chao LY (1976) Mechanism of action of ftorafur in chinese hamster cell (CHC) cultures. Proc Am Assoc Cancer Res 17: 159

55. Sawyer R, Nayak R, Spiegelman S, Martin D (1979) Mechanism of action of 5-fluorouracil (FU) in the chemotherapy of the murine mammary tumor. Proc Am Assoc Cancer Res 20: 263

56. Smolyanskaya AZ, Tugarinov OA (1972) The biological activity of antitumor antimetabolite ftorafur. Neoplasma 19: 341−345

57. Taguchi T, Nakano Y, Fujita M, Tominaga T, Takami M, Usukane M, Takahashi A, Kato T, Tei N, Kitamura M, Maeda T, Ishida T, Shiba S (1972) Clinical studies of anticancer activity of FT-207 (N-1-(2′-tetrahydrofuryl)-5-fluorouracil. Jpn J Cancer Clin 18: 550−553 (This reference is cited in line 23 on p 5. It should read 57 instead of 66)

58. Valdivieso M, Bodey GP, Gottlieb JA, Freireich EJ (1976) Clinical evaluation of ftorafur (pyrimidine-deoxyribose N-1-2′-furanidyl-5-fluorouracil). Cancer Res 36: 1821−1824

59. Vree TB, van der Kleijn E (1976) Rapid determination of 4-hydroxybutyric acid (gamma OH) and 2-propylpentanoate (depakine) in human plasma by means of gas-liquid chromatography. J Chromatogr 121: 150−152

60. Vree TB, van der Kleinja E, van der Bogert AG, Hoes M, Grimere JSF, Gouveia, WA, Tognoni G, van der Kleijn E (1976) Clinical toxicology of central depressant and stimulant drugs. In: Gouveia WA, Tognoni G, van der Kleijn E (eds) Clinical pharmacy and clinical pharmacology. Elsevier, North-Holland, pp 67−87

61. Weeth JB (1979) Ftorafur: Oral tablet trial follows intravenous phase I study. Proc Am Assoc Cancer Res 20: 307

62. Wu AT, Schwandt H-J, Finn C, Sadée W (1976) Determination of ftorafur and 5-fluorouracil levels in plasma and urine. Res Commun Chem Pathol Pharmacol 14: 89−102

63. Wu AT, Au JL, Sadée W (1978) Hydroxylated metabolites of R,S-1-(tetrahydro-2-furnayl)-5-fluorouracil (ftorafur) in rats and rabbits. Cancer Res 38: 210−214

64. Yamayama M, Moriyama A, Unemi N, Hashimoto S, Suzue T (1977) Studies of antitumor agents. I. Resolution of racemic 1-(tetrahydro-2-furanyl)-5-fluorouracil into the R and S isomers and examination of the biological activities of the isomers. J Med Chem 20: 1592−1594

Current Status of Nitrosoureas Under Development in Japan*

M. Ogawa and S. Fujimoto

Division of Clinical Chemotherapy, Cancer Chemotherapy Center,
Japanese Foundation for Cancer Research, Kami-Ikebukuro 1-37-1,
Toshima-ku, J – Tokyo 170

Three nitrosourea compounds [1–4], BCNU, CCNU, and methyl CCNU (MeCCNU) have demonstrated clinical efficacy in a variety of human malignancies including lung cancer, gastrointestinal tumors, lymphomas, melanomas, and brain tumors. But delayed and cumulative hematologic toxicity has been an obstacle to clinical use.

A water-soluble introsourea, streptozotocin [5], which is composed of methylnitrosourea attached to an aminoglucose carrier, showed minimal hematologic toxicity, however the clinical efficacy is rather limited and, in addition, it was reported that renal toxicity is a dose-limiting factor.

Recently, another water-soluble nitrosourea, chlorozotocin, in which the methyl group in the structure of streptozotocin is substituted by a chloroethyl group, has been developed by Schein and co-workers [6–8]. Chlorozotocin induced minimal thrombocytopenia and negligible leukopenia. Furthermore, hyperglycemia and renal and hepatic dysfunction [8, 9] were not observed. Currently phase II study is underway in the United States. Thus, new nitrosourea compounds with reduced hematologic toxicity and wider antitumor spectrum have been undergoing development. This paper reviews the current status of three new analogous compounds of nitrosourea being developed in Japan.

The data reviewed in this paper were summarized from published papers in which the definitions of responses were clearly described. The criteria used for the evaluation of responses was based on similar definitions described by Muggia [10]; however, since most investigators used Karnofsky's criteria, the responses were rearranged as follows:

1–C: complete tumor regression (CR); 1–B: partial regression (PR); 1–A: minor response (MR); 0–C and 0–B: stable disease (SD); and 0–A and 0–0: progressive disease.

Since most data were summarized from the results of phase I and II studies and nearly all patients had had prior chemotherapy, the definition of minor response was included. In hematologic malignancy, the definition of response was based on Kimura's criterion [11, 12].

* This study was supported partially by NCI contract N01-CM-22054 in the United States and by a grant from the Ministry of Health and Welfare 52-12 in Japan

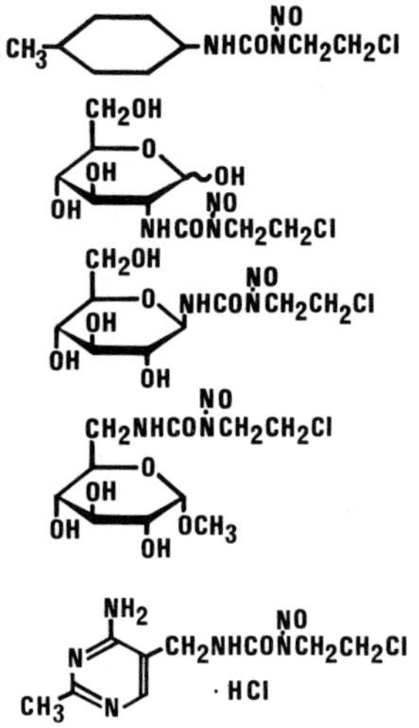

CH₃—⟨⟩—NHCONCH₂CH₂Cl   Methyl–CCNU

Chlorozotocin

G A N U

M C N U

A C N U

Fig. 1. Structure of MeCCNU, chlorozotocin,
ACNU, GANU, and MCNU

ACNU

ACNU   1-(4-amino-2-methylpyrimidin-5-yl)methyl-3-(2-chloroethyl)-3-nitrosourea hydrochloride ACNU was synthesized by Arakawa [13, 14] and co-workers (Sankyo Co., Ltd.) in 1974, and the structure is shown in Fig. 1. ACNU belongs to a water-soluble compound of nitrosourea and thus it is different from BCNU, MeCCNU, and CCNU which are lipophilic. ACNU inhibits DNA and protein synthesis and works on the transition period from postmitotic phase to DNA synthetic phase in cell cycle [15].

After intravenous injection of a radiolabeled compound into tumor bearing mice and rats [16], ACNU showed wide distribution into tissues and organs in the whole body and was rapidly excreted from the kidney; however, significant retention was observed in tumor tissues, liver, and thymus, while the distribution was relatively low level in brain and cerebrospinal fluid. ACNU showed high antitumor activity [13, 14] against L1210 mouse leukemia when it was administered in both early and advanced stages. Furthermore, it was active in a variety of animal tumors [17] including Lewis lung carcinoma, Ehrlich carcinoma, P388, myeloid leukemia C-1498, plasma cell tumor X-5563, mammary tumor N4-102, and others.

Clinical Trials

Phase I study of ACNU [18] was initiated in 1974, involving 20 major institutions. The starting dose [18] of 0.2 mg/kg was based on one-tenth the maximum tolerated dose (MTD) in dogs. A maximum single dose was escalated up to 4 mg/kg and was found that the dose limiting factor was hematologic toxicity.

An optimal single dose was determined to be either 2 mg/kg weekly [18] or 3 mg/kg in 6−8 weeks intervals [19, 20].

Results

The results obtained through phase I-II studies are summarized in Table 1. Among 60 patients with advanced gastric cancer [19, 24], three partial regressions (PR) and three

Table 1. Phase I-II study of ACNU

Diagnosis	No. of patients	Solid tumor				
		CR	PR	MR	SD	PD
Stomach	60	0	3	3	11	43
Colorectal	20	0	1	2	5	12
Pancreas	6	0	0	0	0	6
Gallsladder and hepatoma	9	0	1	1	2	5
Breast	13	0	1	0	2	10
Uterus	12	0	2	1	2	7
Ovary	7	0	0	0	5	2
Head and neck	6	0	2	0	0	4
Sarcoma	14	1	0	2	0	10
Renal cell	2	0	0	0	0	2
Brain	37	5	12	8	0	12
Total	186	6 (3.2%)	22 (11.8%)	17 (9.1%)	27 (21.3%)	113 (60.8%)

minor responses (MR) were reported. Phase II study using either 3 mg/kg of ACNU alone or the same dosage combined with an immunopotentiator picibanil was conducted by the Tokyo Cancer Chemotherapy Cooperative Study Group. They obtained from 16 patients with gastric cancer three PRs (19%). From 20 patients with colorectal cancer they obtained one PR and three MRs. No improvement was obtained in six patients with pancreatic cancer. One PR and one MR were obtained in nine patients with gallsladder cancer or hepatoma. One PR was reported from 13 patients with breast cancer. No response was reported in seven patients with ovarian cancer.

Saijo and co-workers [25, 26] conducted phase II study in pulmonary metastatic patients with cancers and sarcomas, and obtained two PRs out of seven patients with uterine cancer, two PRs out of three patients with head and neck tumors, and on CR and PR each out of seven patients with sarcoma.

Among 37 patients with brain tumors [27, 28] treated by either ACNU alone or in combination with irradiation, there were five responders who showed neurologic improvement and almost total disappearance of brain tumors and 12 responders who showed improvement of neurologic and CT-scan findings. In advanced lung cancer [18−22, 25, 28] each of the three complete (23%) and partial regressions (23%) were obtained out of 13 patients with small cell carcinoma of lung, while only two partial regressions (6%) were reported out of 33 patients with nonoat cell carcinoma, as shown in Table 2.

In hematologic malignancies [18−21, 29, 30] one complete remission and four partial remissions were obtained out of 11 patients with Hodgkin's disease, as shown in Table 3. Both CR and PR were obtained out of 14 patients with non-Hodgkin's lymphomas. No patients responded with acute leukemias. Five CRs were obtained out of ten patients with chronic myelogenous leukemia.

Hematologic improvements were observed in four patients with polycythemia vera, two patients with essential thrombocythemia, and one patient with multiple myeloma.

Table 2. Phase I-II study of ACNU

Histology	No. of patients	Lung cancer				
		CR	PR	MR	SD	PD
Squamous	11	0	1	0	0	10
Adeno	19	0	0	1	1	17
Large cell	3	0	1	0	1	1
Small cell	13	3	3	1	1	5
Unclassified	22	0	0	4	0	18
Total	68	3 (4.4%)	5 (7.3%)	6 (8.8%)	3 (4.4%)	51 (75%)

Table 3. Phase I-II study of ACNU

Diagnosis	No. of patients	Hematologic malignancy		
		CR	PR	NR
Hodgkin's disease	11	1	4	6
Non-Hodgkin lymphoma	14	1	1	12
Acute leukemia	6	0	0	6
CML	10	5	1	4
CLL	1	0	0	1

	No. of patients	Improvement	No improvement
Polycythemia vera	5	4	1
Thrombocythemia	2	2	0
Meyeloma	3	1	2

The results obtained in phase II-III studies in melanoma are summarized in Table 4. No improvements were observed in three patients who used ACNU alone against malignant melanoma.

Only one patient showed minor response to the administered combination of ACNU and Vinca alkaloid [20]. In our preliminary [31] study that combined DTIC 200 mg/m^2 and ACNU 100 mg/m^2 on days 1−5, two partial regressions and three minor responses were observed out of seven patients.

Hematologic and clinical toxicities [19, 25, 26] are summarized in Table 5.

Severity of hematologic toxicity was dose dependent. At a dose of 3 mg/kg, both leukopenia of less than 4 000/mm^3 and thrombocytopenia of less than 7×10^4/mm^3 occurred in about half of the patients. Thrombocytopenia reached a nadir 3−4 weeks later while leukocyte reached its nadir 1 week later than thrombocytopenia. Both needed 2−3 weeks for recovery and the hematologic toxicity appeared to be cumulative. Mild to moderate gastrointestinal disturbances occurred in about one-third of the patients when a dose of 3 mg/kg was administered, but they were well tolerated. Transient and reversible liver dysfunctions were observed in a few cases while no renal dysfunction was reported.

Table 4. Phase II-III study of ACNU

Regimen	No. of patients	Malignant melanoma				
		CR	PR	MR	SD	PD
ACNU alone	3	0	0	0	0	3
ACNU + VCR	6	0	0	1	3	2
ACNU + VLB	1	0	0	0	1	0
ACNU + MTX	1	0	0	0	0	1
ACNU + DIC	7	0	2	3	0	2
ACNU + DIC + VCR	3	0	1	1	0	1
Total	21	0	3	5	4	9
			(14.3%)	(23.8%)	(19.0%)	(42.9%)

Table 5. Toxicity of ACNU

Leukopenia (%)	Thombocytopenia (%)	Clinical (%)
$\geqq 4,000 : 30$ (55)	$\geqq 7 \times 10^4 : 25$ (45)	Anorexia: 11 (32)
$2-4,000 : 30$ (55)	$3-7 \times 10^4 : 17$ (31)	Nausea : 10 (29)
$< 2,000 : \ 8$ (15)	$< 3 \times 10^4 : 13$ (24)	Vomiting : 5 (15)
		Others : 4 (12)
Total: 55	Total: 55	Total: 30

GANU

A water-soluble nitrosourea, GANU 1-(2-chloroethyl)-3-(β-D-glucopyranosyl)-1-nitrosourea was synthesized by Machinami, Suami [32], and co-workers in 1975, and the structure is similar to that of chlorozotocin (Fig. 1.). GANU [33] inhibited incorporation of ^{3}H-thymidine and DNA polymerase in vitro system of L51178Y cells; thus, the result indicated that major mode of action is the inhibition of DNA synthesis. In animal tumor systems [34], GANU was active against L1210 mouse leukemia, sarcoma 180, rat hepatoma A-130, and others.

Aoshima and Sakurai [35] reported that antitumor activity of GANU was comparable to chlorozotocin but it was more myelosuppressive. Similar results were reported by Fox and co-workers [36], that is, that GANU has significant L1210 activity, but was less active than chlorozotocin and was more toxic.

We conducted comparative studies to test antitumor activities of five nitrosourea compounds [38]. ACNU, MeCCNU chlorozotocin (CZT), GANU, and 1-(2-chloroethyl)-3-(methyl α-D-glucopyranos-6-yl)-1-nitrosourea (MCNU) as shown in Fig. 2.

Optimal doses of each drugs were injected IP on day 1 to five randomized groups of BDF_1 mice inoculated 1×10^5 cell/mouse. Five nitrosoureas showed similar antitumor activities. However, when treatment started in advanced stage of L1210 on day 4, ACNU, MeCCNU and MCNU proved superior activities to GANU and chlorozo-

tocin, as shown in Fig. 3. The results [38] were similar when treatments were started on day 5 or day 6.
In preclinical toxicology using mice, rats, and beagle dogs, hematologic, gastrointestinal, and renal toxicities were predicted.

Phase I Study

Phase I study was initiated in October 1978. The starting dose of 10 mg/m^2 in a single injection was determined, based on one-tenth dosage of LD_{10} in mice. Dosages have been escalated up to 70 mg/m^2 at present and until now no significant toxicities were found.

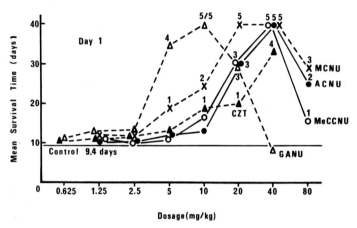

Fig. 2. Comparative activity of ACNU, GANU, MCNU, chlorozotocin (CZT), and MeCCNU against the 1-day-old L1210 leukemia. L1210 ascitic cells (10^5/mouse) were implanted IP into five BDF$_1$ mice per group on day 0 and five drugs were given IP on day 1 only. Dose-response studies were done. Number on each symbol denotes the number of mice (of five mice) which survived for 40 days after implantation of tumor. Mean survival time of the group with 40-day survivors was calculated, including the 40-day survivors as they survived for 40 days

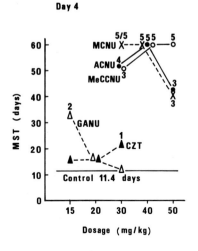

Fig. 3. Comparative activity of ACNU, GANU, MCNU, chlorozotocin (CZT), and MeCCNU against the 4-day-old L1210 leukemia. L1210 ascitic cells (10^5/mouse) were implanted IP into five BDF$_1$ mice per group on day 0 and five drugs were given IP on day 4 only. Three dosages employed for each drug were the LD_{10}, LD_0, and $0.75 \times LD_0$ of each drug against normal BDF$_1$ mice, respectively. Number on each symbol denotes the number of mice (of five mice) which survived for 60 days after implantation of tumor. Mean survival time (MST) of the group with 60-day survivors was calculated, including the 60-day survivors as they survived for 60 days

MCNU

A water-soluble nitrosourea, MCNU 1-(2-chloroethyl)-3-(methyl α-D-glucopyra-nos-6-yl)-1-nitrosourea [37] was synthesized in Research Laboratory of Tokyo Tanabe Co., Ltd. The structure was similar to those of chlorozotocin and GANU (Fig. 1). MCNU inhibited DNA synthesis of L1210 mouse leukemic cells in vitro and did not inhibit RNA synthesis. MCNU showed significant antitumor activities in a variety of animal tumors including L1210, P388, sarcoma 180, B-16 melanoma, Lewis lung carcinoma, and others.

As previously described, MCNU has superior antitumor activity to GANU and chlorozotocin in advanced stages of L1210 mouse leukemia. When a single injection of each optimal dose of five nitrosoureas was initiated IP on day 1 against Lewis lung carcinoma inoculated $(5 \times 10^5$ cells per mouse) subcutaneously, GANU and chlorozotocin did not show prolongation of mean survival time, while MCNU showed significant activity and 90-day survivors were obtained in four of six BDF$_1$ mice (Fig. 4). The results [38] indicated that antitumor activity of MCNU was superior to GANU and chlorozotocin, and it was comparable to ACNU and MeCCNU. Comparing hematologic toxicity of these five nitrosoureas using normal BDF$_1$ mice and injecting them with LD$_{10}$ doses, chlorozotocin showed most minimal decrease of leukocyte count in peripheral blood and rapid recovery, while GANU showed significant decrease of leukocyte count, needing 2 weeks recovery. MeCCNU, MCNU, and ACNU showed similar decreasing pattern of leukocyte count and more than 3 weeks needed for recovery (Fig. 5).

Recently Sekido and co-workers [37] reported that the antitumor activity of MCNU [8] was superior to chlorozotocin or CCNU and comparable to MeCCNU, while the hematologic toxicity was more than that of chlorozotocin but less than that of CCNU.

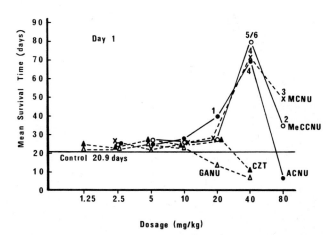

Fig. 4. Comparative activity of ACNU, GANU, MCNU, chlorozotocin (CZT), and MeCCNU against the 1-day-old Lewis lung carcinoma. Trypan blue-excluding Lewis lung carcinoma cells $(5 \times 10^5$/mouse) were implanted SC into six BDF$_1$ mice per group on day 1 and five drugs were given IP on day 1 only. Dose-response studies were done. Number on each symbol denotes the number of mice (of six mice) which survived for 90 days after implantation of tumor. Mean survival time of the group with 90-day survivors was calculated, including the 90-day survivors as they survived for 90 days

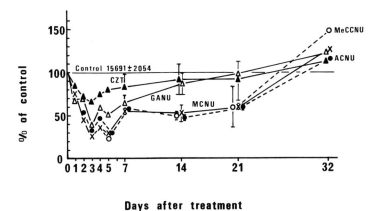

Days after treatment

Fig. 5. Serial white blood cell counts in the peripheral blood of BDF$_1$ mice after the administration of ACNU, GANU, MCNU, chlorozotocin (CZT), and MeCCNU. Thirty-three BDF$_1$ female mice per group were given intraperitoneal injections of 0.2 ml saline containing a LD$_{10}$ dose of each drug (LD$_{10}$ dose of each drug is shown in Fig. 3.). Three mice from each group were bled by lateral tail vein incision at the indicated time after drug administration. Blood (0.01 ml) was diluted with 10 ml saline. After hemolysis with cethyltrimethylammonium chloride, total white blood cells were counted using the Coulter counter Model ZBI. Vertical bars (shown only on days 7, 14, and 21) indicate one standard deviation from mean value of three determinants. This experiment was carried out three times and similar results were obtained in all experiments

Discussion

Throughout phase I study and preliminary phase II study, ACNU proved significant clinical efficacy against gastric cancer, uterine cancer, small cell carcinoma of lung, lymphomas, chronic myelogenous leukemia, malignant melanoma, and brain tumors, while it appeared to be less active against colorectal cancer, breast cancer, ovarian cancer, pancreatic cancer, nonoat cell carcinoma of lung and acute leukemias. In addition, it is of interest that responders were found in hepatoma, head and neck tumors, and sarcomas. However, the majority of patients who entered the study had already had prior chemotherapy and became resistant to conventional agents. Thus, available data of phase II study were insufficient to judge clinical efficacy. Further phase II and III studies will require the establishment of the clinical antitumor spectrum of ACNU.

Severity of hematologic toxicity seems to be similar to those of other nitrosoureas, but gastrointestinal toxicity appeared to be less frequent and milder.

Phase I study of GANU is now in progress. Up to now 70 mg/m^2 mild anorexia and nausea have been observed in a few patients, but no hematologic, hepatic, and renal toxicities have been found. It may need a few escalations of dosages to reach the maximum tolerated dose.

MCNU is an expectant nitrosourea for clinical trials, since it showed superior antitumor activities to GANU and chlorozotocin in experimental animal systems, and less hepatic and renal toxicities in preclinical toxicology. However, the hematologic toxicity appeared to be similar to that of ACNU. MCNU will enter to phase I study in the near future.

References

1. Symposium on the Nitrosoureas. Cancer Chemother Rep (Part 3) 4:1−35
2. Proceedings of the Seventh New Drug Seminar on the Nitrosoureas. Cancer Treat Rep 60:645−807
3. Wasserman TH, Slavik M, Carter SK (1974) Review of CCNU in clinical cancer therapy. Cancer Treat Rev 1:131−151
4. Wasserman TH, Slavik M, Carter SK (1974) Methyl CCNU in clinical cancer therapy. Cancer Treat Rev 1:251−269
5. Schein PS, O'Connel MJ, Blom J, Magrath IT, Bergevin P, Wiernik PH, Ziegler JI, Devita VT (1974) Clinical antitumor activity and toxicity of streptozotocin (NSC-85998). Cancer 34:993−1000
6. Schein PS, Panasci L, Wooley PV, Anderson T (1976) Pharmacology of chlorozotocin (NSC-178248), a new nitrosourea antitumor agent. Cancer Treat Rept 60:801−805
7. Fox PA, Panasci LC, Schein PS (1977) Biological and biochemical properties of 1-(2-chloroethyl)-3-(β-D-glucopyranosyl)-1-nitrosourea (NSC D254157), a nitrosourea with reduced bone marrow toxicity. Cancer Res 37:783−787
8. Hoth D, Schein P, Macdonald J, Buscaglia D, Haller D (1977) Phase I trial and clinical pharmacology of chlorozotocin (CLZ). Proc Am Assoc Cancer Res 18:309
9. Gralla RJ, Tan CTC, Young CW (1979) Phase I trial of chlorozotocin. Cancer Treat Rep 63:17−20
10. Muggia FM (to be published) Clinical trials in cancer; general concepts and methodologies. Cancer Clin Trials
11. Kimura K (1965) Chemotherapy of acute leukemia with special reference to criteria for evaluation of therapeutic effect. In: Advances in chemotherapy of acute leukemia under the Japan-US cooperative science program. Sept. 27−28. Bethesda, USA pp 21−23
12. Kimura K, Sakai Y, Konda C, Kashiwada N, Kitahara, T, Inagaki J, Mikuni M, Sakano T (1969) Chemotherapy of malignant lymphomas. Saishin Igaku 24:816−824
13. Arakawa M, Shimizu F, Okada N (1974) Effect of 1-(4-amino-2-methylpyrimidin-5-yl)-methyl-3-(2-chloroethyl)-3-nitrosourea hydrochloride on leukemia L-1210. Gann 65:191
14. Shimizu F, Arakawa M (1975) Effect of 3-[(4-amino-2-methyl-5-pyrimidinyl)methyl]-1-(2-chloroethyl)-1-nitrosourea hydrochlorize on lymphoid leukemia L-1210. Gann 66:149−154
15. Nakamura T, Sasada M, Tashima M, Yamamoto K, Uchida M, Sawada H, Uchino H (1978) Biological and biochemical mechanism of action of ACNU has been studied in L1210 cells in culture and human leukemic leucocytes obtained from patients with leukemia in vitro. Cancer Chemother 5:991−1000
16. Shigehara E, Tanaka M (1978) Whole body autographic studies on tissue distribution of 3-[(4-amino-2-methyl-5-pyrimidinyl)methyl-1-(2-chloroethyl)-1-nitrosourea hydrochloride in tumor-bearing mice and rats. Gann 69:709−714
17. Shimizu F, Okada N, Arakawa M (1975) Antitumor effect of ACNU (3); Effect on transplantable tumors in mice. Proc Jpn Cancer Assoc 34:302
18. Cooperative Study Group of Phase I Study on ACNU: Phase I study of 1-(4-amino-2-methyl-3-(2-chloroethyl)-3-nitrosourea hydrochloride (ACNU). Jpn J Clin Oncol 6:55−62
19. Saito T, Yokoyama M, Himori T, Ujiie S, Sugawara N, Sugiyama Z, Kitada K (1977) Phase I and preliminary phase II study of 1-(4-amino-2-methyl-5-pyrimidyl)methyl-3-(2-chloroethyl)-3-nitrosourea hydrochloride (ACNU) administered by intermittent dose schedule. Cancer Chemother 4:991−1004
20. Ogawa M, Inagaki J, Horikoshi N, Inoue K, Chinen T, Ueoka H, Nagura E, Fujimoto S, Murakami M, Ota K (1978) A clinical study on a new water-soluble nitrosourea derivative (ACNU). Cancer Chemother 5:105−110

21. Kimura I, Harada H, Ohnoshi T, Urabe Y, Fujii M, Machida K, Murakami N (1978) Clinical trial of 1-(4-amino-2-methyl-5-pyrimidinyl)methyl-3-(2-chloroethyl)-3-nitrosourea hydrochloride (ACNU). Cancer Chemother 5: 767–772

22. Ishii Y, Hattori T (Tokyo Cancer Chemotherapy Cooperative Study) (1978) Cooperative study on comparison between ACNU treatment and combined treatment with ACNU and OK-432. Cancer Chemother 5: 1195–1203

23. Ishiyama K (1978) Clinical results of ACNU on gastrointestinal tumors. Rinsho Kenkyu 55: 309–312

24. Honjo H, Fujii M, Tsuda S, Kimura T, Ohshima K, Yamamoto T, Murakami A (1979) Clinical experience of ACNU against gynecological tumors. Basic Pharmacol Ther 7: 163–171

25. Saijo N, Kawase I, Nishiwaki Y, Suzuki A, Niitani H (1977) Phase II study of ACNU [1-(4-amino-2-methyl-5-pyrimidinyl) methyl-3-(2-chloroethyl)-3-nitrosourea hydrochloride] for primary lung cancer and nodular pulmonary metastases. Cancer Chemother 4: 579–584

26. Saijo N, Nishiwaki Y, Kawase I, Kobayashi T, Suzuki A, Niitani H (1978) Effect of ACNU on primary lung cancer, methothelioma, and metastatic pulmonary tumors. Cancer Treat Rep 62: 139–141

27. Hori M, Nakagawa H, Hasegawa H, Mogami H, Hayakawa T, Nakata Y (1978) Chemotherapy of malignant glioma with the new nitrosourea derivative (ACNU). Cancer Chemother 5: 773–778

28. Saito Y, Nakaya Y, Muraoka K, Fujiwara T (1978) Chemotherapy of brain tumors with nitrosourea derivative (ACNU). Cancer Chemother 5: 779–794

29. Majima H, Oguro M, Takagi T (1978) Treatment of malignant lymphoma with ACNU. Cancer Chemother 5: 355–359

30. Takubo T, Masaoka T, Nakamura H, Ueda T, Shibata H, Yoshitake J (1978) ACNU treatment of blood malignancy. Cancer Chemother 5: 599–603

31. Inoue K, Inagaki J, Horikoshi N, Nagura E, Ueoka H, Murosaki S, Kobayashi T, Sujimoto S, Ogawa M, Saito T (1979) Clinical effect of DTIC containing combination chemotherapy against malignant melanoma and sarcomas. Proc Annu Meet Chemother 149

32. Machinami T, Nishiyama S, Kikuchi K, Suami T (1975) Synthesis of (2-chloroethyl)-nitrosourea derivatives of carbohydrate. Bull Chem Soc Jpn 48: 3763–3764

33. Yoshida K, Hoshi A, Kuretani K (1976) Mechanism of action of 1-(2-chloroethyl)-3-(β-D-glucopyranosyl)-1-nitrosourea (GANU) in vitro. Proc Jpn Cancer Assoc 486

34. Hisamatsu T, Uchida T (1977) Effect of 1-(2-chloroethyl)-3-(β-D-glucopyranosyl)-1-nitrosourea on experimental tumors. Gann 68: 819–824

35. Aoshima M, Sakurai Y (1977) Comparative studies on the antitumor activity and the bone marrow toxicity of 1-(β-D-glucopyranosyl)-3-(2-chloroethyl)-3-nitrosourea and 2-[3-(2-chloroethyl)-3-nitrosoureido)-D-glycopyranose. Gann 68: 247–250

36. Fox PA, Panasci LC, Schein PS (1977) Biological and biochemical properties of 1-(2-chloroethyl)-3-(β-D-glucopyranosyl)-1-nitrosourea (NSC D254157), a nitrosourea with reduced bone marrow toxicity. Cancer Res 37: 783–787

37. Sekido S, Ninomiya K, Iwasaki M (to be publisched) Biological activity of 1-(2-chloroethyl)-3-(methyl-α-D-glucopyranos-6-yl)-1-nitrosourea (MCNU; NSC-D270516); A new antitumor agent. Cancer Treat Rep

38. Fujimoto S, Ogawa M Unpublished work

PCNU Phase I Study
in the Northern California Oncology Group

M. A. Friedman*

University of California, San Francisco Cancer Research Institute, 1282 M,
USA – San Francisco, CA 94143

Introduction

The nitrosoureas are a family of antitumor agents that have been the subject of intensive laboratoy and clinical study for the past decade. In the United States a great many nitrosourreas have been sequentially studied under the sponsorship of the National Cancer Institute. From a large number of possible compounds there have been, however, three principal nitrosoureas extensively investigated in man. The first to be clinically evaluated was urea, 1,3-bis(2-chloroethyl)-1-nitroso, (BCNU), then was urea, 1-(2-chloroethyl)-3-cyclohexyl-1-nitroso, (CCNU), and more recently urea, 1-(2-chloroethyl)-3-(4-methyl cyclohexyl)-1-nitroso, (MeCCNU). Other related drugs have or are undergoing evaluation in the United States (including streptozotocin and chlorozotocin) but will not be discussed here.
BCNU, CCNU, and MeCCNU have had Phase II testing and all have meaningful activity in primary brain tumor and somewhat lesser activity in myeloma, lymphoma, enteric adenocarcinoma, and melanoma patients [2]. This modest general activity has encouraged hopes for greater benefit in analog development. Consequently, nitrosourea analog have been synthesized in attempts to achieve a superior therapeutic index and/or wider clinical spectrum. This research effort has not, however, proved fruitful, and currently there is little to recommend one of these nitrosoureas over another [2]. The search for a more efficacious and/or less toxic nitrosourea continues. PCNU, urea, 1-(2-chloroethyl)-3-(2,6-dioxo-1-piperidyl)-1-nitroso, is one of the newer compounds vying for the title of "best nitrosourea". PCNU (NSC 95466) has been undergoing Phase I-II testing in the United States and it will be my purpose here to report on the background and preliminary data of these trials.

Background

In general, nitrosoureas have been selected for clinical trials on the basis of animal tumor screening and pharmacologic properties. Leukemia L1210 has been the initial

* The author would like to acknowledge the assistance of E. A. Chevlen, MD and RM Hammers, RN. This study was supported in part by American Cancer Society Clinical Fellowship 4285 and Northern California Oncology Group Study NIH 1 R10 CA 21744/02-002b

screen for these drugs and it was their activity against intracerebrally (IC) inoculated L1210 that presaged activity in human brain tumors. In addition to intraperitoneal (IP) and IC L1210, more resistant rodent tumors (Lewis lung, for example) were added to the screening process. It has been hoped that greater effectiveness in animal tumors would correlate positively with greater efficacy in humans. This process has helped select CCNU and MeCCNU for clinical investigation.

The chemical and pharmacologic features of the nitrosourea family have also been studied in attempts to identify those properties which confer clinical utility and efficacy. The three principal nitrosoureas are relatively lipophilic and it is this characteristic that is thought to be associated with IC antitumor effectiveness in animals and similar benefits for central nervous system (CNS) tumors in man. Until recently, these drugs have been designed to have greater lipophilicity — so that BCNU < CCNU < MeCCNU — in hopes of improving the delivery of drug to patients with CNS tumors.

Moreover, although the nitrosoureas have both alkylating and carbamoylating activity, selection for clinical study was initially made without a clear appreciation of these functions. Wheeler et al. in 1974 [3] studied animals bearing L1210 and suggested that antitumor effectiveness correlated well with alkylating activity and increased as lipid solubility decreased. Carbamoylating activity, on the other hand, has not been clearly related to effectiveness. Recognizing the relationships between form and function, newer nitrosoureas have been selected for their effectiveness in animal tumor screens and their relative alkylating/carbamoylating activity.

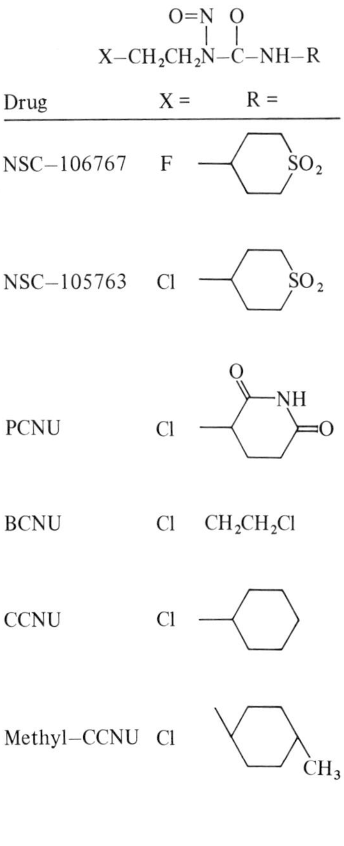

Fig. 1. The structures of the major nitrosoureas

Rationale for PCNU Evaluation

PCNU is a N-(2-chloroethyl)-N-nitrosourea similar in structure to the other major nitrosoureas. Recognizing the number of similar, currently available compounds, there needs to be persuasive reasons for choosing a particular nitrosourea to test clinically. The rationale for evaluating PCNU may be summarized as follows:

1) In tests performed by the NCI against IC, IP, and IM tumors (including L1210, 9L rat sarcoma, murine ependymoblastoma, P388 lymphoid leukemia, colon 26, B16 melanocarcinoma, CD8F mammary, and colon 38 tumors) PCNU was generally superior to other nitrosoureas.

2) The in vitro alkylating activity of PCNU is higher and the carbamoylating activity lower than several other nitrosoureas tested [1]. This data is summarized in Table 1.

3) Finally, Levin and Kabra [1] mathematically analyzed the chemical characteristics that would predict the most effective agent against CNS tumors. They described the log P value's (octanol/water partition coefficient) relation to antitumor effectiveness as a parabolic function. They predicted that the ideal log P would be between -0.20 and 1.34. PCNU's log P was 0.37 are within these limits while the other nitrosoureas had the following values:

BCNU, 1.53; CCNU, 2.83; and Methyl CCNU 3.30.

They theorized that the optimum log P for an effective drug against solid tumors in the brain would be 0.4 − a value close to that for PCNU (0.37).

Therefore, there seems abundant reason to study PCNU in the clinical setting.

Phase I Trial

The animal toxicology data on PCNU from the National Cancer Institute indicated organ system damage qualitatively similar to other nitrosoureas. Principal toxicities were hematologic, but less significant dysfunction was noted in liver and kidneys also. Moreover, there is now an enormous experience with the spectrum of toxicity of the nitrosoureas so that Phase I testing was embarked upon with a confidence rarely seen in clinical oncology.

There are several concurrent Phase I trials ongoing in the United States. Table 2 summarizes the institutions testing the drug and the schedule employed:

In the Northern California Oncology Group we have employed the following criteria to identify a patient appropriate for this study:

Table 1. The antitumor alkylating and carbamoylating activities of several nitrosoureas

Drug	Antitumor activity	Alkylating activity	Carbamoylating activity
PCNU	100[a]	100	100
BCNU	48	75	285
CCNU	21	28	417
MeCCNU	15	28	379

[a] The activity of PCNU was arbitratily assigned to be 100 for purposes of comparing the other drugs

Table 2. Current Phase I trials of PCNU in the United States

Institutions	Schedule
University of California, San Francisco	D1 + 2 every 6 weeks
M.D. Anderson	D1 every 6 weeks
Memorial Sloan-Kettering	D1 + 2 + 3 + 4 + 5 every 6 weeks
University of Wisconsin	D1 + 2 + 3 + 4 + 5 every 6 weeks
Georgetown University	D1 + 2 + 3 every 6 weeks

Table 3. The routine phase I evaluation

Parameters	On study entry	Weekly	every 3 weeks	Before each cycle (every 6 weeks)
PE	×			×
Visit date	×	×	×	×
Weight	×	×	×	×
Nausea and vomiting				×
Other toxicities			×	×
WBC	×	×		×
Hematocrit/Hemoglobin	×	×		×
Platelets	×	×		×
Differential	×	×		
Calcium	×		×	
BUN	×		×	
Uric acid	×		×	
Total protein	×		×	
Albumin	×		×	
Bilirubin	×		×	
Alkaline phosphatase	×		×	
LDH	×		×	
SGOT	×		×	
Creatinine	×		×	
Chest X-ray	×	As clinically indicated		

1) Biopsy proven cancer.
2) Incurable by any modality.
3) Karnofsky Performance Status $\geq 40\%$.
4) Age ≤ 70 years.
5) Life expectancy ≥ 10 weeks.
6) Informed consent.
7) Adequate physiologic function: a) WBC $\geq 4\,000$ cells/mm^3; b) Platelets $\geq 100\,000$ cells/mm^3; c) Creatinine < 2.5 mg/dl; and d) Bilirubin < 2.0 mg/dl (see Table 3).

Table 4. Results indicating toxicity after PCNU therapy

Dosage × 2d	Number of patients	Toxicity
12 mg/m²	3	PLT = 91,000 on day 8 (increased to 171,000 throughout the rest of cycle)
24 mg/m²	4	PLT = 77,000 on day 21
36 mg/m²	2	
48 mg/m²	2	PLT = 33,000 on day 21

The following criteria exclude a patient from PCNU therapy:
1) Prior treatment with another nitrosourea.
2) Prior radiation or chemotherapy within 3 weeks.
3) Patients with hematologic malignancy.

Results and Future Plans

We initiated our PCNU at a dosage of 12 mg/m² IV on 2 consecutive days every 6 weeks. Our data to date is.

To date no significant leukopenia or anemia has been noted; nor has there been evidence of cumulative toxicity. Three patients have had platelet counts less than 100 000 cells/mm³. No nausea or vomiting has been noted nor any hepatic or renal dysfunction. Unfortunately, no therapeutic benefit has been apparent either.

As with the other nitrosoureas, patients previously treated with radiation and other chemotherapy will probably be more sensitive to PCNU. We plan to continue to evaluate 96 mg/m² every 6 weeks to confirm the presence of reproducible hematotoxicity, or until another dose-limiting toxicity is apparent.

Our future plans for PCNU include detailed pharmacology studies as an integral part of our Phase I assessment. Further, we intend to test this agent in patients with brain, enteric, lymphoid, and breast malignancies. The relative effectiveness of this agent (compared to BCNU, CCNU, MeCCNU, or other nitrosoureas) will become apparent only if unique solid tumor activity or less systemic toxicity are noted. Future comparative trials will be aimed at assessing the value of this new agent.

References

1. Levin VA, Kabra P (1974) Effectiveness of the nitrosoureas as a function of their lipid solubility in the chemotherapy of experimental rat brain tumors. Cancer Chemother Rep (Part 1) 58: 787–792
2. Wasserman TH, Slavik M, Carter SK (1975) Clinical comparison of the nitrosoureas. Cancer 36: 1258–1268
3. Wheeler GP, Bowdon BJ, Grimsley JA, Harris HH (1974) Interrelationships of some chemical, physicochemical, and biological activities of several 1-(2-halo-ethyl)-1-nitroso-ureas. Cancer Res 34: 194–200

Molecular Pharmacology of Nitrosoureas

K. D. Tew, M. E. Smulson, and P. S. Schein

Georgetown University Medical Center, 3800 Reservoir Road, N.W.,
USA – Washington, DC 20007

Introduction

The development of a wide range of aliphatic nitrosamides has followed the original observation that 1-methyl-1-nitroso-3-nitrosoguanidine had reproducible antitumor activity against murine L1210 leukemia [7]. The resultant synthesis of new *N*-nitroso containing compounds has produced two general classes of drug, the methyl and chloroethyl nitrosoureas. Both groups of drugs have the potential to alkylate and carbamoylate cellular macromolecules under physiologic conditions with no preliminary enzymatic activation required. In addition, the original observation that 1-methyl-1-nitrosourea (MNU) increased the life span of mice bearing intercranially implanted L1210 cells [25] was correlated with the lipid solubility of the drug and its potential to cross the blood brain barrier. This property instigated the development and clinical use of a series of chloroethyl nitrosoureas, including, 1,3-bis(2-chloroethyl)-1-nitrosourea (BCNU) [11], 1-(2-chloroethyl)-3-cyclohexyl-1-nitrosourea (CCNU) and eventually methyl-CCNU. These drugs have established clinical antitumor activity for a broad range of human malignancies including acute lymphocytic leukemia, lymphomas, myeloma, melanoma, gliomas, and gastrointestinal neoplasms [32]. Unfortunately, these same agents produce delayed and cumulative bone marrow toxicity which is a serious limitation to their therapeutic efficacy. The attachment of MNU to the C-2 position of glucose (streptozotocin) greatly reduced this myelosuppression and further led to the synthesis of a chloroethyl derivative, 2-[3-(2-chloroethyl)-3-nitrosoureido]-D-glucopyranose or chlorozotocin [12] which, similarly exhibited minimal myelotoxicity [24]. This article is designed to provide comparative analysis of the biochemical pharmacology of methyl and chloroethyl nitrosoureas and to relate these properties to the interaction of these drugs with chromatin, encompassing the potential importance of drug-induced nuclear modifications at the molecular level.

Metabolism

A spontaneous decomposition of nitrosoureas occurs under physiologic conditions [2, 17] (Fig. 1). At pH 7.4 in phosphate buffered saline the individual chemical half-lives range from 7 min to 2 h. During degradation a series of alkylating moieties are formed,

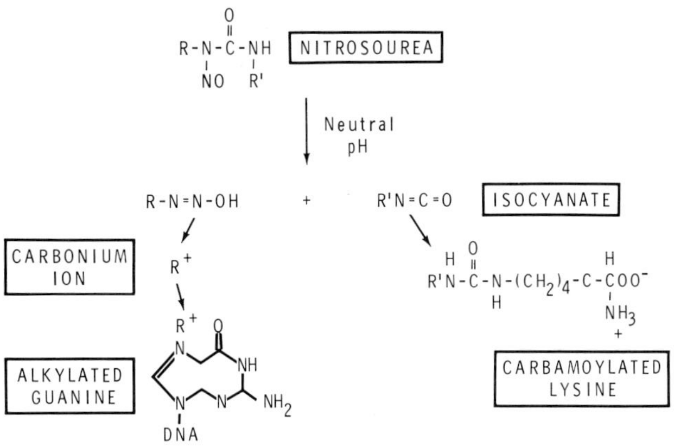

Fig. 1. Physiologic decomposition of nitrosoureas

of which an alkyldiazohydroxide precursor and methyl or chloroethyl carbonium ion are considered of premier importance. In addition, organic isocyanate moieties are generated and these are responsible for carbamoylating cellular proteins. Generally, amino, carboxyl, sulphydryl, and phosphate groups are susceptible to alkylation. Carbamoylation of amino acids by the organic isocyanate occurs at sites of "active" hydrogen groups, such as the amino group of lysine or arginine.

CCNU is now known to be metabolized by the liver microsomal mixed function oxidase system to more polar hydroxylated products that retain both the cyclohexyl ring structure and the cytotoxic nitrosoureido moiety [16, 23]. Studies with CCNU in man have shown that 75% of the plasma drug concentration following a 1 h slow infusion was in the form of hydroxylated products [31]. Two-thirds appeared as trans-4-hydroxy CCNU and one-third as the cis-4-isomer. It is thought that the rate of metabolic hydroxylation of CCNU exceeds the rate of chemical dissociation, and as a result, the hydroxylated metabolites are the immediate precursors of the therapeutic and toxic moieties. In addition to the hydroxylation of the nitrosourea ring structure, it has been shown that both BCNU and MNU are denitrosated by microsomal enzymes [10]. All nitrosoureas shown in Table 1, except ACNU, elicit greater mutagenic activity (12%−40%) after incubation with S9 liver microsomal fractions than before [4]. Although there is no linear relationship between in vitro alkylating activity and mutagenic potential, results suggest that after S9 activation, nitrosoureas possess mutagenic activity equivalent to metabolized 3-methylcholanthrene [4]. Therefore such metabolism may have relevance in regard to potential carcinogenic activity in man.

Alkylation and Carbamoylation

Table 1 shows the comparative alkylating and carbamoylating potential of a series of methyl and chloroethyl nitrosoureas. Although alkylation is widely accepted as the principal mechanism of cytotoxicity, previous studies have failed to demonstrate a linear correlation between NBP alkylating activity and antitumor activity against murine L1210 leukemia [8, 19]. Similarly, other studies have failed to show a correlation between carbamoylating activity and antitumor activity [34], granulocyte suppression [18] or lethal toxicity [9]. Both chlorozotocin and streptozotocin possess

Table 1. Comparitive alkylating and carbamoylating activity of some nitrosoureas

Drug	Structure	Alkylating activity (% CNU)	Carbamoylating activity (% CNU)
CNU	R-H	100	100
GANU		86	44
Chloro-zotocin		64	4
BCNU	R-CH$_2$CH$_2$Cl	41	49
ACNU		38	3.5
CCNU		10	94
MNU	R'-H	20	105
Strepto-zotocin		5	3

$$R = \overset{H}{\underset{\underset{O}{\|}}{N}}\overset{O}{\overset{\|}{C}}NCH_2CH_2Cl$$

$$R' = \overset{H}{\underset{\underset{O}{\|}}{N}}\overset{O}{\overset{\|}{C}}NCH_3$$

neglible carbamoylating potential because of internal attack of the carbon-1- hydroxyl group by the isocyanate [18]. Since both elicit antitumor efficacy, it is likely that the contribution of carbamoylation to overall cytotoxicity is minor. Finally, chloroethyl nitrosoureas have the potential to cause cross links in DNA [13] (inter or intrastrand) or between DNA and nuclear proteins by an initial chloroethylation of the nucleophilic site on one strand, followed by a gradual displacement of Cl$^-$ by a second nucleophilic site. Most plausibly, a combination of alkylation, carbamoylation, and cross-linking contribute to ultimate cytotoxicity.

Interaction with Chromatin

At the molecular level chromatin is composed of nucleosomes, composed of a double tetrameric core of histones H2a, H2b, H3 and H4, surrounded by a helical turn of 140

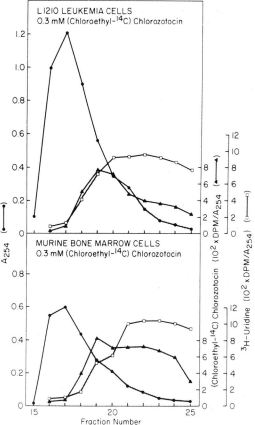

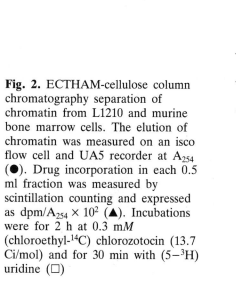

Fig. 2. ECTHAM-cellulose column chromatography separation of chromatin from L1210 and murine bone marrow cells. The elution of chromatin was measured on an isco flow cell and UA5 recorder at A_{254} (●). Drug incorporation in each 0.5 ml fraction was measured by scintillation counting and expressed as dpm/A_{254} × 10^2 (▲). Incubations were for 2 h at 0.3 mM (chloroethyl-^{14}C) chlorozotocin (13.7 Ci/mol) and for 30 min with (5−^{3}H) uridine (□)

base pairs of DNA [30]. Histone Hl is associated with the linker region of DNA which connects the nucleosomes and is approximately 60 base pairs in length. The complex superhelical structure is thought to be stabilized by Hl interaction and by an important, but as yet undefined, nonhistone protein involvement. Although the repetitive nucleosome structure is believed to occur in both transcriptionally active and inactive regions of chromatin [3], it is proposed that the constrained superhelical structure is "relaxed" and extended in transcriptional chromatin in order to permit access for the enzymes involved in the transcriptional process [15].

Using radiolabeled nitrosoureas, it has been possible to consider their alkylating and carbamoylating properties at various levels of chromatin complexity. Figure 2 shows a chromatin separation based on the technique of Reeck et al. (1972) [22] using ECTHAM-cellulose column chromatography. Incorporation of ^{3}H-uridine into the latter eluting chromatin fractions confirmed the in vitro transcriptional activity of these fractions. In both the L1210 and bone marrow samples, alkylation by chlorozotocin was restricted to this transcriptional chromatin. These data are in concordance with similar studies in HeLa cells using either chlorozotocin (Fig. 3) or CCNU [28] and confirmed that extended chromatin was a preferential target for alkylation by chloroethyl nitrosoureas.

In addition, DNase I is known to cleave preferentially transcriptional DNA [5, 14, 33]. The limit digest data (Fig. 4) showed that early digestion of HeLa cell chromatin by

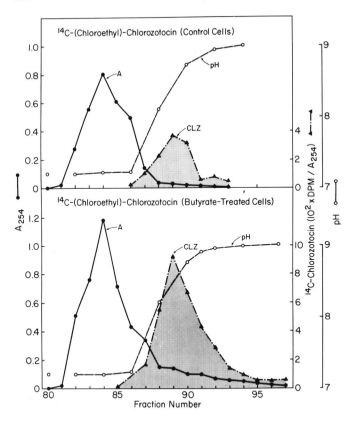

Fig. 3. As for Fig. 2, in normal and sodium butyrate (5 m*M* for 24 h) treated HeLa cells. Chlorozotocin was for 2 h at 30 μ*M*. The alteration of pH after buffer change (Reeck et al. 1972) was monitored for representative 0.5 ml fractions. Tew et al. (1978) Cancer Res 38: 3371–3378

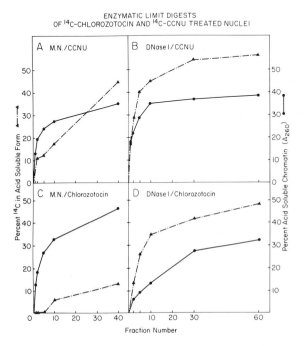

Fig. 4. A, B Limit digest of HeLa cell nuclei treated with 0.3 m*M* chlorozotocin (chloroethyl-^{14}C) or 0.3 m*M* CCNU (chloroethyl-^{14}C). Micrococcal nuclease (**A** and **C**) and DNase I (**B** and **D**) were used as described elsewhere (Tew et al. 1978). The release of TCA soluble ^{14}C was monitored (▲) and compared with the digestion of nuclear chromatin (●). Abscissa, time in minutes. Tew et al. (1978) Cancer Res 38: 3371–3378

DNase I released proportionally greater amounts of alkylated material (both for chlorozotocin and CCNU) and therefore, provided further confirmatory data that a nonrandom alkylation of chromatin occurred, preferentially localizing in the transcriptionally active regions. Figure 4 also shows a similar experimental approach utilizing micrococcal nuclease, an enzyme which cleaves DNA initially between nucleosomes, i.e., linker DNA. As with DNase I, such enzymatic degradation creates small segments of chromatin which may be separated, and therefore, distinguished from bulk chromatin, by differential solubilization in acid. The data for HeLa cells (Fig. 4) is in agreement with L1210 cells (Fig. 5) treated with three concentrations of chlorozotocin.

In both L1210 and HeLa cells, the solubilization of chromatin, as measured at A_{254} was greater than the concomitant release of alkylated material. These data demonstrated a preferential alkylation of the DNA which was inaccessible to micrococcal nuclease, namely the DNA associated with the nucleosome core particle. Conversely, the release of alkylated chromatin was higher than that of bulk chromatin in murine bone marrow. This showed a preferential alkylation of linker DNA in these cells. This differential may be germane to the nonmyelotoxic properties of chlorozotocin, since there are reports of an increased repair potential within internucleosomal, linker DNA [1, 21]. Using similar techniques, we have previously demonstrated that although

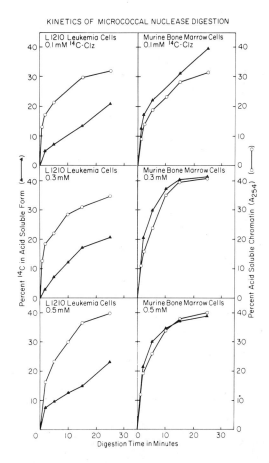

Fig. 5. Limit digest of L1210 and murine bone marrow cells treated with 0.1, 0.3 and 0.5 mM (chloroethyl-^{14}C) chlorozotocin. The release of acid soluble ^{14}C was monitored (▲) and compared with digestion of bulk chromatin (○). For experimental details see Fig. 4

CCNU preferentially alkylates nucleosome core DNA (Fig. 4), MNU preferentially alkylates linker DNA in HeLa cells [26]. Such differences may contribute to the differential cytotoxic and carcinogenic properties of these drugs.

Although alkylation of cytoplasmic RNA forms a major proportion of total cellular alkylation (Table 2), nuclear RNA contributed only between 10% and 20% of the nuclear alkylation by chlorozotocin and CCNU (Table 3). T2 RNase attacks nonspecifically at all phosphodiester bonds and splits RNA into 3' nucleotides which may be solubilized in acid. By prelabeling with ^{3}H-uridine it was found that 90% of the nuclear RNA was solubilized by the nuclease. Control experiments using ^{3}H-thymidine showed that approximately 10% DNA was digested, suggesting either some ^{3}H-thymidine was converted to ribothymine and incorporated into RNA [29] or there was DNase contamination of the T2 RNase or an intrinsic DNase was activated during the incubation. Thus it is not possible definitively to quantitate nuclear RNA alkylation.

Table 2. In vitro alkylation of cellular DNA, RNA, and protein following a 2-h incubation with 0.1 mM (chloroethyl-^{14}C) nitrosourea

L1210 leukemia	CCNU[a] (ethyl-U-^{14}C)	Chlorozotocin[a] (ethyl-1-^{14}C)
DNA	24.4 ± 5.3	56.5 ± 1.7
RNA	103 ± 34.3	239 ± 34.3
Protein	98 ± 9.2	139 ± 32
Murine bone marrow		
DNA	41.5 ± 2.3	44.9 ± 4.7
RNA	88.0 ± 12.5	140 ± 17.8
Protein	118 ± 12.7	198 ± 65.8

[a] Data expressed as picomoles of ethyl-^{14}C group/mg DNA, RNA, or protein ± SD

Table 3. Nuclear RNA Alkylation

	^{3}H-Uridine	^{14}C-CLZ	^{14}C-CCNU	^{3}H-TdR
Whole Chromatin	87.9 ± 2.8	18.7 ± 4.3	15.0 ± 3.0	7.5 ± 2.7
DNase II Digest	86.3 ± 2.6	21.0 ± 4.6	12.7 ± 3.5	15.4 ± 3.9

Data expressed as %TCA PPT radioactivity released by T2 RNase.
Values are mean ± for 3 experiments.
Log phase cells were treated with 0.2 mM (^{14}C-chloroethyl)-CLZ or (^{14}C-chloroethyl)-CCNU for 2 h or with 3uCi/ml ^{3}H-uridine or ^{3}H-TdR for 1 h. Samples of whole chromatin were treated either directly with 50 units of T2 RNase or were first digested with DNase II (see Gottesfeld and Partington, 1977) and solubilized in MgCl^2 prior to T2 RNase digestion. After digestion with T2 RNase, samples were precipitated with cold 5% TCA and counted for radioctivity. The percent released by digestion was calculated by comparison with the acid insoluble radioactivity in the original samples

Cytoplasmic proteins also constitute a major proportion of total cellular alkylation (Table 2). However, at the nuclear level, the alkylation by CCNU or chlorozotocin of histone or nonhistone proteins was found to be extremely low at physiologic drug concentrations [28]. At high drug concentrations (2.2 mM) MNU was found to alkylate histones H2a and H1, plus a number of nonhistone proteins [20]. At lower concentrations, carbamoylation of nuclear proteins by both MNU and CCNU was

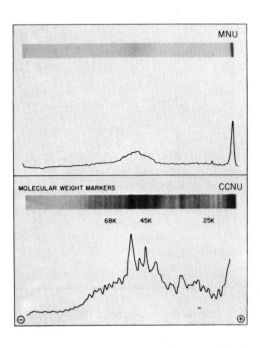

Fig. 6. Above: Modification of nuclear proteins by (carbonyl-^{14}C) MNU and (cyclohexyl-^{14}C) CCNU. HeLa cells (5×10^7) in 1 ml were incubated with 30 μCi of (carbonyl-^{14}C) MNU (7.9 Ci/mol) and (cyclohexyl-^{14}C) CCNU (8.3 Ci/mol) for 1 and 2 h respectively. Nuclei were isolated, proteins extracted with 0.4 N H_2SO_4 and analyzed on Triton-acetic acid-urea slab gels. **Above:** Autoradiograph of MNU-modified histones and densitometer scan; **below** same as **above**, of CCNU-modified proteins. Sudkakar et al. (1979) Cancer Res 39: 1411–1417

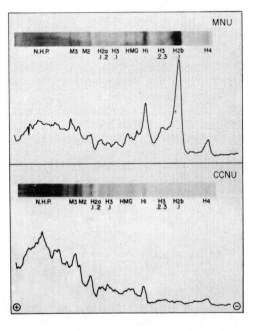

Fig. 7. As for Fig. 6. except using SDS gel electrophoresis. Sudkakar et al. (1979) Cancer Res 39: 1411–1417

detectable (Figs. 6 and 7). Using triton-acetic acid-urea gel electrophoresis [27] followed by gel autoradiography, it was shown that MNU carbamoylation of H2b and H1 predominated, with lower levels of H4 and nonhistone protein modification. By comparison, CCNU carbamoylated mainly nonhistone proteins (Fig. 7) with slight H1 modification (Fig. 6). Using sodium dodecyl sulfate (SDS) gel electrophoresis (Fig. 7) CCNU was found to carbamoylate a wide range of nonhistone proteins within both high and low molecular weight range. Since both histone and nonhistone proteins are integral in maintaining structure and function of chromatin, carbamoylation may contribute to eventual cytotoxicity either per se or in conjunction with nucleic acid alkylation.

Perspectives

Studies of nitrosourea/chromatin interactions are of potential significance, not only as a means of determining the mechanism of drug action, but also as an approach to the understanding of chromatin structure and function. The dual capacity of nitrosoureas to alkylate and carbamoylate nuclear material contributes to their unique potential as probes in the elucidation of the molecular biology of chromatin. Additionally, these chromatin modifications may contribute to an understanding of the molecular phenomenon leading to cytotoxicity and carcinogenesis. These studies may provide an approach to drug selectivity and design of novel anticancer agents.

References

1. Bodell WJ, Banerjee MR (1979) The influence of chromatin structure on the distribution of DNA repair synthesis studied by nuclease digestion. Nucleic Acids Res 6: 359–370
2. Colvin M, Brundrett RB, Cowens W, Jardin I, Ludlum DB (1976) A chemical basis for the antitumor activity of chloroethylnitrosoureas. Biochem Pharmacol 25: 695–699
3. Felsenfeld C (1978) Chromatin. Nature 271: 115–122
4. Franza B, Schein P, Saslaw L, Oeschger M (1978) Basal mutagenic activity (BMA) of clinical chloroethylnitrosoureas (NU), and the effect of microsomal activation. Proc Am Assoc Cancer Res 19: 234
5. Garel A, Axel R (1976) Selective digestion of transcriptionally active ovalbumin genes from oviduct nuclei. Proc Natl Acad Sci USA 73: 3966–3970
6. Gottesfeld JM, Partington GA (1977) Distribution of messenger RNA-coding sequences in fractionated chromatin. Cell 12: 953–962
7. Greene MO, Greenberg J (1960) The activity of nitrosoguanidines against ascites tumors in mice. Cancer Res 20: 1166–1171
8. Heal JM, Fox PA, Doukas D, Schein PS (1978) Biological and biochemical properties of the 2-hydroxyl metabolites of 1-(2-chloroethyl)-3-cyclohexyl-1-nitrosourea. Cancer Res 38: 1070–1074
9. Heal JM, Fox PA, Sinks L, Schein P (1978) Effect of carbamoylation on repair of nitrosourea alkylated DNA in L1210 cells. Proc Am Assoc Cancer Res 19: 202
10. Hill DL, Kirk MC, Struck RF (1975) Microsomal metabolism of nitrosoureas. Cancer Res 25: 296–301
11. Johnston TP, McCaleb GS, Montgomery JA (1963) Synthesis of antineoplastic agents. 32. N-nitrosoureas 1. J Med Chem 6: 669–681

12. Johnston TP, McCaleb GS, Montgomery JA (1975) Synthesis of chlorozotocin, the 2-chloroethyl analog of the anticancer antibiotic streptozotocin. J Med Chem 18: 104–106

13. Kohn KW (1977) Interstand cross-linking of DNA by 1,3-bis(2-chloroethyl)-1-nitrosourea and other 1-(2-haloethyl)-1-nitrosoureas. Cancer Res 37: 1450–1454

14. Levy WB, Dixon GH (1977) Complementary to cytoplasmic polyadenylated RNA from rainbow-trout testis accessibility of transcribed genes to pancreatic DNASE. Nucleic Acids Res 4: 883–898

15. Matthews HR (1977) The structure of transcribing chromatin. Nature 267: 203–204

16. May HE, Boose R, Reed DJ (1974) Hydroxylation of the carcinostatic 1-(2-chloro-ethyl)-3-cyclohexyl-1-nitrosourea (CCNU) by rat liver microsomes. Biochem Biophys Res Commun 57: 426–433

17. Montgomery JA, James R, McCaleb GS, Kirk MC, Johnston TP (1975) Decomposition of N-(2-chloroethyl)-N-nitrosoureas in aqueous media. J Med Chem 18: 568–571

18. Panasci LC, Fox PA, Schein PS (1977) Structure-activity studies of methylnitrosourea antitumor agents with reduced murine bone marrow toxicity. Cancer Res 37: 3321–3328

19. Panasci LC, Green DC, Nagourney R, Fox PA, Schein PS (1977) A structure-activity analysis of chemical and biological parameters of chloroethylnitrosoureas in mice. Cancer Res 37: 2615–2618

20. Pinsky SD, Tew KD, Smulson ME, Woolley PV (1979) Modification of L1210 cell nuclear proteins by 1-methyl-1-nitrosourea and 1-methyl-3-nitro-1-nitrosoguanidine. Cancer Res 39: 923–928

21. Ramanathan R, Rajalakshmi S, Sarma DS, Farber E (1976) Non-random nature of in vivo methylation by dimethylnitrosamine and the subsequent removal of methylated products from rat liver chromatin DNA. Cancer Res 36: 2073–2079

22. Reeck GR, Simpson RT, Sober HA (1972) Resolution of a spectrum of nucleoprotein species in sonicated chromatin. Proc Natl Acad Sci USA 69: 2317–2321

23. Reed DJ, May HE (1975) Alkylation and carbamoylation intermediates from the carcinostatic 1-(2-chloroethyl)-3-cyclohexyl-1-nitrosourea (CCNU). Life Sci 16: 1263–1270

24. Schein PS, Bull JM, Doukas D, Hoth D (1978) Sensitivity of human and murine hematopoietic precursor cells to 2-[3-(2-chloroethyl)-3-nitrosoureido]-D-glucopyranose and 1,3-bis(2-chloroethyl)-1-nitrosourea. Cancer Res 38: 257–260

25. Skipper HE, Schabel FM, Trader MW, Thomson JR (1961) Experimental evaluation of potential anticancer agents VI. Anatomical distribution of leukemic cells and failure of chemotherapy. Cancer Res 21: 1154–1164

26. Sudhakar S, Tew KD, Smulson ME (1979) Effect of 1-methyl-1-nitrosourea on poly (adenosine diphosphate-ribose) polymerase activity at the nucleosomal level. Cancer Res 39: 1405–1410

27. Sudhakar S, Tew KD, Schein PS, Woolley PV, Smulson ME (1979) Nitrosourea interaction with chromatin and effect on poly (adenosine diphosphate ribose) polymerase activity. Cancer Res 39: 1411–1417

28. Tew KD, Sudhakar S, Schein PS, Smulson ME (1978) Binding of chlorozotocin and 1-(2-chloroethyl)-3-cyclohexyl-1-nitrosourea to chromatin and nucleosomal fractions of HeLa cells. Cancer Res 38: 3371–3378

29. Tew KD, Taylor DM (1978) The relationship of thymidine metabolism to the use of fractional incorporation as a measure of DNA synthesis and tissue proliferation. Eur J Cancer 14: 153–168

30. Thomas JO, Kornberg RD (1975) An octamer of histones in chromatin and free in solution. Proc Natl Acad Sci USA 72: 2626–2630

31. Walker MD, Hilton J (1976) Nitrosourea pharmacodynamics in relation to the central nervous system. Cancer Treat Rep 60: 725–728

32. Wasserman TH, Slavik M, Carter SK (1975) Clinical comparison of the nitrosoureas. Cancer 36: 1258–1268
33. Weintraub H, Groudine M (1976) Chromosomal subunits in active genes have an altered conformation. Science 193: 848–856
34. Wheeler GP, Bowden BJ, Grinsley JA, Lloyd HH (1974) Interrelationships of some chemical physiochemical, and biological activities of several 1-(2-haloethyl)-1-nitrosoureas. Cancer Res 34: 194–200

Mechanistic Approaches to New Nitrosourea Development

K. W. Kohn

Laboratory of Molecular Pharmacology, Developmental Therapeutics Program, Division of Cancer Treatment, National Cancer Institute, National Institutes of Health, USA — Bethesda, MD 20205

The 1-chloroethyl-1-nitrosoureas are highly active against nearly all experimental tumors that have been extensively tested in mice, rats, and hamsters [39]. The benefits against the human disease, however, have been relatively modest [4]. Although the activity in man has so far been disappointing, the high activity in animals suggests that there is greater potential to be tapped. The nitrosoureas are known to react with DNA, as well as with other cellular macromolecules [5, 31, 33, 34, 41, 43, 44]. If DNA is the critical target, some key mechanistic questions may yield to presently available experimental techniques. Some current concepts and results along this line of approach will be reviewed.

Reactions with Macromolecules: Alkylation and Carbamoylation

The nitrosoureas are unstable molecules that decompose by splitting to form two types of reactive intermediates (Fig. 1) [43, 44]. One cleavage product, chloro-ethyldiazohydroxide, is an alkylating agent that can add chloroethyl groups to various nucleophilic sites (X: in Fig. 1) [3, 7, 8, 38]. The resulting adducts could undergo nucleophilic displacement of Cl^- to form a cross-bridge to a second nucleophilic site (Y: in Fig. 1). The other cleavage product is an isocyanate that can react with nucleophiles such as primary amines to form carbamoyl products [40, 45]. The nitrosoureas thus produce two different types of chemical actions of possible biologic significance.

Both types of adduct formation — alkylation and carbamoylation — can occur on biologically important macromolecules. The alkylating intermediate, however, is much more reactive than the isocyanates and, therefore, reacts at a wider variety of sites. Alkylation occurs at several sites on nucleic acids and proteins, but carbamoyl-ation is restricted to the more reactive protein sites and does not occur on nucleic acids [5]. Some chloroethylnitrosoureas have little or no ability to carbamoylate because of intramolecular inactivation of the isocyanate group shortly after its forma-tion [35, 37, 47]. Derivatives of this type — notably chlorozotocin and some hydroxy-CCNU derivatives — have hydroxyl groups in positions that allow these groups to react with the isocyanate function. The noncarbamoylating derivatives lack some of the bio-chemical effects of other nitrosoureas, but retain the antitumor activity; the antitumor activity in fact depends mainly on the presence of a haloethyl alkylating function [35].

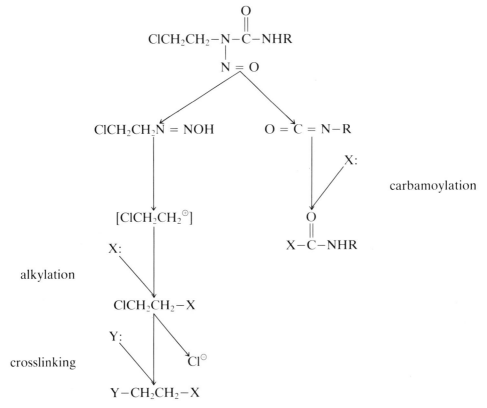

Fig. 1. Reactions of chloroethylnitrosourea with macromolecules. X and Y are nucleophilic groups on DNA, proteins etc.

The carbamoylating function, however, does have biochemical effects of possible importance. Of greatest potential significance is an inhibition of the rejoining of DNA single-strand breaks, a key step in the repair of DNA damage. This inhibition has been demonstrated for the case of single-strand breaks produced by X ray [11, 22] and for the case of single-strand breaks generated during excision repair in human cells irradiated with ultraviolet light [16]. The inhibition of strand rejoining could also influence the repair of alkylation damage, possibly including that produced by the nitrosoureas themselves [19]. Nitrosoureas lacking carbamoylation activity do not inhibit the rejoining of DNA single-strand breaks (Kann HE, Jr, personal communication).

Other actions related to carbamoylating activity include inhibition of DNA replication [2, 6, 21] and inhibition of RNA strand scission steps in the maturational processing of ribosomal RNA and possibly also in high molecular weight nucleoplasmic RNA [1, 23].

Since carbamoylating activity is not required for antitumor activity, it could be advantageous to separate it from the alkylating activity that is the primary source of the antitumor activity. It is not known whether the effects of carbamoylation are beneficial or detrimental. Specific toxicities such as myelosuppression, however, appear to be unrelated to carbamoylation [17, 18, 36]. Carbamoylation may produce either desirable or undesirable effects. This problem could be attacked by utilizing separate agents to provide alkylating and carbamoylating actions, so that the extent of each effect can be controlled both in magnitude and in timing. Compounds are now available that have alkylating or carbamoylating activity almost exclusively. Alkylation with little or no carbamoylation is provided for example by *cis*-2-OH-CCNU, a metabolite of 1-(2-chloroethyl)-1-nitroso-3-cyclohexylurea (CCNU) [46]. The OH group of this compound is so placed that it can react with the isocyanate group formed in the same molecule. In other isomers, such as *trans*-4-OH-CCNU, the OH group is so placed that it cannot access the isocyanate function of the same molecule; therefore, carbamoylating ability is retained. The two isomers otherwise resemble each other chemically and physically, so that direct comparisons between them would be revealing. Chlorozotocin is another noncarbamoylating derivative, but it is less attractive because it lacks activity against intracerebral tumors and has lost the activity against the Lewis lung tumor (screening data, Division of Cancer Treatment, National Cancer Institute, Bethesda, Maryland).

Carbamoylation with little or no alkylating activity can be provided by compounds such as bis-cyclohexylnitrosourea. This compound inhibits the rejoining of DNA single-strand breaks but is much less toxic than the haloethylnitrosoureas (Kann HE, Jr, personal communication). The prospect thus exists for using two compounds to administer the alkylating and carbamoylating functions of the nitrosoureas separately and at will.

Interstrand Crosslinking in Purified DNA

The first indication that chloroethylnitrosoureas may produce bifunctional adducts to nucleic acids was the identification of an ethylene bridged cytosine product in the reaction of 1,3-bis(2-chloroethyl) nitrosourea (BCNU) with poly C [31, 34]. The formation of this and other products showed that chloroethylation could occur at a heterocyclic nitrogen, cytosine N_3, and then react further with the primary amino group of cytosine with elimination of chloride. The result is an intramolecular ethylene bridge between the two cytosine nitrogens. This shows that the cytosine amino group, although a weak nucleophile, can engage in nucleophilic displacement of a suitably placed alkyl chloride.

An analogous sequence of reactions could, in principle, give rise to an ethylene crosslink between paired DNA strands (Fig. 2), provided that the hypothetical nucleophilic atoms, X and Y, are close enough to be linked by an ethylene bridge. The formation of interstrand crosslinks was examined by testing for an inhibition of the ability of the paired strands to be separated by alkali [24, 25, 30]. Figure 3 illustrates an experiment that demonstrates the inhibition of strand separation in calf thymus DNA treated with CCNU [25]. Qualitatively similar results were obtained with BCNU, 1-(2-chloroethyl)-1-nitrosourea (CNU), and chlorozotocin, but not with methylnitrosourea which lacks the chloride that would be required for the second step of the crosslinking reaction. The fluoro analog of CCNU produced a small but significant degree of reaction that increased after longer reaction times. The slower reaction of the fluoro analog may be due to the weak leaving-group capabilities of fluoride compared to chloride.

The chloride displacement reaction which forms crosslinks in the case of chloroethylnitrosoureas (Fig. 2) occurs slowly over a period of several hours at 37° C and pH

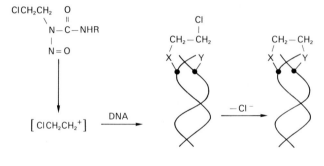

Fig. 2. Proposed mechanism of formation of an ethylenebridge crosslink between strands of a DNA helix. X and Y are nucleophilic sites on DNA (Kohn 1977)

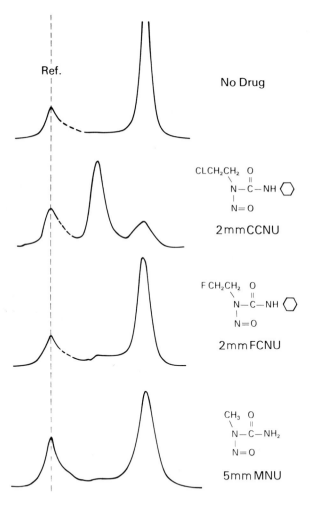

Fig. 3. Demonstration of interstrand crosslinking by CCNU. *E. coli* DNA was incubated with or without drug for 9 h at 37° C and then treated with alkali to separate the strands. Upon neutralization, only crosslinked strands reassociate to a double helix. Double helical DNA (middle band) is then separated from single-strand DNA (right band) by equilibirium sedimentation in CsCl. FCNU, 1-(2-fluoroethyl)-1-nitroso-3-cyclohexylurea; MNU, 1-methyl-1-nitrosourea (Kohn 1977)

7. This was determined by first reacting DNA with drug for 1 h, then removing the drug and further incubating the DNA in the absence of drug (Fig. 4). The rate of this second step in the crosslinking reaction appears to be independent of the type of chloroethylnitrosoureas used, since BCNU and CNU, although reacting at different rates in the first reaction step, form crosslinks at the same rate during postincubation

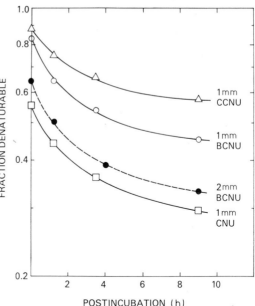

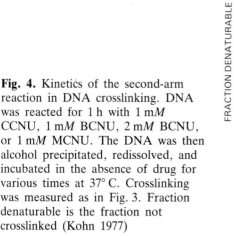

Fig. 4. Kinetics of the second-arm reaction in DNA crosslinking. DNA was reacted for 1 h with 1 m*M* CCNU, 1 m*M* BCNU, 2 m*M* BCNU, or 1 m*M* MCNU. The DNA was then alcohol precipitated, redissolved, and incubated in the absence of drug for various times at 37° C. Crosslinking was measured as in Fig. 3. Fraction denaturable is the fraction not crosslinked (Kohn 1977)

(lower two curves in Fig. 4). This is as expected since the second step should be identical for all chloroethylnitrosoureas.

Fluoroethyl groups, as already mentioned, should react much more slowly than chloroethyl in the crosslinking step in which the halogen is displaced. Perhaps surprisingly, the fluoroethylnitrosoureas are as active as chloroethylnitrosoureas against experimental tumors in mice. Perhaps this is because crosslinks formed many hours after the initial fluoroethylation reaction are still effective in killing cells. This presumes that the haloethyl adducts are not removed during this time. This is a reasonable possibility for rodent cells that do not have active excision repair, but it is less likely for human cells.

The two-step kinetics of interstrand crosslink formation in purified DNA by chloroethylnitrosoureas has been confirmed using a fluorometric technique, and the comparative effects of several derivatives have been studied [32].

DNA Lesions in Cells

Studies of the effects of DNA damaging agents in mammalian cells have been facilitated by the use of the alkaline elution technique [15, 26−29]. Variations of this technique can be used to measure interstrand crosslinks, DNA-protein crosslinks, single-strand breaks, and alkali-labile sites.

The effects of BCNU on the DNA of L1210 cells are illustrated in Fig. 5 [14]. Log-phase cells, previously labeled with ^{14}C-thymidine for 20 h, were exposed to 50 μM BCNU for 1 h. This treatment yielded 0.1% survival of colony-forming ability. After washing to remove drug, the cells were postincubated for various times in fresh medium. The cells were then chilled and deposited on filters (2 μM pore size polyvinylchloride membranes) and washed with cold phosphate-buffered saline. The

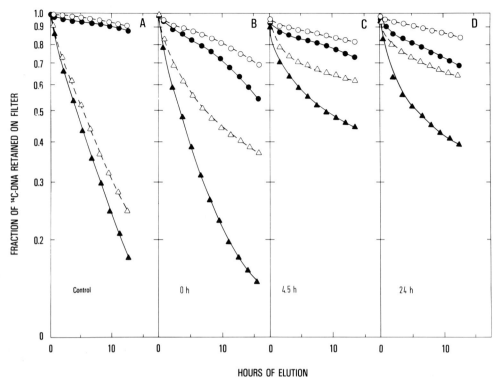

HOURS OF ELUTION

Fig. 5A−D. Effects of BCNU on DNA in L1210 cells measured by alkaline elution. L1210 cells were labeled with (^{14}C) thymidine for 20 h and then treated with 50 μM BCNU for 1 h. Cells were analyzed 0 h (**B**), 4.5 h (**C**), or 24 h (**D**) after removal of drug; (**A**), results with untreated cells. Assays: 0, no X ray, no proteinase; △, 300 R, no proteinase; ●, no X ray, with proteinase; ▲, 300 R, with proteinase (Ewig and Kohn 1977)

cells were then lysed with 0.2% sodium lauroyl sarkosinate, 2 M NaCl, 0.02 M EDTA, pH 10. The lysis solution was removed by rinsing with 0.02 M EDTA, pH 10, after which alkaline elution was carried out by pumping a solution of 0.02 M tetrapropylammonium hydroxide-EDTA, pH 12.1, through the filter at a rate of 2 ml/h. Fractions were collected at 1.5 h intervals and assayed for radioactivity.

The DNA of untreated cells was retained to the extent of 90% after 15 h of elution (Fig. 5A, *open circles*). Immediately after treatment with BCNU, there is a significant increase in elution rate (Fig. 5B, *open circles*), indicating the presence of single-strand breaks. For measurement of crosslinks, the assay procedure included an exposure of the cells to 300 R of X ray, delivered to the chilled cells prior to the alkaline elution procedure. The X ray produces single-strand breakage that increased the elution rate to that shown in Fig. 5A (*open triangles*). The drug-treated cells, however, showed slower elution than this control (Fig. 5B, *open triangles*), a result that is attributable to interstrand crosslinks and/or DNA-protein crosslinks. Interstrand crosslinks reduce elution by increasing the effective strand lengths [26, 29]. DNA-protein crosslinks reduce elution due to the adsorption of proteins to the filters under alkaline conditions [28]. The effect of DNA-protein crosslinks can largely be reversed by including an incubation with proteinase-K during the lysis step [15]. The proteinase treatment has little effect on the DNA elution of control cells in either of the assays, with or without X ray (Fig. 5A, *closed circles* and *closed triangles*, respectively). After BCNU treatment, however, both assays are markedly affected by proteinase (Fig. 5B, *closed circles* and *closed triangles*). The crosslinking effect in cells immediately following the BCNU treatment is seen to be totally reversed by proteinase, meaning that only crosslinks of the DNA-protein type are detected at this time. The proteinase method also gives a better measure of strand breaks (Fig. 5B, *solid circles*), since the effect of the breaks may be partially obscured by the filter retention of protein-linked DNA strands.

After postincubation (Fig. 5C and D), the extent of crosslinking increases and the effect becomes partially resistant to proteinase, indicating the appearance of interstrand crosslinks. The delayed formation of interstrand crosslinks agrees with the findings with purified DNA, and was also observed in L1210 cells with CCNU and chlorozotocin [15]. The crosslinks in mouse L1210 cells decreased only to a small extent in a 24-h period allowed for repair. Chinese hamster V-79 cells, however, may be more capable of removing crosslinks [12].

Thus a full description of three categories of DNA lesions measurable by alkaline elution − single-strand breaks, interstrand crosslinks, and DNA-protein crosslinks − requires four types of assays: with and without X ray, and with and without proteinase. A fourth category of lesions − alkalilabile sites − is in principle distinguishable by determining the effect of elution pH [29]. Alkali-labile sites, produced for example by methylnitrosourea, also produce a characteristic convex shape to the elution curves, as if breaks were accumulating during the alkaline assay [14]. The chloroethylnitro-soureas may produce strand breaks and alkali-labile lesions in addition to crosslinks [10].

Relations Between DNA Lesions and Cell Killing

Having determined some categories of DNA lesions produced by nitrosoureas, the next problem is to relate DNA lesions with cell lethality. This more difficult problem will require comparative studies of many different cell types. The variables that must be considered include cell type, lesion type, drug identity, drug dose, and time after treatment. Clearly, a great deal of work will be needed to determine the relationships between lesions and lethality under different circumstances. Initial results however have been promising, and some of these will be summarized.

One set of studies compared human colon tumor lines of different sensitivities to MeCCNU. The tumors were grown as xenografts in immunodeficient nude mice [42], and related cell lines were grown in culture [13]; in both systems, the tumor or cell line designated "BE" was more sensitive than line "HT" (Figs 6 and 7). The production of DNA crosslinks by 1-(2-chloroethyl)-1-nitroso-3-(trans-4-methylcyclohexyl) urea (MeCCNU) was determined at various times after a single injection of the drug in mice bearing the two tumor types implanted, one on each side, in the flank (Fig. 8). In the analogous experiment in cell culture, the two cell types were exposed to MeCCNU for 1 h (Fig. 9). Both in vivo and in vitro, the sensitive BE tumor exhibited more DNA crosslinking at various times following MeCCNU than did the resistant HT tumor. In the in vivo experiments, the difference between the cell types was already evident during the first few hours following treatment, and the difference persisted at least 19 h. In the cell culture experiments, however, the initial formation of crosslinks was

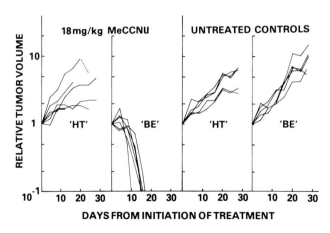

Fig. 6. Effect of MeCCNU on human colon tumor xenografts in nude mice. Mice carried colon tumor lines BE and HT on opposite flanks and were treated with a single IP dose of 18 mg MeCCNU/kg (Thomas et al. 1978)

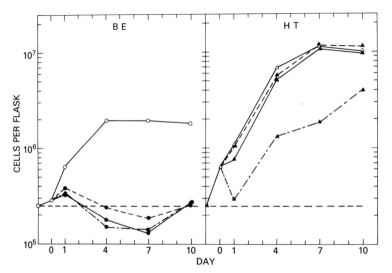

Fig. 7. Effect of MeCCNU on cell cultures of human colon tumor lines BE and HT. Cells were treated with 50, 100, or 200 μM MeCCNU for 1 h on day 0 (solid symbols). Open symbols, untreated controls (Erickson et al. 1978)

comparable in the two cell types; the resistant HT cells then proceeded to remove the crosslinks while the sensitive BE cells did not (Fig. 9). It may be that the HT cells are better able to repair crosslinks or to remove monoadducts before they go on to form crosslinks. Only the total crosslink assay was used in these experiments, the role of interstrand and DNA-protein crosslinks remains to be determined.

Another study compared a normal with a transformed line of human embryo cells [9]. The normal cell strain (IMR-90) was uniformly less sensitive to several nitrosoureas than the transformed line (VA-13), whether assayed by rate of increase in cell number or by colony-forming ability. The magnitude of the difference between these cell types was greater for CNU and CHLZ than for BCNU and CCNU (Fig. 10). Alkaline elution measurements of total crosslinking (i.e., without the use of proteinase) disclosed only small differences. There was thus no great difference between these cell

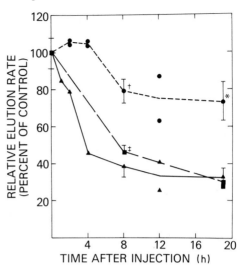

Fig. 8. DNA crosslinking in human colon tumor xenografts as a function of time after an intraperitoneal injection of 18 mg MeCCNU/kg. Total crosslinking was measured by alkaline elution using 300 R without proteinase (Fig. 5.). Relative elution rate is inversely related to crosslinking. Tumor lines: ▲ BE (sensitive); ● HT (resistant); ■ CA (intermediate responsiveness) (Thomas et al. 1978)

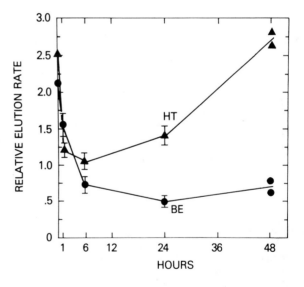

Fig. 9. DNA crosslinking in human colon tumor cell culture lines BE and HT treated with 100 μM MeCCNU for 1 h. Total crosslinking was measured by alkaline elution using 300 R without proteinase (Fig. 5). Relative elution rate is inversely related to crosslinking (Erickson et al. 1978)

types in the combined measure of interstrand and DNA-protein crosslinking. Using the proteinase method, however, a marked difference emerged. The crosslinking effect in the IMR-90 cells was completely reversible by proteinase: interstrand crosslinking was undetectable in these cells. The VA-13 line, on the other hand, exhibited substantial interstrand crosslinking (Fig. 11). The difference in sensitivity of the cells is not due to a difference in drug uptake or to differences in general reactivity with intracellular targets because there was no great difference in DNA-protein crosslinking. Possible explanations for the sensitivity difference are that IMR-90 cells remove chloroethyl DNA adducts so rapidly that interstrand crosslinks are not formed, or that the crosslinks are removed so quickly that they never become evident. Another difference between the two cell types that might reflect a difference in DNA repair is in the appearance of single-strand breaks following nitrosourea treatment [10].

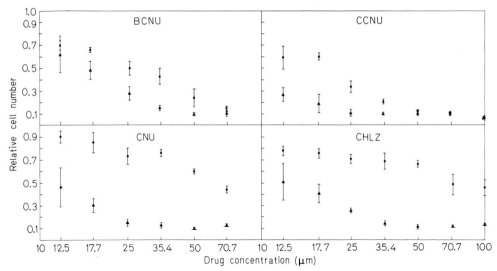

Fig. 10. Effects of chloroethylnitrosoureas on proliferation of normal and transformed human embryo cells. Normal cells (IMR-90, ●) or transformed cells (VA-13, ▲) were exposed to various concentrations of drug for 2 h. Cell number relative to control was determined after 3 days (Data of Erickson LC, Ducore J, and Kohn KW)

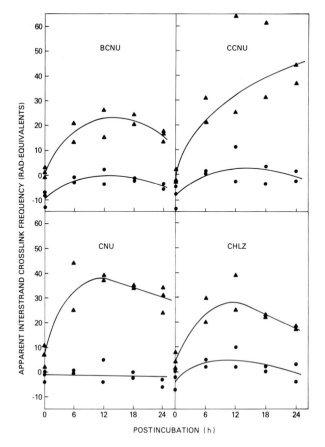

Fig. 11. DNA interstrand crosslinking as a function of time after treatment of IMR-90 (●) or VA-13 (▲) cells with 50 μM of various chloroethylnitrosoureas for 2 h. Assays were by alkaline elution using 300 R of X ray and proteinase (Data of Erickson LC, Ducore J, and Kohn KW)

Summary

Because of their broad range of effectiveness against experimental tumors in rodents, nitrosoureas could have a greater potential against human cancer than has so far been achieved with these agents. Greater effectiveness against human cancer might be attained from an understanding of the mechanisms by which these drugs kill cells. Some clues to possible mechanisms have been obtained and can be pursued using existing experimental techniques. The most promising leads center on the chemical effects of nitrosoureas on DNA. Several types of nitrosourea-induced DNA damage have been identified, including interstrand crosslinks, DNA-protein crosslinks and single-strand breaks. These DNA lesions can be sensitively measured in mammalian cells by the alkaline elution technique. The experimental results so far support the idea that cell killing is related to the formation and repair of DNA lesions. Antitumor activity would then depend on differences in sensitivity of neoplastic versus normal cells in regard to certain types of DNA damage and/or differences in the ability to repair this damage.

References

1. Abelson HT, Karlan D, Penman S (1974) Biochim Biophys Acta 349: 389−401
2. Baril BB, Baril EF, Laszlo J, Wheeler GP (1975) Cancer Res 35: 1−5
3. Brundrett RB, Cowens JW, Colvin M (1976) J Med Chem 19: 958−961
4. Carter SK (ed) (1976) Proceedings of the 7th New Drug Seminar: Nitrosoureas. Cancer Treat Rep 60: 645−811
5. Cheng CJ, Fujimura S, Grunberger D, Weinstein IB (1972) Cancer Res 32: 22−27
6. Chuang RY, Laszlo J, Keller P (1976) Biochim Biophys Acta 425: 463−468
7. Colvin M, Brundrett RB, Cowens W, Jardine I, Ludlum DB (1976) Biochem Pharmacol 25: 695−699
8. Colvin M, Cowens JW, Brundrett RB, Kramer BS, Ludlum DB (1974) Biochem Biophys Res Commun 60: 515−520
9. Erickson LC, Bradley MO, Ducore J, Kohn KW (1980) Proc Natl Acad Sci USA 70: 467−471
10. Erickson LC, Bradley MO, Kohn KW (1977) Cancer Res 37: 3744−3750
11. Erickson LC, Bradley MO, Kohn KW (1978) Cancer Res 38: 672−677
12. Erickson LC, Bradley MO, Kohn KW (1978) Cancer Res 38: 3379−3384
13. Erickson LC, Osieka R, Kohn KW (1978) Cancer Res 38: 802−808
14. Ewig RAG, Kohn KW (1977) Cancer Res 37: 2114−2122
15. Ewig RAG, Kohn KW (1978) Cancer Res 38: 3197−3203
16. Fornace AJ Jr, Kohn KW, Kann HE jr (1978) Cancer Res 38: 1064−1069
17. Fox PA, Panasci LC, Schein PS (1977) Cancer Res 37: 783−787
18. Heal JM, Fox PA, Doukas D, Schein PS (1978) Cancer Res 38: 1070−1074
19. Heal JM, Fox PA, Schein PS (to be published) Cancer Res
20. Inaba M, Sakurai Y (1977) Gann 68: 15−19
21. Kann HE jr (1978) Cancer Res 38: 2363−2366
22. Kann HE jr, Kohn KW, Lyles JM (1974) Cancer Res 34: 398−402
23. Kann HE jr, Kohn KW, Widerlite L, Gullion D (1974) Cancer Res 34: 1982−1988
24. Kohn KW (1976) Fed Proc 35: 1708
25. Kohn KW (1977) Cancer Res 37: 1450−1454
26. Kohn KW (1979) In: DeVita VT jr, Busch H (eds) Methods in cancer research, vol XVI. Academic Press, New York pp 291−345
27. Kohn KW, Erickson LC, Ewig RAG, Friedman CA (1976) Biochemistry 15: 4629−4637

28. Kohn KW, Ewig RAG (1979) Biochim Biophys Acta 562:32−40
29. Kohn KW, Ewig RAG, Erickson LC, Zwelling LA (1980) In: Friedberg E, Hanawalt P (eds) DNA repair: A laboratory of manual of research procedures. Dekker, New York
30. Kohn KW, Spears CL, Doty P (1966) J Mol Biol 19:266−288
31. Kramer BS, Fenselau CC, Ludlum DB (1974) Biochem Biophys Res Commun 56:783−788
32. Lown JW, McLaughlin LW, Chang Y-M (1978) Bioorg Chem 7:97−100
33. Ludlum DB (1975) In: Sartorelli AC, Johns DG (eds) Handbook of experimental pharmacology, vol 38, part 2. Springer, Berlin Heidelberg New York, pp 6−17
34. Ludlum DB, Kramer BS, Wang J, Fenselau CC (1975) Biochemistry 14:5480
35. Montgomery JA (1976) Cancer Treat Rep 60:651−664
36. Panasci L, Fox PA, Schein PS (1977) Cancer Res 37:3321−3328
37. Panasci L, Green DC, Nagourney R, Fox P, Schein PS (1977) Cancer Res 37:2615−2618
38. Reed DJ, May HE, Boose RB, Gregory KM, Beilstein MA (1975) Cancer Res 35:568−576
39. Schabel FM jr (1976) Cancer Treat Rep 60:665−698
40. Schmall B, Cheng CJ, Fujimura S, Gersten N, Grunberger D (1973) Cancer Res 33:1921−1924
41. Singer B (1975) Prog Nucleic Acid Res Mol Biol 15:219−284
42. Thomas CB, Osieka R, Kohn KW (1978) Cancer Res 38:2448−2454
43. Wheeler GP (1975) In: Sartorelli AC, Johns DG (eds) Handbook of experimental pharmacology, vol 38, part 2. Springer Berlin Heidelberg New York, pp 65−79
44. Wheeler GP (1975) In: Sartorelli AC (ed) Cancer chemotherapy. ACS Symposium 30. American Chemical Society, Washington D.C, pp 87−119
45. Wheeler GP, Bowdon BJ, Struck RF (1975) Cancer Res 35:2974−2984
46. Wheeler GP, Johnston TP, Bowdon BJ, McCaleb GS, Hill DL, Montgomery JA (1977) Biochem Pharmacol 26:2331−2336
47. Wheeler KT, Deen DF, Wilson CB, Williams ME, Sheppard S (1977) Int J Radiat Oncol Biol Phys 2:79−88

New Natural Products Under Development at the National Cancer Institute

J. Douros and M. Suffness

Natural Products Branch, Developmental Therapeutics Program, Division of Cancer Treatment, National Cancer Institute, USA — Bethesda, MD

Summary

Twenty-six new agents of natural products origin which are under preclinical development as potential antitumor agents at the National Cancer Institute are discussed with reference to their sources, structures, antitumor activity, current status, and future potential as clinically effective drugs.

Introduction

Since 1956 the Cancer Chemotherapy National Service Center, now incorporated into the Developmental Therapeutics Program (DTP), Division of Cancer Treatment, has had a comprehensive drug development program that includes the screening of compounds obtained from natural products [7]. Since the inception of the program, approximately 178,802 microbial cultures have been isolated and fermented and 103,272 plants extracted. The fermentation broths and plant extracts have been tested for their cell cytotoxicity and in vivo activity against various animal tumors using standard protocols [10]. During the last 3 years the fermentation broths in many cases have first been tested in various in vitro prescreens (e.g., enzyme inhibition, tubulin binding, phage induction, antimicrobial and antiyeast screens) [6]. Approximately 7 years ago a concentrated effort to evaluate animal products (primarily marine) was initiated and to date 13,751 extracts have been screened and 0.7% showed confirmed in vivo activity.

Many compounds have been isolated from the above-mentioned programs and in addition many natural products are obtained from the NCI worldwide surveillance program which includes agreements with industrial companies, research institutes, universities, and scientists. Some of the more interesting compounds in preclinical drug development that will be discussed are listed in Table 1. Many of the compounds discussed are analogs of earlier compounds which have been prepared in an effort to discover second generation drugs which retain the activity of the parent molecule and have less toxicity.

Table 1. Natural products undergoing preclinical drug development at NCI

Compound	NCI No.
Actinomycin pip 1β	107660
Azetomycin 1	244392
Actinomycin S_3	296940
Pepleomycin	276382
Bleomycin BAPP	294979
Tallysomycin A	279496
Aclacinomycin A	208734
7-0-methyl nogarol	269148
Nogamycin	265450
Echinomycin	526417
Valinomycin	122023
Largomycin	237020
Aphidicolin	234714
Neothramycin	285223
Rapamycin	226080
CC-1065	298223
Borrelidin	216128
Eriofertopin	283439
Homoharringtonine	141633
Tripdiolide	163063
Taxol	125973
Baccharin	269757
Isobaccharin	269760
Phyllanthoside	266492
Fagaronine	157995
Psorospermin	266491

Methodology

Natural products, when purified (> 90%), are assigned NSC numbers which are identification codes used by NCI for all compounds studied. NCI prefers materials to be at least 98% pure before assigning NCS numbers; however, because proteins, peptides, polysaccharides, and some other antibiotics do not lend themselves to easy purification or are extremely costly to purify to a state of > 90% purity, they are assigned NSC numbers also. The various protocols for screening these drugs have been established by the Drug Evaluation Branch, NCI [10]. Normally the P388 leukemia assay in mice is the first in vivo test in which a natural product compound is evaluated. However, rational selection can result in using another in vivo tumor as the first screen if there is information on organ distribution, lipophilicity, selective tissue effects, or other antitumor data that indicate that other testing is preferable.

In most cases a material is tested initially against the P388 leukemia (PS) to determine toxicity data even though this may not be the test tumor of greatest interest. If reproducible activity is demonstrated in PS as evidenced by an increase in life span (ILS) of 20% or greater and if the compound has a novel structure, it is tested against a panel of tumors (Table 2). Close analogs of known compounds are tested under special

Table 2. Division of Cancer Treatment (DCT) panel of antiserum screens

Tumor	Parameter	Activity criteria	Route inoculation	Tissue and level of inoculation	
Mouse colon 38 (C8)	Tumor inhibition	T/C ≤ 42%	IP	Brei	1 : 100
Mouse Breast (CD)	Tumor inhibition	T/C ≤ 42%	SC	Brei	5×10^6
Human colon xenograft	Tumor inhibition	T/C ≤ 42%	SC	Fragment	14 mg
Mouse breast xenograft	Tumor inhibition	T/C ≤ 42%	SC	Fragment	14 mg
Mouse lung xenograft	Tumor inhibition	T/C ≤ 42%	SC	Fragment	14 mg
Mouse B16 melanosarcoma (B 16)	Survival	T/C ≥ 125%	IP	Brei	1 : 10
Mouse Lewis lung carcinoma (LL)	Survival	T/C ≥ 140%	IP	Cells	10^5
Mouse L1210 leukemia (LE)	Survival	T/C ≥ 125%	IP	Cells	10^5

protocols in comparison with the parent compound. Rational bypass can be used to expedite testing in tumor panel systems or to screen against tumors that are not part of the tumor panel, including, for example, brain tumors for compounds that are known to cross the blood brain barrier or hormone dependent tumors for compounds with endocrine activity.

If the compound has sufficient activity and is a novel structure or an analog deemed of interest to NCI, it will now be reviewed by the Decision Network (DN) Committee and, if approved, is scheduled for formulation studies. When a clinical formulation is obtained, the agent is tested for schedule dependency and oral route activity. The DN group then determines if the compound should progress into toxicology studies. While toxicology studies are being done, the pharmacology group determines pharmacokinetics and tissue distribution of this drug. The DN Committee reviews the toxicology results and determines if the drug is suitable for Phase I clinical trials. After Phase I trials are completed, the DN group again reviews the results and determines if the drug should be a candidate for Phase II clinical trials against the panel of human tumors selected by NCI:

1. Breast
2. Colon
3. Lung
4. Melanoma
5. Acute leukemia
6. Lymphoma, Hodgkin's disease

Natural products, whether derived from microbes, plants, or animals, are all evaluated in the same way. Thorough discussions of the methodologies used in development of fermentation-derived compounds and plant-derived compounds are found in the paper by Douros [6] and Suffness and Douros [26].

Results

The following drugs derived from natural sources are now in some phase of preclinical drug development at NCI:

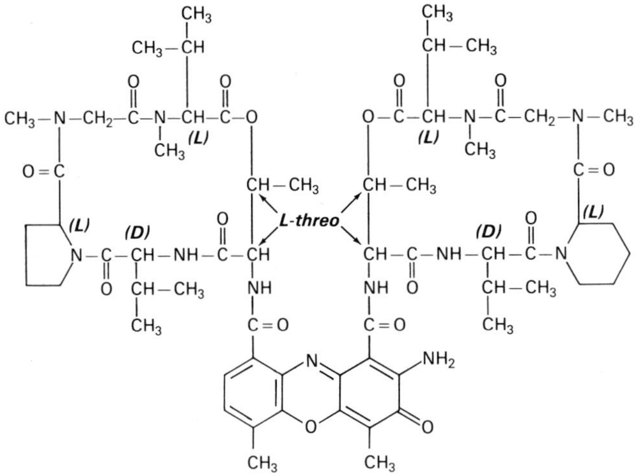

Fig. 1. Structure of actinomycin pip 1β (NSC 107660)

Actinomycin pip 1β (NSC-107660) (Fig. 1) is a peptide antibiotic with a phenoxazine chromophore that is produced by *Streptomyces parvulus*. This antibiotic differs from actinomycin D in that the proline residue in the *beta* peptide chain is replaced with pipecolic acid. The production of actinomycin pip 1β and actinomycins in general by precursor feeding has been extensively studied by Katz and co-workers [8, 12]. There is interest in evaluation of a new actinomycin in clinical trial if the compound gives indication of a broader or different spectrum of activity, less toxicity, or a better chemotherapeutic index than actinomycin D. More than 100 actinomycins have been evaluated in NCI's program and three seem to have activities of interest. Actinomycin pip 1β is being compared with actinomycin D in gastrointestinal toxicity tests and in the NCI tumor panel. Actinomycin pip 1β has shown good activity in murine tumors against colon 38 (C8) giving 91% inhibition, mammary carcinoma (CD) 99% inhibition, colon 26 (C6) 84% increased life span (ILS), B16 melanoma 66% ILS, L1210 leukemia (LE) 59% ILS, P388 leukemia (PS) 105% ILS. These activities are quite similar to those of actinomycin D. The critical data will be whether gastrointestinal toxicity is considerably less than that of actinomycin D and whether some xenograft activity is found with this analog. If actinomycin pip 1β is superior to actinomycin D in these tests it will be presented to DN. A comparison of the various actinomycin activities can be found in Table 3.

Azetomycin I (NSC-244392) (Fig. 2) is an analog of actinomycin D and is also obtained by precursor fermentation [8]. This antibiotic differs from actinomycin D in that one of the prolines is replaced with azetidine. This compound has shown good activity against P388 giving 166% ILS, 51% ILS against LE, 52% against B16, 100% inhibition of CD, 57% ILS against C6 (Table 3). This drug has also shown activity against an actinomycin D-resistant leukemia. One additional actinomycin is being tested, actinomycin S₃ (NSC-296940) [9]. The spectrum of antitumor activity in the few tests evaluated is inferior to that of actinomycin D (Table 3). The comparison of actinomycin D, azetomycin I, and actinomycin pip 1β antitumor data shows that thus far none has an advantage over the other and thus the comparative toxicity data becomes the crucial factor on whether one of the analogs is developed towards clinical trials.

Table 3. Typical activities of actinomycin derivatives in murine tumor systems[a]

Tumor	Actinomycin D NSC-3053		Actinomycin pip 1β NSC-107660		Azetomycin I NSC-244392		Actinomysin S₃ NSC-296940	
	% T/C	O.D.[b]	% T/C	O.D.[b]	% T/C	O.D.[b]	% T/C	O.D.[b]
PS31 P388 lymphocytic leukemia	279	100	205	400	266	50	72	10
LE21 L1210 lymphoid leukemia	158	60	159	750	151	300	[115][c]	20
B132 B16 melanocarcinoma	200	25	166	1100	152	75	186	10
C631 Colon 26	153	500	184	2880	157	750	–[d]	–[d]
C872 Colon 38	22	300	9	4500	27	1200	[110][c]	20
CD72 CD8F₁ mammary tumor	0	300	1	3000	0	600	36	5

[a] Data are typical for each system and testing is not in direct comparison
[b] O.D., optimal dose in micrograms/kg/inj
[c] [ ], activity criteria not met in this system
[d] –, not tested

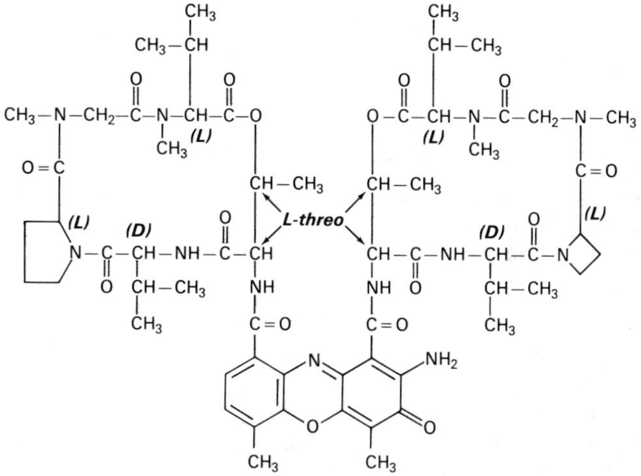

Fig. 2. Structure of azetomycin 1 (NSC 244392)

Pepleomycin (NSC-276382). Many bleomycins have been tested by NCI and in Japan. In the last 18 months the Japanese have renewed NCI's interest in the bleomycins by presenting to NCI their data on several bleomycin analogs including pepleomycin and bleomycin BAPP (Figs. 3 and 4). Pepleomycin (Fig. 3), developed in Japan, differs from bleomycin in the terminal amine group. According to the Japanese data this drug shows less pulmonary toxicity in human clinical trials than does bleomycin, which would make this a second generation drug (less toxicity but equal activity) [22]. This drug is awaiting completion of pulmonary toxicity tests and tumor panel evaluation at NCI in direct comparison with bleomycin, and if results are favorable will be presented to DN late in 1979. Table 4 shows the data obtained with the various bleomycins that are presently of interest to NCI.

Bleomycin BAPP (NSC-294979) (Fig. 4) is another fermentation-derived analog of bleomycin that shows less pulmonary toxicity than bleomycin in the mouse test [22].

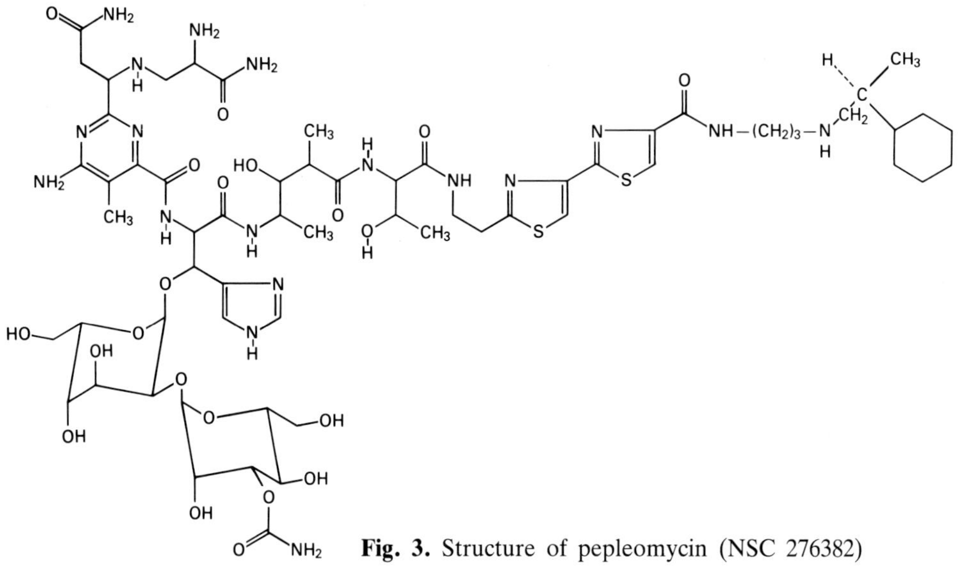

Fig. 3. Structure of pepleomycin (NSC 276382)

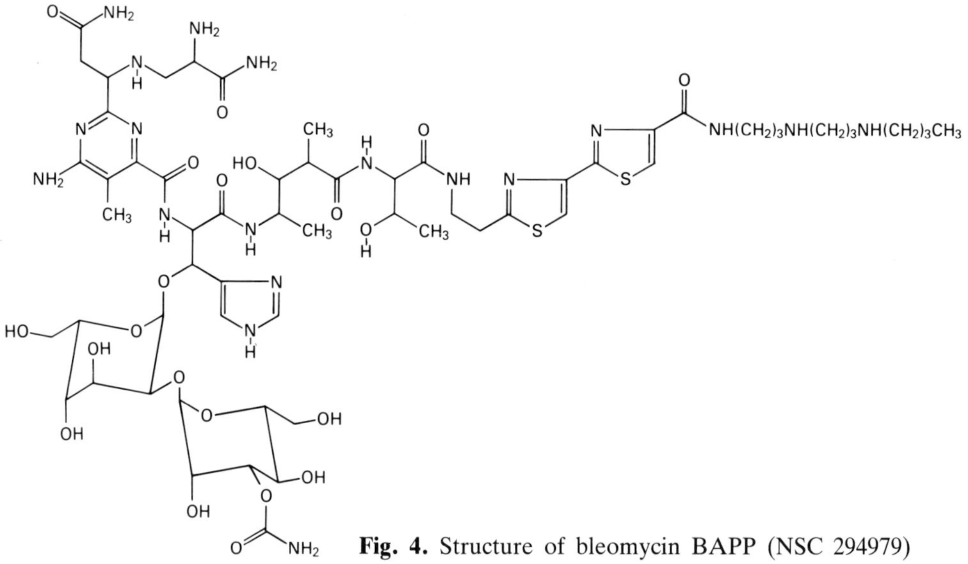

Fig. 4. Structure of bleomycin BAPP (NSC 294979)

BAPP is being tested in comparison with bleomycin in the entire tumor panel. The antitumor data for bleomycin BAPP is presented in Table 4.

Tallysomycin (NSC-279496) (Fig. 5) is a bleomycin analog similar to phleomycin that is being developed by Bristol Laboratories [13, 15]. The drug is being compared with bleomycin, bleomycin BAPP, and pepleomycin at NCI. The NCI Bleomycin Analog Committee will make recommendations to NCI scientists on the above analogs of bleomycin when testing is completed. Bristol Laboratories have several other derivatives of tallysomycin that are at present being evaluated against selected NCI murine tumor systems.

Table 4. Typical activities of bleomycin derivatives in murine tumor systems[a]

Tumor	Bleomycin NSC-125066		Pepleomycin NSC-276382		Bleomy-cin BAPP NSC-294979		Tallysomycin A NSC-279496	
	% T/C	O.D.[b]	% T/C	O.D.[b]	% T/C	O.D.[b]	% T/C	O.D.[b]
PS31 P388 lymphocytic leukemia	146	12	127	2	132	10	[119][c]	8
LE21 L1210 lymphoid leukemia	[119][c]	2.5	[123][c]	1	[114][c]	10	[104][c]	4
B132 B16 melanocarcinoma	185	8	184	1	158	5	—[d]	—[d]
C631 Colon 26	[119][c]	15	[121][c]	8	161	20	—[d]	—[d]
C872 Colon 38	11	64	29	32	[48][c]	30	12	32
CD72 CD8F$_1$ mammary tumor	9	32	16	16	16	64	10	32
LL39 Lewis lung carcinoma	159	32	[138][c]	8	—[d]	—[d]	—[d]	—[d]

[a] Data is typical for each system and testing is not in direct comparison
[b] Optimal dose in mg/kg/inj
[c] [ ], activity criteria not met in this system
[d] —, not tested

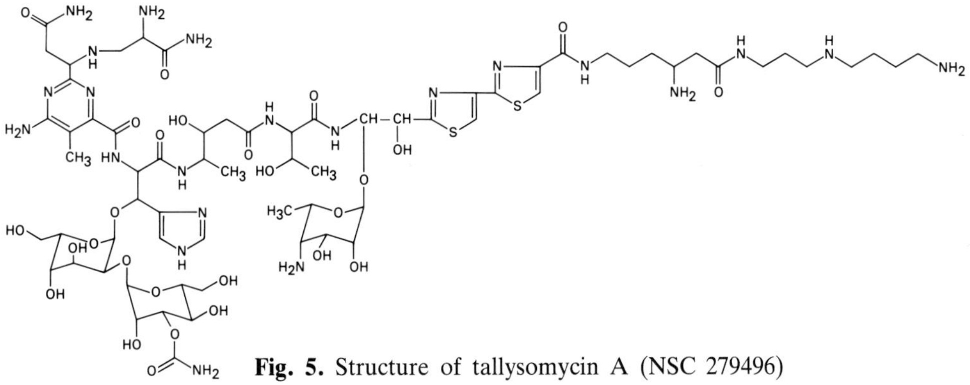

Fig. 5. Structure of tallysomycin A (NSC 279496)

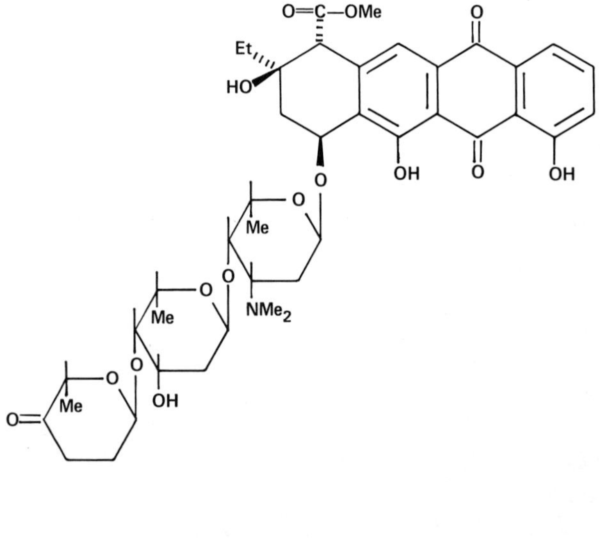

Fig. 6. Structure of aclacinomycin A (NSC 208734)

Table 5. Antitumor activity of aclacinomycin A NSC-208734

Tumor systems		Activities	
		% T/C[a]	Opt. dose mg/kg/inj.
PS	P388 lymphocytic leukemia	236	8
LE	L1210 lymphoid leukemia	141	25
B16	B16 melanocarcinoma	148	3
C6	Colon 26	(123)	12
C8	Colon 38	40	6
CD	CD8F$_1$ mammary	1	15
LL	Lewis lung carcinoma	(125)	3
PA	Adriamycin resistant PS	138	15
C2G5	CX-1 Colon renal capsule	9	1
C9G5	CX-5 Colon renal capsule	(76)	2
C9H2	CX-5 Colon xenograft	(49)	9.38
LKG5	LX-1 Lung renal capsule	42	2
LKH2	LX-1 Lung xenograft	(62)	9.38
MBG5	MX-1 Breast renal capsule	20	2
MBH2	MX-1 Breast xenograft	(53)	9.38

[a] T/C values in parentheses do not meet minimum criteria for activity

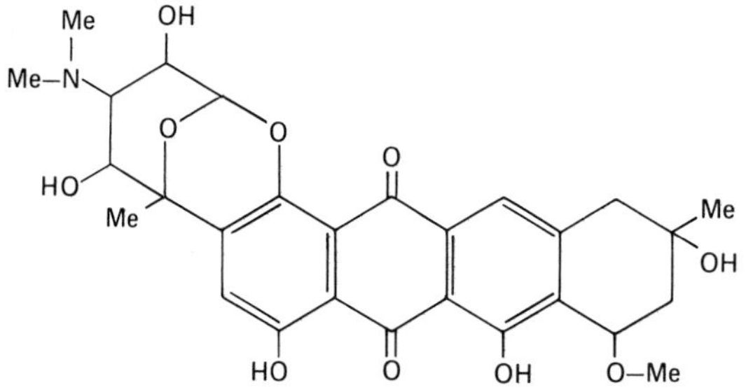

Fig. 7. Structure of 7-O-methylnogarol (7-Omen) (NSC 269148)

Table 6. Antitumor activity of 7-0-methylnogarol NSC-269148

Tumor systems		Activities	
		% T/C[a]	Opt. dose mg/kg/inj.
PS	P388 lymphocytic leukemia	240	12.5
LE	L1210 lymphoid leukemia	240	12.5
B16	B16 melanocarcinoma	209	12.5
C6	Colon 26	206	25
C8	Colon 38	21	25
CD	CD8F$_1$ mammary	1	25
LL	Lewis lung carcinoma	187	12.5
PA	Adriamycin resistant P388	(116)	30

[a] T/C values in parentheses do not meet activity criteria

Aclacinomycin A (NSC-208734) (Fig. 6) is a cinerubin-like anthracycline was isolated by Dr. Umezawa's research group at the Institute of Microbial Chemistry in Japan and has been developed by the Sanraku Ocean Company [23]. This compound is scheduled for clinical trials in the United States in 1979. The drug was chosen for clinical trials by NCI because it showed less alopecia and cardiotoxicity when evaluated in Phase I and Phase II clinical trials in Japan [25]. Phase III clinical studies in Japan have confirmed that this drug causes less cardiac toxicity than adriamycin and NCI's cardiac toxicity test in rabbits likewise indicated a lower cardiac toxicity. NCI feels that this is a second generation anthracycline that will provide clinical advantages over adriamycin due to less human cardiac toxicity and less alopecia. Aclacinomycin is highly active in NCI murine tumor tests (Table 5).

7-0-Methyl nogarol (NSC-269148) (Fig. 7) was obtained from the Upjohn microbial chemical biotransformation program [28]. This nogalomycin derivative showed broad activity against murine tumors (Table 6). Another nogalomycin analog from the Upjohn program is nogamycin (NSC-265450) (Fig. 8). This compound has shown superior activity to 7-0-methyl nogarol against B16 (Table 7).

Echinomycin (NSC-526417) (Fig. 9) *and valinomycin* (NSC-122023) (Fig. 10) are two cyclic peptides presently of interest to NCI [21]. Echinomycin showed very selective

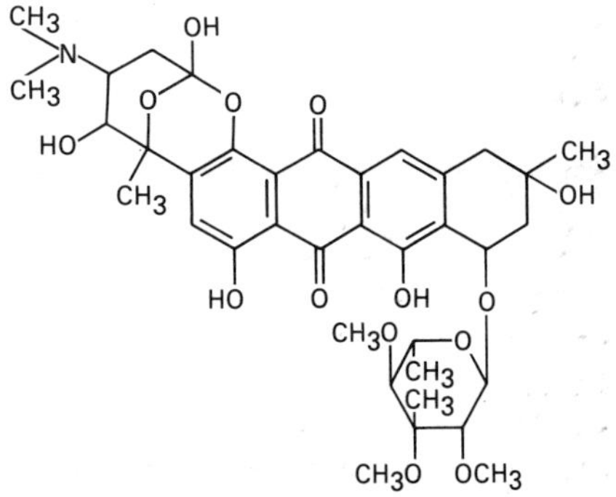

Fig. 8. Structure of nogamycin (Nogalomycin C) (NSC 265450)

Table 7. Antitumor activity of nogamycin (nogalomycin C) NSC-265450

Tumor systems		Activities	
		% T/C[a]	Opt. dose mg/kg/inj.
PS	P388 lymphocytic leukemia	193	5
LE	L1210 lymphoid leukemia	127	1.25
B16	B16 melanocarcinoma	357	5
C6	Colon 26	(102)	5
C8	Colon 38	(53)	0.62
CD	CD8F$_1$ mammary	(57)	10
LL	Lewis lung carcinoma	(119)	0.63
PA	Adriamycin resistant P388	120	10

[a] T/C values in parentheses do not meet activity criteria

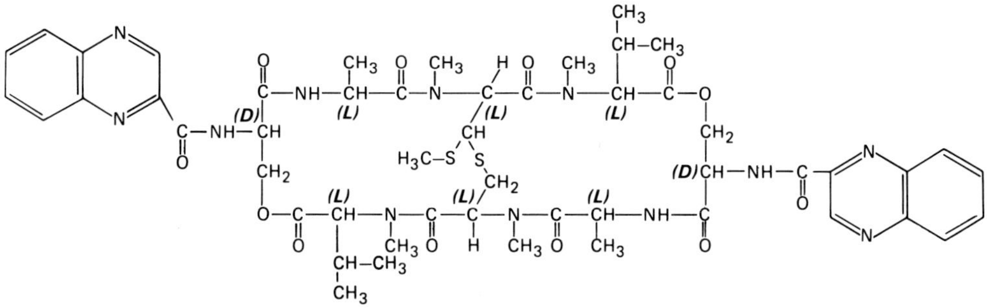

Fig. 9. Structure of echinomycin (NSC 526417)

Table 8. Antitumor activity of echinomycin (quinomycin A) NSC-526417

Tumor systems		Activities	
		% T/C[a]	Opt. dose mg/kg/inj.
PS	P388 lymphocytic leukemia	2050.06	
LE	L1210 lymphoid leukemia	126	0.03
B16	B16 melanocarcinoma	189	0.12
C6	Colon 26	(104)	0.06
C8	Colon 38	(123)	0.015
CD	CD8F$_1$ mammary	(67)	0.0075
LL	Lewis lung carcinoma	(111)	0.015
LKG5	Lung renal capsule	(52)	0.12
MBH2	Breast xenograft	(54)	0.03
C2G5	Colon renal capsule	21	0.24
C2H2	Colon xenograft	(78)	0.03
C9G5	CX-5 colon renal capsule	(55)	0.012
C9H2	CX-5 Colon xenograft	(56)	0.1
LKH2	LX-1 lung xenograft	(85)	0.1
MBG5	Breast renal capsule	(55)	0.24

[a] T/C values in parentheses do not meet activity criteria

activity, being highly active against B16 and P388 and showing activity against the colon renal capsule xenograft (Table 8). Valinomycin shows superior activity against the murine tumors to echinomycin. Murine antitumor data for valinomycin is presented in Table 9.

Largomycin (NSC-237020), a protein originally isolated in Japan [29, 30, 31], was obtained through the NCI literature surveillance program and is highly active against murine tumors (Table 10). Largomycin is one of the few natural products showing activity against the Lewis lung carcinoma. In addition, activity was observed against C6 and C8. Production methods for this drug are being developed at the Frederick Cancer Research Center (FCRC).

Aphidicolin (NSC-234714) (Fig. 11), which was obtained from Imperial Chemical Industries (ICI), passed DN2 because of its excellent C6 activity (ILS 129%) [2, 3, 5].

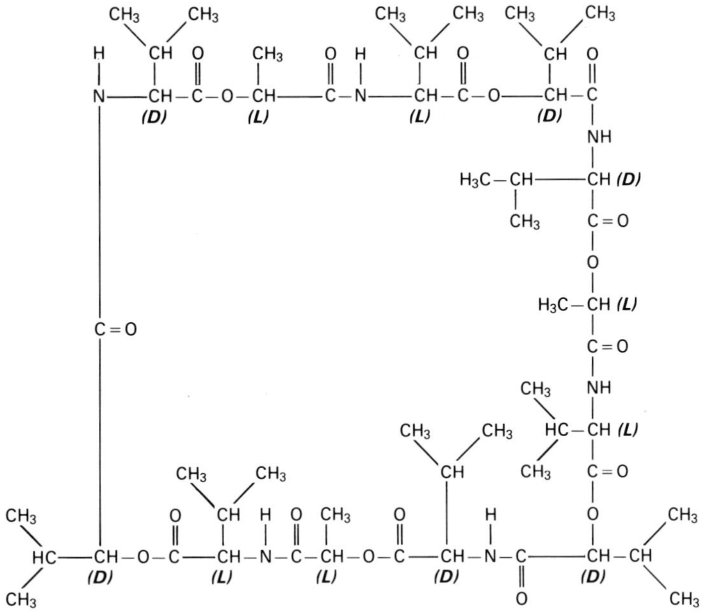

Fig. 10. Structure of valinomycin (NSC 122023)

Table 9. Antitumor activity of valinomycin NSC-122023

Tumor systems		Activities	
		% T/C[a]	Opt. dose mg/kg/inj.
PS	P388 lymphocytic leukemia	183	10
LE	L1210 lymphoid leukemia	131	5
B16	B16 melanocarcinoma	183	5
C6	Colon 26	200	3
C8	Colon 38	25	20
CD	CD8F$_1$ mammary	(49)	1
LL	Lewis lung carcinoma	145	6
C2G5	CX-1 colon renal capsule	(47)	40
C9H2	CX-5 colon xenograft	(64)	3
C9G5	CX-5 colon renal capsule	(54)	5
LKH2	LX-1 lung xenograft	(88)	12
LKG5	LX-1 lung renal capsule	(99)	5
MBH2	MX-1 breast xenograft	(97)	24
MBG5	MX-1 breast renal capsule	(52)	20

[a] T/C values in parentheses do not meet activity criteria

This diterpene has been superior to the seven analogs tested against C6 and is scheduled for formulation studies. Aphidicolin also showed activity against the lung renal capsule xenograft, B16, and P388 (Table 11). Aphidicolin was originally selected for screening because of its antiviral activity.

Table 10. Antitumor activity of largomycin NSC-237020

Tumor systems		Activities	
		% T/C[a]	Opt. dose mg/kg/inj.
PS	P388 lymphocytic leukemia	225	4.4
LE	L1210 lymphoid leukemia	(112)	1
B16	B16 melanocarcinoma	200	8
C6	Colon 26	184	4
C8	Colon 38	32	16
CD	CD8F$_1$ mammary	18	8
LL	Lewis lung carcinoma	151	2

[a] T/C values in parentheses do not meet activity criteria

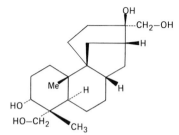

Fig. 11. Structure of aphidicolin (NSC 234714)

Table 11. Antitumor activity of aphidicolin NSC-234714

Tumor systems		Activities	
		% T/C[a]	Opt. dose mg/kg/inj.
PS	P388 lymphocytic leukemia	155	75
LE	L1210 lymphoid leukemia	(122)	100
B16	B16 melanocarcinoma	176	150
C6	Colon 26	229	200
C8	Colon 38	(65)	100
CD	CD8F$_1$ mammary	(44)	400
LL	Lewis lung carcinoma	(126)	100
MBH2	Breast xenograft	(83)	400
LKG5	Lung renal capsule	26	100
LKH2	LX-1 lung xenograft	(86)	200
C2G2	CX-1 colon renal capsule	(73)	50
C2H2	CX-1 colon xenograft	(95)	400
C9G5	CX-5 colon renal capsule	(45)	200
C9H2	CX-5 colon xenograft	(78)	200

[a] T/C values in parentheses do not meet activity criteria

Neothramycin (NSC-285223) (Fig. 12) is an anthramycin-like compound obtained from Japan. Our results are similar to those of the Meiji Seika Company and at the present time NCI is evaluating this compound against rat tumors. The Japanese indicated that neothramycin was superior to most drugs against rat tumors but that it is only marginally active against mouse tumors. This drug has shown minimal activity against P388 and L1210 leukemias in mice and has shown no activity in any other murine tumor systems (Table 12).

Rapamycin (NSC-226080) (Fig. 13) was obtained from Ayerst Laboratories where it was originally developed as an anti-*Candida* drug. This triene fermentation product has shown marked activity against ependymoblastoma, mammary, colon 38, and colon 26 tumors (Table 13). This drug is undergoing formulation studies and hopefully will be available for toxicologic evaluations in late 1979. It passed DN in April, 1979 and is

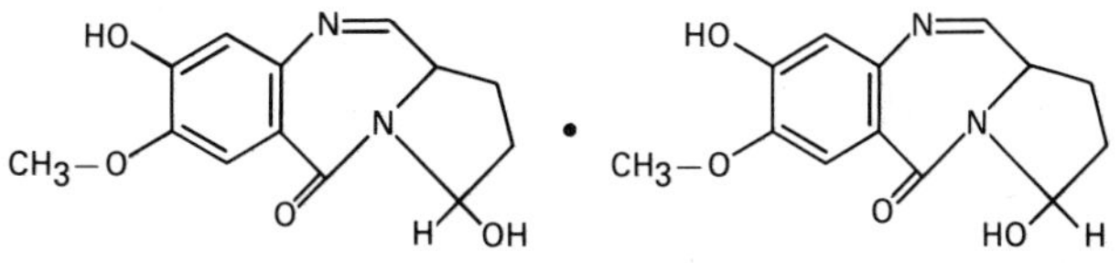

Fig. 12. Structure of neothramycin (NSC 285223)

Table 12. Antitumor activity of neothramycin NSC-285223

Tumor systems		Activities	
		% T/C[a]	Opt. dose mg/kg/inj.
PS	P388 lymphocytic leukemia	150	4
LE	L1210 lymphoid leukemia	126	4
B16	B16 melanocarcinoma	(119)	4
C6	Colon 26	(102)	0.6
C8	Colon 38	(62)	1.1
CD	CD8F$_1$ mammary	(79)	4
LL	Lewis lung carcinoma	(121)	1
EM	Ependymoblastoma	(95)	2

[a] T/C values in parentheses do not meet activity criteria

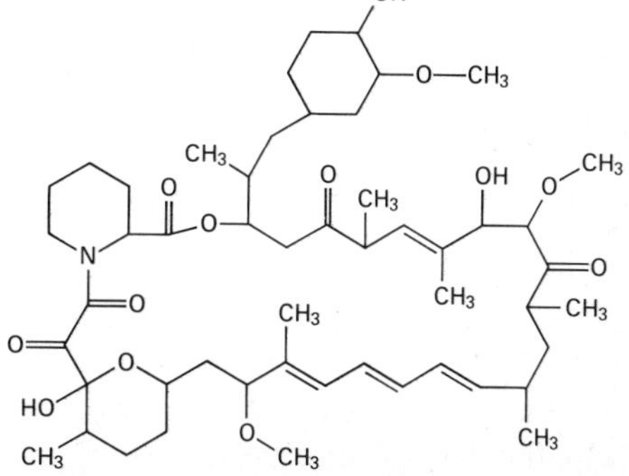

Fig. 13. Structure of rapamycin (NSC 226080)

Table 13. Antitumor activity of rapamycin NSC-226080

Tumor systems		Activities	
		% T/C[a]	Opt. dose mg/kg/inj.
PS	P388 lymphocytic leukemia	142	25
LE	L1210 lymphoid leukemia	(120)	400
B16	B16 melanocarcinoma	146	12.5
C6	Colon 26	159, 205	12.5, 6.25
C8	Colon 38	26, 19	25, 25
CD	CD8F$_1$ mammary	29, 4	12.5, 12.5
LL	Lewis lung carcinoma	(107)	400
EM	Ependymoblastoma	243, 211	200, 50

[a] T/C values in parentheses do not meet activity criteria

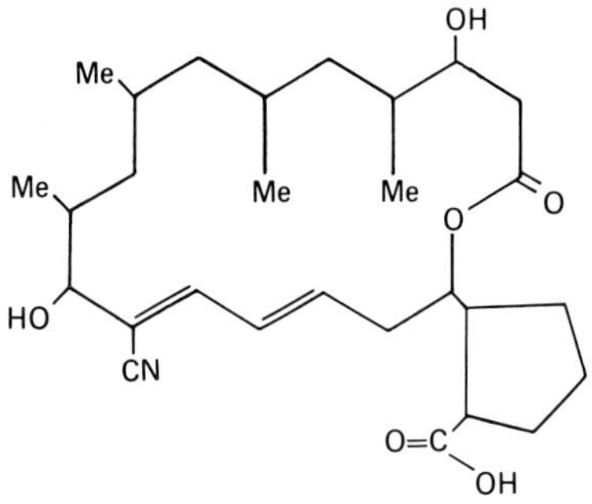

Fig. 14. Structure of borreledin (NSC 216128)

at present being tested in the entire tumor panel (Table 17). NCI is trying to obtain a clinical formulation for this highly insoluble material. The drug was identified as being of potential interest from our worldwide surveillance program.

Borrelidin (NSC-216128) (Fig. 14) was obtained from Bristol Laboratories fermentations [1, 14]. This compound has shown activity against Lewis lung, CD mammary, B16, and P388 (Table 14). At present this macrocylic lactone is being evaluated in the tumor panel.

CC-1065 (NSC-298223) is an Upjohn fermentation product which is undergoing structure elucidation studies [11]. Sufficient structural information has been obtained to insure that this is a novel antitumor agent. This highly toxic material is quite effective against murine tumors (Table 15). The drug has been found active against PS, LE, B16, C6, C8, and CD and minimally active against an adriamycin-resistant leukemia. It is currently being evaluated in NCI xenograft tumors.
The following drugs of preclinical interest are higher plant products:

Eriofertopin (NSC-283439) (Fig. 15), a sesquiterpene lactone, has been isolated from *Eriophyllum confertiflorum* which is found in California [18]. This compound has shown activity against both murine leukemias and B16 (Table 16). At present it is scheduled for tumor panel testing.

Table 14. Antitumor activity of borrelidin NSC-216128

Tumor systems		Activities	
		% T/C[a]	Opt. dose mg/kg/inj.
PS	P388 lymphocytic leukemia	169	0.5
LE	L1210 lymphoid leukemia	(109)	3
B16	B16 melanocarcinoma	159	1
C6	Colon 26	(111)	3
C8	Colon 38	(69)	2
CD	CD8F$_1$ mammary	14	16
LL	Lewis lung carcinoma	154	1.56

[a] T/C values in parentheses do not meet activity criteria

Table 15. Antitumor activity of CC-1065 (U-56314) NSC-298223

Tumor systems		Activities	
		% T/C[a]	Opt. dose mg/kg/inj.
PS	P388 lymphocytic leukemia	190	0.01
LE	L1210 lymphoid leukemia	148	0.3
B16	B16 melanocarcinoma	181	0.01
C6	Colon 26	150	0.05
C8	Colon 38	37	0.1
CD	CD8F$_1$ mammary	38	0.03
LL	Lewis lung carcinoma	(104)	0.04
PA	Adriamycin restistant P388	120	0.1

[a] T/C values in parentheses do not meet activity criteria

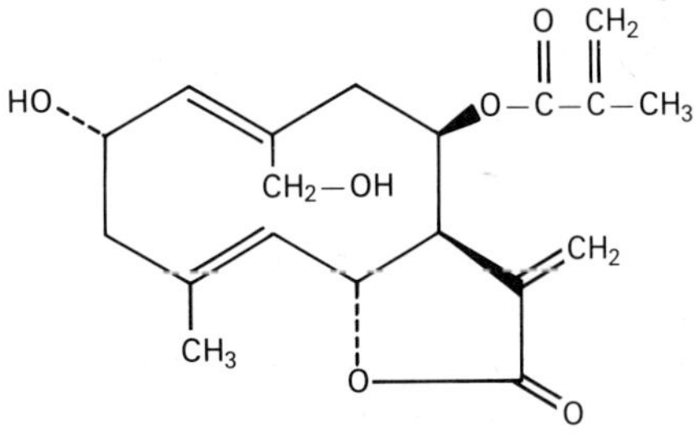

Fig. 15. Structure of eriofertopin (NSC 283439)

Homoharringtonine (NSC-141633) (Fig. 16) is a cephalotaxine ester isolated from *Cephalotaxus harringtonia* var. *drupacea* [24]. This evergreen is a native of the China mainland and procurement of this plant has been difficult. At present several grams of homoharringtonine have been obtained from the People's Republic of China. This compound shows good activity against murine leukemia and is highly active against C8 and CD tumors (Table 17). Some Lewis lung and colon capsule activity has been

Table 16 Anticancer activity of eriofertopin NSC-283439

Tumor systems		Activities	
		% T/C[a]	Opt. dose mg/kg/inj.
PS	P388 lymphocytic leukemia	167	20
LE	L1210 lymphoid leukemia	129	20
B16	B16 melanocarcinoma	126	20
C8	Colon 38	(105)	2.5

[a] T/C values in parentheses do not meet activity criteria

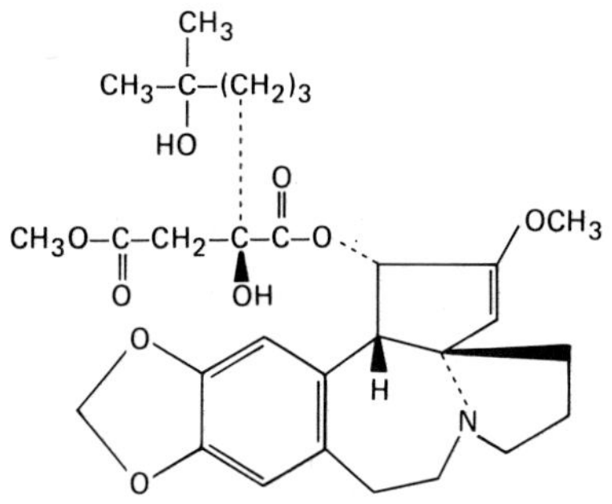

Fig. 16. Structure of homoharringtonine (NSC 141633)

Table 17. Antitumor activity of homoharringtonine NSC-141633

Tumor systems		Activities	
		% T/C[a]	Opt. dose mg/kg/inj.
PS	P388 lymphocytic leukemia	327	1
LE	L1210 lymphoid leukemia	150	2
B16	B16 melanocarcinoma	137	2
C6	Colon 26	(113)	1
C8	Colon 38	8	4
CD	CD8F$_1$ mammary	7	4
LL	Lewis lung carcinoma	142	0.5
EM	Ependymoblastoma	(103)	0.25
PA	Adriamycin resistant P388	(103)	1.2
PV	Vincristine resistant P388	(100)	0.72
16	Mammary adenocarcinoma C3H	185	1.9
CY	Colon 36	181	3
CZ	Colon 51	(106)	1.2
C2G5	CX-1 colon renal capsule	38	0.5
C9G5	CX-5 colon renal capsule	(44)	2
LKG5	LX-5 lung renal capsule	(74)	1
MB65	Mx-1 breast renal capsule	(103)	1

[a] T/C values in parentheses do not meet activity criteria

observed. The drug has been reported to be active against various leukemias in clinical trials conducted in China [4]. Formulation studies are now underway at NCI.

Tripdiolide (NSC-163063) (Fig. 17) is a diterpene triepoxide which was isolated from *Tripterygium wilfordii* in 1972 [16]. The selection of tripdiolide as a candidate for preclinical development was made on the basis of its activity in the L1210 leukemia system. Tripdiolide is also active against the B16 melanoma and the P388 leukemia (Table 18). A great deal of difficulty has been encountered in isolating large amounts of this material but at present 12 000 lb of plant have been obtained and are being extracted. Tumor panel testing must be completed and a clinical formulation obtained before this compound is ready to be presented for toxicology.

Taxol (NSC-125973) (Fig. 18) is a diterpene of the taxane type which is unusual in that it has large and complex ester groupings that have been shown to be related to its

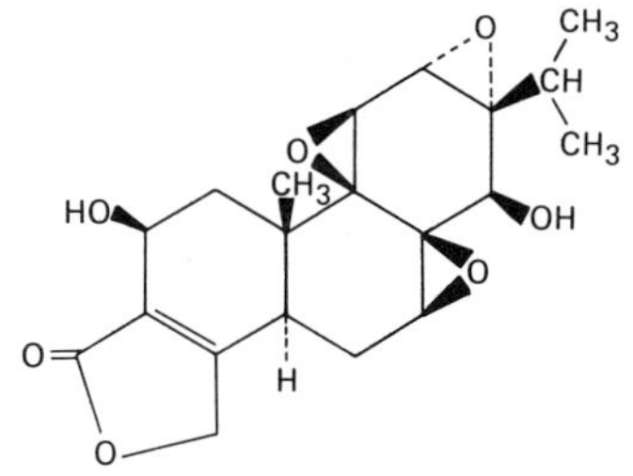

Fig. 17. Structure of tripdiolide (NSC 163063)

Table 18. Antitumor activity of tripdiolide NSC-163063

Tumor systems		Activities	
		% T/Cᵃ	Opt. dose mg/kg/inj.
PS	P388 lymphocytic leukemia	158	250
LE	L1210 lymphoid leukemia	207	250
B16	B16 melanocarcinoma	134	100
C6	Colon 26	(103)	250
LL	Lewis lung carcinoma	(138)	25

ᵃ T/C values in parentheses do not meet activity criteria

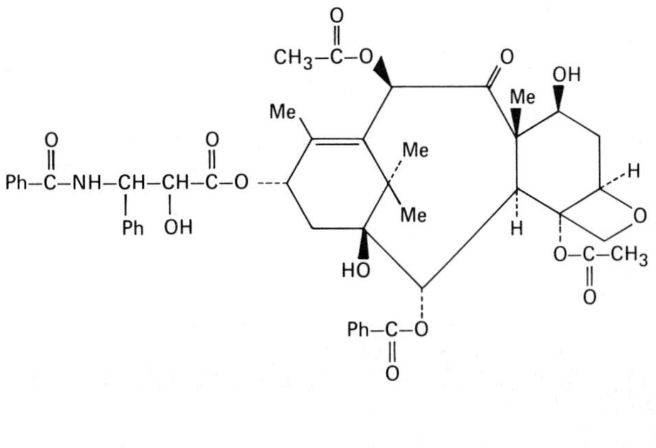

Fig. 18. Structure of Taxol (NSC 125973)

activity [27]. This compound was isolated from several species of *Taxus*. The best source appears to be stem bark of *Taxus brevifolia*, the western yew, a small evergreen native to the Pacific northwest. Taxol has shown antitumor activity in the B16 melanoma, P388, L1210, C6, P1534 leukemia, and in the breast and colon capsule xenograft tests (Table 19). A clinical formulation is being tested at this time. If a satisfactory formulation is developed the compound will proceed to toxicology studies.

Table 19. Antitumor activity of taxol NSC-125973

Tumor systems		Activities	
		% T/C[a]	Opt. dose mg/kg/inj.
PS	P388 lymphocytic leukemia	190	20
LE	L1210 lymphoid leukemia	139	15
B16	B16 melanocarcinoma	226	10
C6	Colon 26	161	30
C8	Colon 38	(69)	7.5
CD	CD8F$_1$ mammary	(57)	15
LL	Lewis lung carcinoma	(113)	4
EM	Ependymoblastoma	(106)	10
PA	Adriamycin resistant P388	(103)	25.9
PV	Vincristine resistant P388	(98)	21.6
P4	P-1534 leukemia	300	188
C2H2	CX-1 colon xenograft	(94)	5
C2G5	CX-1 colon renal capsule	9	50
C4H2	CX-2 colon xenograft	(85)	60
C9H2	CX-5 colon xenograft	(175)	5
C9G5	CX-5 colon renal capsule	14	100
LKH2	LX-1 lung xenograft	(93)	5
MBH2	MX-1 breast xenograft	(94)	6.25
MBG5	MX-1 breast renal capsule	4	100

[a] T/C values in parentheses do not meet activity criteria

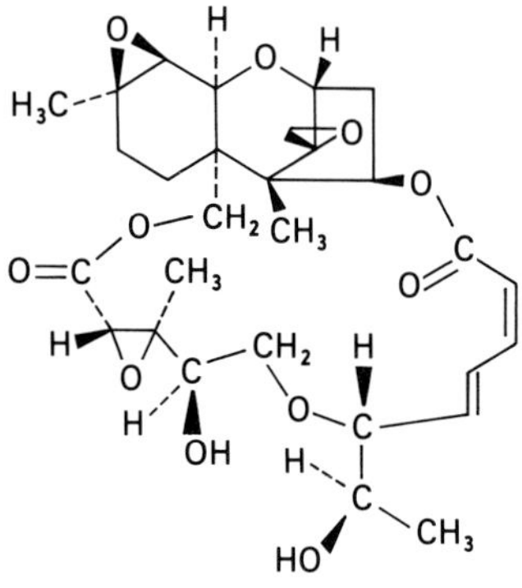

Fig. 19. Structure of baccharin (NSC 269757)

Baccharin (NSC-269757). Many trichothecanes have been evaluated in our program and two of the more interesting have been isolated from the Brazilian plant *Baccharis megapotamica* [17]. Baccharin (Fig. 19) has shown good activity against PS and LE and the adriamycin-resistant leukemia. In addition, activity has been observed against B16 and the ovarian carcinoma (Table 22).

Table 20. Antitumor activity of baccharin NSC-269757

Tumor systems		Activities	
		% T/C[a]	Opt. dose mg/kg/inj.
PS	P388 lymphocytic leukemia	311	10
LE	L1210 lymphoid leukemia	157	40
B16	B16 melanocarcinoma	158	2.5
C6	Colon 26	(123)	3.24
C8	Colon 38	(66)	20
CD	CD8F$_1$ mammary	(76)	20
LL	Lewis lung carcinoma	(105)	5
M5	Ovarian carcinoma	131	0.75
PA	Adriamycin resistant P388	158	7.2
PV	Vincristine resistant P388	(106)	3.24

[a] T/C values in parentheses do not meet activity criteria

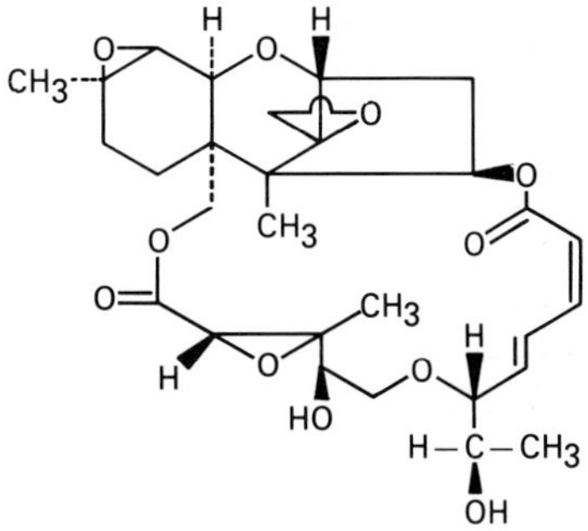

Fig. 20. Structure of isobaccharin (NSC 269760)

Table 21. Antitumor activity of isobaccharin NSC-269760

Tumor systems		Activities	
		% T/C[a]	Opt. dose mg/kg/inj.
PS	P388 lymphocytic leukemia	239	5
LE	L1210 lymphoid leukemia	151	5
B16	B16 melanocarcinoma	238	2.5
C6	Colon 26	(123)	4

[a] T/C values in parentheses do not meet activity criteria

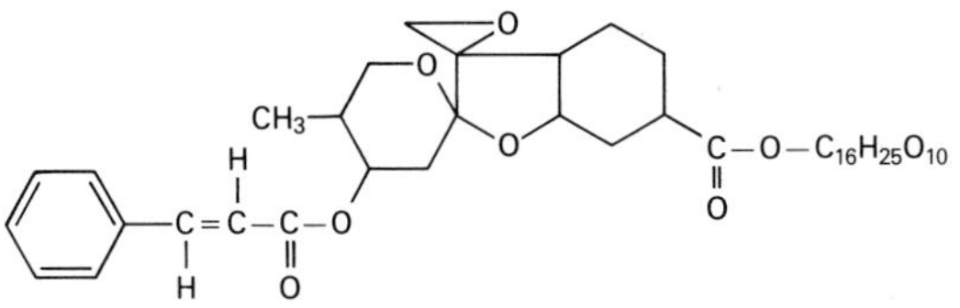

Fig. 21. Structure of phyllanthoside
(NSC 266492)

Table 22. Antitumor activity of phyllanthoside NSC-266492

Tumor systems		Activities	
		% T/C[a]	Opt. dose mg/kg/inj.
PS	P388 lymphocytic leukemia	149	8
B16	B16 melanocarcinoma	158	8
C6	Colon 26	(116)	48
LL	Lewis lung carcinoma	(103)	4

[a] T/C values in parentheses do not meet activity criteria

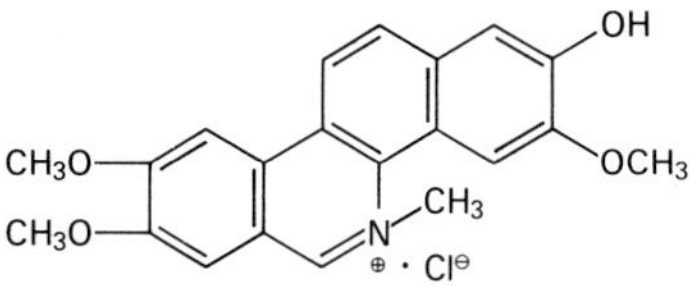

Fig. 22. Structure of fagaronine (NSC 157995)

Table 23. Antitumor activity of fagaronine NSC-157995

Tumor systems		Activities	
		% T/C[a]	Opt. dose mg/kg/inj.
PS	P388 lymphocytic leukemia	270	160
LE	L1210 lymphoid leukemia	159	80
B16	B16 melanocarcinoma	(108)	50
C6	Colon 26	138	320

[a] T/C values in parentheses do not meet activity criteria

Isobaccharin (NSC-269760) (Fig. 20) has shown superior B16 and less PS activity than baccharin [20] (Table 21). Both of these compounds will be obtained in sufficient quantity to complete tumor panel testing.

Phyllanthoside (NSC-266492) (Fig. 21) is a terpenoid glycoside obtained from *Phyllanthus braziliensis* that has shown sufficient B16 and PS activity to be tested in the entire tumor panel (Table 22) [19].

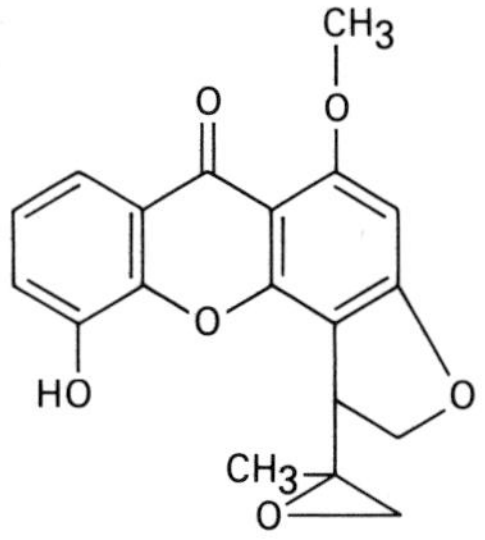

Fig. 23. Structure of psorospermin (NSC 266491)

Table 24. Antitumor activity of psorospermin NSC-266491

Tumor systems		Activities	
		% T/C[a]	Opt. dose mg/kg/inj.
PS	P388 lymphocytic leukemia	164	4
B16	B16 melanocarcinoma	(88)	2
C6	Colon 26	135	4
CD	CD8F$_1$ mammary	36	8
LL	Lewis lung carcinoma	(111)	0.5

[a] T/C values in parentheses do not meet activity criteria

Fagaronine (NSC-157993) (Fig. 22) is a benzophenanthridine alkaloid similar to nitidine that is obtained from *Fagara macrophylla*. This compound has shown PS, LE, and C6 activity (Table 23). This compound is scheduled for tumor panel testing.

Psorospermin (NSC-266491) (Fig. 23) is a xanthone that is obtained from *Psorospermum febrifugum*. This compoundd has shown activity in CD, C6, and P388 and is scheduled for tumor panel evaluation (Table 24).

Discussion

The NCI has had a very active natural products program that has constantly supplied novel potential antineoplastic agents to the clinicians for evaluation. Twenty-six compounds are now in various stages of preclinical evaluation at NCI (Table 1). In order to maintain the supply of novel anticancer agents in the program several changes have been made in the natural products program in the last 4 years and the major ones are listed:
1) Increased use of in vitro prescreens (tubulin binding, enzyme inhibition, phage induction, microbial mutants etc.) to evaluate fermentation broths. It is hoped that in the next two years this type of prescreening can be initiated to evaluate crude extracts in the plant and animal programs.
2) Isolation of unusual microbes.
3) Fermentation of unusual organisms under varied conditions.

4) Development of more efficient dereplication methods to rule out reisolation of known drugs more quickly.
5) Utilization of chromatographic dereplication earlier in the fermentation program.
6) More genetic mutational work with microbes.
7) Increased worldwide surveillance of all natural products.
8) Plant collection in the rain forests of the tropics.
9) Larger recollections of interesting plant leads.
10) A contract for a pilot plant laboratory to process large amounts of plant material.
11) A literature surveillance contract to obtain more novel compounds.
12) Aqueous extraction of fresh plants to search for water-soluble active components.
13) Larger collections of marine animal leads.

The above are a few of the modifications that will keep the natural products program at NCI highly viable. Many other potential natural product anticancer drugs are in early stages of testing and new leads for clinical trials will continue to be forthcoming.

References

1. Berger J, Jampolsky IM, Goldberg MW (1949) Borrelidin, a new antibiotic with anti-borrelia activity and penicillin enhancement properties. Arch Biochem Biophys 22: 476−478
2. Brundret KM, Dalziel W, Hesp B, Jarvis JAJ, Neidle S (1972) X-ray crystallographic determination of the structure of the antibiotic aphidicolin: a tetracyclic diterpenoid containing a new ring system. J Chem Soc Chem Commun 1972: 1027−1028
3. Bucknall RA, Moores H, Simms R, Hesp B (1973) Antiviral effects of aphidicolin, a new antibiotic produced by cephalosporium aphidicola. Antimicrob Agents Chemother 4: 294−298
4. Cephalotaxus Research Coordinating Group (1976) Cephalotaxine esters in the treatment of acute leukemia: A preliminary clinical assessment. Chin Med J [Engl] 2: 263−272
5. Dalziel W, Hesp B, Stevenson KM, Jarvis JAJ (1973) The structure and absolute configuration of the antibiotic aphidicolin: a tetracyclic diterpenoid containing a new ring system. J Cehm Soc [Perkin I] pp 2841−2851
6. Douros JD (1978) National Cancer Institute's fermentation development program. In: Carter SK, Umezawa H, Douros J, Sakurai Y (eds) Recent results in cancer research, vol 63. Springer, Berlin Heidelberg New York, pp 34−48
7. Douros J, Suffness M (1978) New natural products of interest under development at the National Cancer Institute. Cancer Chemother Pharmacol 1: 91−100
8. Formica JV, Shatkin AJ, Katz E (1968) Actinomycin analogues containing pipecolic acid: relationship of structure to biological activity. J Bacteriol 95: 2139−2150
9. Furukawa M, Inoue A, Asand K, Kawamata J (1968) Chemical studies on actinomycin S. II. chemical structures of actinomycin S_2 and S_3. J Antibiot (Tokyo) 21: 568−570
10. Geran RL, Greenberg NH, MacDonald MM, Schumacher AM, Abbott BJ (1972) Protocols for screening chemical agents and natural products against animal tumors and other biological systems (3rd ed). Cancer Chemother Rep Part 33: 1−103
11. Hanka LJ, Dietz A, Gerpheide SA, Kuentzel SL, Martin DG (1978) CC-1065 (NSC-298223) a new antitumor antibiotic. Production, in vitro biological activity, microbiological assays and taxonomy of the producing organism. J Antibiot (Tokyo) 31: 1211−1217

12. Katz E (1960) Biogenesis of the actinomycins. Ann NY Acad Sci 89: 304–322
13. Kawaguchi H, Tsukiura H, Tomita K, Konishi M, Saito K, Kobaru S, Numata K, Fujisawa K, Miyaki T, Hatori M, Koshiyama H (1977) Tallysomycin, a new antitumor antibiotic complex related to bleomycin. I. Production, isolation and properties. J Antibiot (Tokyo) 30: 779–788
14. Keller-Schierlein W (1966) Die Konstitution des Borrelidins. Experientia 22: 355–363
15. Konishi M, Saito K, Numata K, Tsuno T, Asama K, Tsukiura H, Naito T, Kawaguchi H (1977) Tallysomycin, a new antitumor antibiotic complex related to bleomycin. II. Structure determination of tallysomycins A and B. J Antibiot (Tokyo) 30: 789–805
16. Kupchan SM, Court WA, Dailey RG, jr, Gilmore CJ, Bryan RF (1972) Triptolide and tripdiolide, novel antileukemic diterpenoid triepoxides from *Tripterygium wilfordii*. J Am Chem Soc 94: 7194–7195
17. Kupchan SM, Jarvis BB, Dailey RG, jr, Bright W, Bryan RF, Shizuri Y (1976) Baccharin, a novel potent antileukemic trichothecenetriepoxide from *Baccharis megapotamica*. J Am Chem Soc 98: 7092–7093
18. Kupchan SM, Ashmore JW, Sneden AT (1977) Eriofertopin and 2-0-acetyleriofertopin, new tumor inhibitory germacradienolides from *Eriophyllum confertiflorum*. Phytochemistry 16: 1834–1835
19. Kupchan SM, Lavoie EJ, Branfman AR, Fei BY, Bright WM, Bryan RF (1977) Phyllanthocin, a novel bisabolane aglycone from the antileukemic glycoside, phyllanthoside. J Am Chem Soc 99: 3199–3201
20. Kupchan SM, Streelman DR, Jarvis BB, Dailey RG, jr, Sneden AT (1977) Isolation of potent new antileukemic trichothecenes from baccharis megapotamica. J Org Chem 42: 4221–4225
21. Martin DG, Mizsak SA, Biles C, Stewart JC, Baczynskyj L, Meulman PA (1975) Structure of quinomycin antibiotics. J Antibiot (Tokyo) 28: 332–336
22. Matsuda A, Yoshioka O, Yamashita T, Ebihara K, Umezawa H, Miura T, Katayama K, Yokoyama M, Nagai S (1978) Fundamental and clinical studies on new bleomycin analogs. In: Carter SK, Umezawa H, Douros J, Sakura Y (eds) Recent results in cancer, vol 63. Springer, Berlin Heidelberg New York, pp 191–210
23. Oki T, Matsuzawa Y, Yoshimoto A, Numata K, Kitamura I, Hori S, Takamatsu A, Umezawa H, Ishizuka M, Naganawa H, Suda H, Hamada M, Takeuchi T (1975) New antitumor antibiotics, aclacinomycins A and B. J Antibiot (Tokyo) 28: 830–834
24. Powell RG, Weisleder D, Smith CR, Jr, Rohwedder WK (1970) Structures of harringtonine, isoharringtonine, and homoharringtonine. Tetrahedron Lett 1970: 815–818
25. Sakano T, Okazaki N, Ise T, Kitaoka K, Kimura K (1978) Phase 1 study of aclacinomycin A. Jpn J Clin Oncol 8: 49–53
26. Suffness M, Douros J (1979) Drugs of plant origin. In: Devita VT, Jr, Busch H (eds) Methods in cancer research, vol XVI A. Academic Press, New York, pp 73–126
27. Wani MC, Taylor HL, Wall ME, Coggon P, MCPHAII AT (1971) Plant antitumor agents. VI. The isolation and structure of taxol, a novel antileukemic and antitumor agent from taxus brevifolia. J Am Chem Soc 93: 2325–2327
28. Wiley PF, Johnson JL, Houser DJ (1977) Nogalomycin analogs having improved antitumor activity. J Antibiot (Tokyo) 30: 628–629
29. Yamaguchi T, Furumai T, Sato M, Okuda T, Ishida N (1970) Studies on a new antitumor antibiotic, largomycin. I. Taxonomy of the largomycin-producing strain and production of the antibiotic. J Antibiot (Tokyo) 23: 369–372
30. Yamaguchi T, Kashida T, Nawa K, Yajima T, Miyagishima T, Ito Y, Okuda T, Ishida N, Kumagi K (1970) Studies on a new antitumor antibiotic, largomycin. II. Isolation, purification and physicochemical properties. J Antibiot (Tokyo) 23: 373–381
31. Yamaguchi T, Sato M, Omura Y, Arai Y, Enomoto K, Ishida M, Kumogai K (1970) Studies on a new antitumor antibiotic, largomycin. III. Biological properties and antitumor activity of largomycin F-II. J Antibiot (Tokyo) 23: 382–387

A Prospective Screening Program: Current Screening and its Status

A. Goldin and J. M. Venditti

Division of Cancer Treatment, National Cancer Institute, USA – Bethesda, MD

The new prospective screening program of the Division of Cancer Treatment, National Cancer Institute, initiated in 1975, started slowly, primarily because of the need to increase supplies of athymic mice and logistic problems pertaining to the maintenance of the health of the animals. But more recently, the program has gathered momentum and a steady flow of antitumor test data on new drugs is becoming available. It is worthwhile to review these data with reference to the questions that have been addressed prospectively to the new screen. The schema for the flow of drugs through the Division of Cancer Treatment screens is presented in Fig. 1 and the tumor panel systems are shown in Table 1 [4, 6–8, 13, 14, 16].

In the broadest sense the primary purpose of antitumor screening programs is to discover new and more effective antitumor agents for the treatment of clinical neoplasia. This involves an increase in the number of true positive compounds identified, namely compounds active in the screens and active in the clinic; reduction in the number of false positives, compounds active in the screen but not active in the clinic; a reduction of false negatives, compounds inactive in the screen but active in the clinic; and proper identification of true negatives, compounds inactive in the screen that would also be inactive in the clinic. In relation to the above it is of interest to list the types of questions that have been addressed prospectively to the new screen [4]:

1) Does the new screen increase the yield of active and more effective compounds for development for the clinic, and does this result in an increased armamentarium of more effective drugs for the treatment of the cancer patient?
2) Does broad spectrum activity in the screening panel result in greater probability of clinical antitumor effectiveness? Does it reduce the number of false negatives relative to the previous "limited" screen?
3) To what extent do human tumor xenografts and animal tumor screens select the same or different drugs as active?
4) Are the human tumor xenografts more effective than the animal tumors in predicting for clinical antitumor activity? Do they increase the likelihood of selection of "true positives" for the clinic? Are the xenograft positives more effective in the clinic than those selected by animal screens?
5) What is the extent of correspondence of activity against animal tumors and/or human tumor xenografts with respect to clinical therapeutic activity for tumors of different organ systems or differing histologic types?

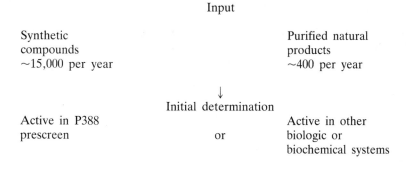

Input

| Synthetic compounds ~15,000 per year | | Purified natural products ~400 per year |

↓
Initial determination

| Active in P388 prescreen | or | Active in other biologic or biochemical systems |

↓
500–1000 Compounds
↓
Panel

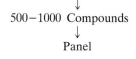

Mouse	Human tumor xenografts
Lung	Lung
Colon	Colon
Breast	Breast
Leukemia	
Melanoma	

Fig. 1. Flow of drugs in the new screen of the division of cancer treatment, NCI

6) Are compounds that have bypassed the prescreen on the basis of activity in other screening programs or in selected biochemical or biologic assays more effective in the screening panel or in the clinic than compounds initially selected for further testing by the prescreen?

7) What contribution will the data of the new screening panel make to predict the clinical effectiveness of new drugs, utilizing multivariate discriminant analysis type, and other types of pertinent mathematical procedures?

In previous studies it had been indicated that compounds that are active in a number of screening tumor systems in rodents may have more likelihood of being active against hematologic malignancies and solid tumors in man. Also, the higher the response in the tumor systems the greater the possibility would appear to be that the compounds would demonstrate clinical antitumor activity. This indication that high, broad spectrum activity in the screening panel will result in greater probability of clinical antitumor effectiveness is fortified considerably by the data emerging in the new screening panel. This generalization would indicate that the new screen does indeed have the potentiality for increasing the number of true positives, reducing the number of false positives and false negatives, and presumably also the ability to identify true negatives appropriately.

Table 1. Tumor panel systems

	L-1210	B-16 Melanoma	Lewis lung	P-388	Colon 26	Colon 38	Colon xenograft CX-1	Colon xenograft CX-2	Colon xenograft CX-5	Mammary xenograft MX-1	CD8F1 mammary	Lung xenograft LX-1
Host	CDF$_1$ or BDF$_1$	BDF1 or B6C3	BDF$_1$	CDF$_1$ or BDF$_1$	CDF$_1$	BDF$_1$	Nu/Nu Swiss	Nu/Nu Swiss	Nu/Nu Swiss	Nu/Nu Swiss	CD8F$_1$	Nu/Nu Swiss
Inoculum	10^5 Ascites	1:10 Homogenate	1×10^5 Viable cells	10^6 Ascites	1% Brei	Fragment	Fragment	Fragment	Fragment	Fragment	5×10^5 cells	Fragment
Site	IP	IP	IV	IP	IP	SC	SC	SC	SC	SC	SC	SC
Parameter	Mean survival time	Median survival time	Tumor weight inhibition ⟶									
Activity Criteria	T/C $\geq 125\%$	T/C $\geq 140\%$	T/C $\geq 140\%$	T/C $\geq 120\%$	T/C $\geq 130\%$	T/C $\leq 42\%$	T/C $\leq 42\%$	T/C $\leq 42\%$	T/C $\leq 42\%$	T/C $\leq 42\%$	T/C $\leq 42\%$	T/C $\leq 42\%$
Computer code	3LE21	3B131	3L139	3PS31	3C631	3C872	3C282	3C482	3C9H2	3MB82	3CD72	3LK82

The screening data as presented in the report of Goldin et al. [5] for a number of clinically active drugs is summarized in Table 2 and the experimental data in the new screen for the same compounds is given in Table 3. The screening data for the xenograft models were obtained by Houchens D and Ovejera T at the Battelle Columbus Laboratories. The clinical activity for individual types of tumors for the same compounds is summarized in Table 4 [15, 17].

A comparison of the activity in animal tumors in the initial screen and in the new screening panel with the activity in the clinic is presented in Table 5.

In the initial retrospective analysis (Table 2) the clinically established antitumor agents in general showed activity in a high percentage of the animal tumor systems, ranging from a low of 17% for actinomycin D to a high of 80% for procarbazine. Similarly, in the new screen (Table 3), the clinically active drugs showed broad spectrum activity, ranging from 36% of the tumor systems for methotrexate to 91% for melphalan. Overall there was good correspondence between the percentage of experimental tumor systems in which the drugs were active for the initial screening system and the new panel. However, in general there was an increased incidence of experimental systems in which the new screen predicted acctivity for the clinic. In the new panel the incidence of tumor systems in which drugs were active was increased markedly for actinomycin D, from 17% to 89%, and for melphalan from 58% to 91%. Increased incidence was also observed for 5-fluorouracil (5-FU), from 67% to 75%, for vincristine from 45% to 70%, and chlorambucil from 42% to 67%. Reduction in incidence of active systems was observed only for Methotrexate (MTX), from 50% to 36%, and for procarbazine from 80% to 67%.

Similarly, for the various human tumor types including instances where it was judged that there was adequate evaluation, or combining the instances where there was either adequate evaluation or evidence of drug activity, there was broad spectrum activity in the various clinical categories (Table 4). In general, the broader the spectrum of activity in the animal tumor systems the broader the spectrum of activity observed against the clinical tumors.

For the human tumor xenografts, in most instances, activity was observed in one or more systems. 6-Mercaptopurine, however, was inactive in 0 of 3 of the xenograft systems in which it was tested. Procarbazine and actinomycin D showed activity in 2 of 2 of the test systems in which studies were conducted.

Comparison of the experimental data for specific tumor types, including human tumor xenografts, with corresponding human tumor categories is of interest (Tables 6–8).

For clinical mammary tumors, the CD8F1 mammary tumor provided true positive prediction for clinical activity in 6 of 6 instances, namely for cyclophosphamide, MTX, melphalan, 5-FU, vincristine and chlorambucil (Table 6). The MX-1 mammary xenograft gave true positive prediction for five of the drugs, but for 5-FU the prediction was false negative.

For human colon tumors the animal carcinomas C26 and C38 and the human colon xenograft CX-2 gave true positive prediction for cyclophosphamide and 5-FU but all three systems failed to identify activity for MTX (Table 7). False positive prediction for a number of the clinically inactive drugs (6 MP, procarbazine, actinomycin D, and vincristine) was high for the C26 and C38 systems, but data were not available for these drugs in most instances with the human xenograft systems.

The CX-1 mammary xenograft was a true positive predictor only for 5-FU. It gave a false negative rating for MTX but was a true negative predictor for melphalan and

Table 2. Activity in animal tumors for clinically established antitumor agents

		Cyclo	MTX	Melphalan (L-PAM)	5-FU	6-MP	Pro-carbazine	Act D	Vin-cristine (vcr)	Chlor-ambucil
L1210 Early	(ST)	80	100	75	60	50	45	45	39	31
L1210 Advanced	(ST)	100	100	28	39	50	21	33	17	0
P1534	(ST)	27	27	89	>133	10	NT	37	>200	32
P1798	(TWI)	68	95	71	76	45	NT	44	97	27
LPC-1 Plasma advanced	(ST)	100	23	75	152	12	81	0	0	36
Dunning ascites	(ST)	>200	87	160	77	78	NT	22	83	200
Walker 256 SC	(TWI)	100	33	100	59	99	NT	53	NT	100
Walker 256 IM	(TWI)	90	95	95	72	86	75	65	80	84
Ca 755	(TWI)	90	66	71	77	95	NT	90	46	75
S 180	(TWI)	96	39	80	80	65	84	66	43	65
Lymphoma 8	(ST)	37	100	35	77	45	NT	25	35	25
Lewis lung	(TWI)	90	28	50	65	49	NT	55	40	40
Murine systems in which active		9/12 75%	6/12 50%	7/12 58%	8/12 67%	6/12 50%	4/5 80%	2/12 17%	5/11 45%	5/12 42%

Criteria for activity
Early leukemia L1210 ≥ 30% increase in survival time (ILS) over controls
Advanced leukemia L1210 ≥ 50% increase in survival time relative to the MTX standard
P-1534, LCP 1 plasma cell, Dunning ascites, lymphoma 8 ≥ 50% increase in survival time over controls
P-1798, Walker 256 SC, Walker 256 IM, Ca 755, S 180, Lewis Lung ≥ 75% inhibition of tumor
    Weight (TWI) relative to controls at maximum tolerated dose

Table 3. Activity in the new screening panel for clinically established antitumor agents

	Cyclo	MTX	Melphalan (L-PAM)	5-FU	6-MP	Pro-carbazine	Act D	Vin-cristine (vcr)	Chlor-ambucil
L1210	236	272	237	180	263	188	168	147	149
P388	>300	296	281	220	150	180	>300	300	171
B16 melanoma	176	<140	257	140	<140	168	212	189	140
Lewis lung IV	222	<140	154	150	<140	<140	<140	<140	<140
Colon 26	165	106	>309	200	246	115	146	130	190
Colon 38	9	76	8	0	10	37	22	23	59
CD8F1	0	20	1	0	21	102	9	7	16
CX-1	> 42	> 42	> 42	+	*	*	*	Neg	*
CX-2	+	> 42	+	+	> 42	*	*	**	*
CX-5	Neg	*	*	> 42	*	*	*	*	*
MX-1	+ +	+	+ + (++)	> 42	> 42	+ (+)	+	+ +	+ +
LX-1	> 42	> 42	+	> 42	> 42 (> 42)	+ +	+	> 42	> 42
Total									
Animal tumors	7/7	3/7	7/7	7/7	5/7	4/7	6/7	6/7	5/7
Xenografts	2/5	1/4	3/4	2/5	0/3	2/2	2/2	1/3	1/2
Animal tumors plus xenografts	9/12	4/11	10/11	9/12	5/10	6/9	8/9	7/10	6/9
	75%	36%	91%	75%	50%	67%	89%	70%	67%

Negative = T/C <140 for B16 or L L
T/C <125 for L1210 or P388

Criteria for activity:
L1210 T/C ≥125%
P388 T/C ≥120%
B16, Lewis lung T/C ≥ 140% Neg = < 140%
Colon 26 T/C ≥ 130%
Colon 38, CD8F1 mammary T/C ≤ 42%
Xenografts CX-1, CX-2, CX-5, MX-1, LX-1

+ + Elicits tumor regression. Relative tumor weight (RW) < 1%
+ Retards relative rate of tumor growth TRW/CRW ≤ 42%
Neg Inactive TRW/CRW ≥ 42%
* not evaluated
** test inadequate

Table 4. Activity in human tumors for clinically established antitumor agents

	Cyclophos.	MTX	Melphalan (L-PAM)	5-FU	6-MP	Pro-carbazine	Actino-mycin D	Vin-cristine	Chlor-ambucil
Colon	⊕	⊕	−	+	−	−	−	−	−
Melanoma	⊕	−	⊕	−	−	−	⊕	−	−
Lung (small cell)	+	+	−	−	−	⊕		⊕	⊕
Breast	+	+	+	+				+	⊕
Ovary	+	⊕	+	+				−	+
Cervix	+	⊕	⊕	⊕				⊕	⊕
Prostate	⊕			⊕	⊕				
Choriocarcinoma		+					+		
Pancreas				+					+
Larynx									
Stomach				+					
Kidney									
Wilms	+							+	
Head and neck	+	+		+			+		
Brain		⊕			⊕	⊕		⊕	⊕
Bladder	⊕			⊕					
Neuroblastoma	+								
Retinoblastoma	+							+	+
Myeloma	+		+						
Sarcoma	+	+	⊕				+		+
Testes	+	+	+				+	+	⊕
Leukoses	+	+			+	+	⊕	+	+
Lymphomas	+	+	+			+	+	+	+
Totals	13/17	8/13	5/10	6/11	1/6	2/6	5/8	6/12	6/12
(per cent)	(76%)	(62%)	(50%)	(55%)	(16%)	(33%)	(63%)	(56%)	(50%)
+ and ⊕	17/17 (100%)	12/13 (92%)	8/10 (80%)	9/11 (82%)	3/6 (50%)	4/6 (67%)	7/8 (88%)	9/12 (75%)	10/12 (83%)

+ Adequate evaluation. Drug active
⊕ Evidence of drug activity but not already established
− Inactive

Table 5. Comparison of activity in animal tumors and in the clinic: number of test systems in which active

	Cyclo-phosphamide	MTX	Melphalan	5-FU	6-MP	Procar-bazine	Act D	VCR	Chlorambucil
Initial animal tumor systems (see table 2)	9/12 (75%)	6/12 (50%)	7/12 (58%)	8/12 (67%)	6/12 (50%)	4/5 (80%)	2/12 (17%)	5/11 (45%)	5/12 (42%)
New screening panel (see table 3)	7/7	3/7	7/7	7/7	5/7	4/7	6/7	6/7	5/7
Animal tumors Human tumor xenografts	2/5	1/4	3/4	2/5	0/3	2/2	2/2	1/3	1/2
Total (and percent)	9/12 (75%)	4/11 (36%)	10/11 (91%)	9/12 (75%)	5/10 (50%)	6/9 (67%)	8/9 (89%)	7/10 (70%)	6/9 (67%)
Clinical (see Table 4) +	13/17 (76%)	8/13 (62%)	5/10 (50%)	6/11 (55%)	1/6 (16%)	2/6 (33%)	5/8 (63%)	6/12 (50%)	6/12 (50%)
+ and ⊕	17/17 (92%)	12/13 (92%)	8/10 (80%)	9/11 (82%)	3/6 (50%)	4/6 (67%)	7/8 (88%)	9/12 (75%)	10/12 (83%)

A. Goldin and J. M. Venditti

Table 6. Comparison of activity screening panel and clinic: Breast cancer

	Animal		Clinic
	CD8F1	MX1	
Cytoxan	T +	T +	+
MTX	T +	T +	+
Melphalan	T +	T +	+
5-FU	T +	F −	+
6-MP	+	−	
Procarbazine	−	+	
Act D	T +	+	
Vincristine	+	T +	+
Chlorambucil	T +	T +	⊕

T +, True positive
T −, True negative
F −, False negative

Table 7. Comparison of activity screening panel and clinic: Colon cancer

	Animal					Clinic colon
	C26	C38	CX1	CX2	CX5	
Cyclophosphamide	T +	T +	F −	T +	F −	⊕
MTX	F −	F −	F −	F −	*	⊕
Melphalan	F +	F +	T −	F +	*	−
5-FU	T +	T +	T +	T +	F −	+
6-MP	F +	F +	*	F −	*	−
Procarbazine	F +	F +	*	*	*	−
Act D	F +	F +	*	*	*	−
Vincristine	F +	F +	T −	*	*	−
Chlorambucil	T −	T −	*	*	*	−

T +, True positive
F +, False positive
T −, True negative
F −, False negative
 *, Not evaluated

vincristine. The CX-5 system improperly classified cyclophosphamide and 5-FU as negative.

For small cell carcinoma of the lung the Lewis lung IV system predicted activity only for cyclophosphamide, and the LX-1 system predicted activity only for procarbazine (Table 8). False negative prediction occurred with both systems for methotrexate and vincristine.

Both systems were false positive predictors for melphalan but true negative predictors for 6 MP. 5-FU was rated as a true negative by the LX-1 tumor and as a false positive by the Lewis lung system. Utilization of the requirement of activity in either one of the

Table 8. Comparison of activity screening panel and clinic: Lung cancer

	Animal		Clinic
	LL IV	LX-1	Lung (small cell)
Cyclophosphamide	T +	F –	+
MTX	F –	F –	+
Melphalan	F +	F +	–
5-FU	F +	T –	–
6-MP	T –	T – (–)	–
Procarbazine	F –	T + +	⊕
Act D	–	+	
Vincristine	F –	F –	⊕
Chlorambucil	–	–	

T +, True positive
F +, False positive
T –, True negative
F –, False negative

experimental systems as an indicator for clinical activity would result in positive prediction of two of the four compounds, namely cyclophosphamide and procarbazine.

Thus, the CD8F1 and MX-1 mammary tumors rated the drugs relatively accurately for activity against mammary tumor in the clinic. The prediction for activity against human colon tumor was reasonably correct, but at the expense of one false negative and a number of false positives. The predictability for activity against small cell lung tumor appeared to be the least accurate, although the utilization of the criterion of activity in either one of the two systems did improve the capability for prediction. This analysis, although conducted with established antitumor agents suggests the possibility that specific types of animal tumors may predict for activity in corresponding types of tumors in the clinic. A definitive analysis awaits the accumulation of a more extensive data base.

It is clear that there is variation in response for different lines of tumor of the same histologic type and it is possible that the testing of compounds in a number of lines of the same histologic type may provide additional important prognostic information. Osieka et al. [13] for example demonstrated that one human tumor xenograft line BE was highly sensitive to treatment with MeCCNU, while two other lines, CA and HT were highly resistant.

Additional drugs that are of interest for the clinic, as related to activity in the new screening panel are listed in Table 9. The acridine derivative 4′-(9-acridinylamino) methanesulfon-m-anisidide (AMSA) [1] had broad spectrum activity in the new screening panel, including activity against leukemia L1210, leukemia P388, B16 melanoma, Lewis lung carcinoma, colon carcinomas 26 and 38, and CD8F1 mammary tumor in mice. It showed no definite activity against the human tumor xenografts. In initial studies in the clinic, AMSA has shown activity against leukemia, breast, ovarian and renal cell tumors.

Phosphonacetyl-L-aspartic acid (PALA), an inhibitor of aspartate transcarbamylase [2], was not active in the treatment of leukemia L1210 and demonstrated borderline

Table 9. Activity of additional drugs of clinical interest in tumor panel systems

NSC	Name	L1210	P388	B16 Melanoma	Lewis lung	Colon 26	Colon 38	CX-1	CX-2	CX-5	MX-1	CD8F1	LX-1
249992	AMSA	+	+	+	+	+	+	NT	−	−	−	+	−
224131	PALA	−	±	+	+	+	±	−	−	−	+	+	−(+)
119875	Cis-pt II	+	+	+	+	+	+	NT	NT	−	+	+	−
125066	Bleomycin	+	+	+	−	−	−	+	+	NT	+	+	−
178248	Chlorozotocin	+	+	+	±	+	+	NT	+	±	±	+	−
13875	Hexamethylmelamine	±	−	±	+	±	±	−	−	+	+	±	−
7365	DON	±	±	−	−	+	±	−	+	+	+	+	+
163501	AT 125	+	+	−	−	−	−	−	−	NT	+	−	+
141537	Anguidine	+	+	+	−	−	+	NT	−	NT	−	+	−
153858	Maytansine	+	+	+	−	−	−	NT	−	NT	−	−	NT

NT, Not tested

activity in the treatment of leukemia P388. However it was active against Lewis lung carcinoma [9] and also active against B16 melanoma, colon 26, mammary CD8F1, and the mammary xenograft tumor MX-1. It had borderline activity against colon 38 and unconfirmed activity against the lung tumor LX-1. In addition, PALA has demonstrated broad spectrum activity against a number of experimental solid tumors [10, 16]. PALA is currently in Phase I clinical trial.

Cis-dichloro-diammine platinum II (Cis-platinum II) also demonstrated broad spectrum activity in the new screen. It had activity against leukemia L1210, leukemia P388, B16 melanoma, Lewis lung carcinoma, colon 26, colon 38, and CD8F1 mammary tumor. In the xenograft systems it was active against mammary tumor MX-1. Activity has already been demonstrated with this drug against testicular tumors, ovarian carcinoma, head and neck carcinoma, bladder carcinoma, carcinoma of the penis, cervical carcinoma, and osteosarcoma.

Bleomycin showed activity against leukemias L1210 and P388, B16 melanoma, and CD8F1 mammary tumor. It was active against the colon xenograft CX-1 and the mammary xenograft MX-1. In the clinic it has been observed to be active against Hodgkin's disease, non-Hodgkin's lymphoma, head and neck carcinoma, testicular tumors, and superficial squamous cell tumors including penile cancer.

Chlorozotocin was active against six of the murine tumors in the new screen and showed marginal activity against Lewis lung carcinoma and the mammary xenograft MX-1. It had activity against the colon tumor CX-2. In preliminary clinical studies it has shown activity against non-Hodgkin's lymphoma.

Hexamethylmelamine was not definitely active against leukemia L1210 or B16 melanoma and was inactive in the treatment of P388 leukemia. It did show activity against Lewis lung carcinoma and the mammary xenograft MX-1. It had borderline activity for colon 26, colon 38, and mammary carcinoma CD8F1. Based on the data in the new screen plus the reports of activity against human colon, bronchus, ovary, and kidney tumors in mice that were thymectomized at birth and then reconstituted with syngeneic bone marrow [3, 12], clinical interest was generated in this compound. In the clinic hexamethylmelamine has demonstrated activity against lung carcinoma, ovarian carcinoma, and Bilharzial bladder cancer.

There has been renewed clinical interest in 6-diazo-5-oxo-L-norleucine (DON), a glutamine antagonist [11], because of activity in the new screen against the human tumor xenografts colon CX-2, mammary MX-1, and lung LX-1. It also demonstrated activity in the new screen against CD8F1 mammary carcinoma and colon carcinoma 26.

Thus, although the new screening panel has not been in operation for an extensive period there have already emerged examples where clinical interest in a new compound has been generated based on the demonstration of requisite activity.

A listing of the screening data in the new panel for compounds in development is presented in Table 10. Many of these have broad spectrum activity and, with the exception of 2'deoxycoformycin, a "by pass" compound related to biochemical interest, and dichloroallyl lawsone, all of the drugs have demonstrated activity in at least two of the tumors of the screening spectrum.

In general, there would appear to be greater activity against the murine tumors than against the human tumor xenografts growing in athymic mice and it may be of interest to focus attention on drugs such as DON that have demonstrated activity in the human tumor xenografts. DON, as indicated above, was active against the xenografts CX-2, MX-1, and LX-1. Also of potential interest is diazonia-bicycloheptane mustard with

Table 10. Data in the new screening panel for compounds in development (data of Ovejera and Houchens)

NSC	Name	L1210	P388	B16 Melanoma	Lewis lung	Colon 26	Colon 38	CX-1	CX-2	CX-5	MX-1	CD8F1	LX-1
7365	D-O-Norleucine	189	190	115	128	170	10	–	++	*	++(++)	17	++
29630	Dichloromethotrexate	234	R	116	111	147	R	–	–	*	–	35	+(–)
51143	Dihydroimidazopyrazole	144	120	106	169	120	50	*	*	–	–	46	–
57198	Diazoniabicyclo-heptane mustard	190	213	157	NT	272	47	+	*	–	++	6	+
71795	Ellipticine	>495	204	147	147	263	0	–	*	+	–	9	–
95466	PCNU	NT	118	193	219	346	12	*	*	++	+	3	*
118742	Pentamethylmelamine	119	138	130	127	121	22	–	+	–	+(++)	13	–
122023	Valinomycin	131	183	183	–	200	40	–	*	–	–	49	–
125973	Taxol	139	190	226	98	161	69	–	*	–(–)	–(–)	57	*
126771	Dichloroallyl lawsone	113	120	120	117	107	45	*	*	–	–	52	*
126840	3-Deazauridine	164	124	125	124	112	73	*	*	*	–	66	*
127755	Dihydrotriazine benzene-sulfonyl fluoride	146	241	200	142	175	26	–	*	–	–	5	*
132319	Indicine-N-oxide	147	262	182	115	176	5	–	*	–	+(+)	21	–
135758	2,5-Piperazinedione	>470	223	141	126	171	R	*	–	–	++(++)	R	–
137679	Selenoguanosine	229	247	136	145	179	R	–	*	–	–	12	+
139490	5-Methyl-tetrahydro-homofolic acid	155	149	127	138	147	64	–	*	–	–	26	+
153353	L-Alanosine, Na-salt	161	178	117	125	141	53	*	–	–(–)	–(–)	30	–
154020	Tricyclic nucleoside	215	156	123	113	125	75	–(–)	*	–(–)	++	0	9
163501	AT-125	191	250	131	147	144	69	–	–	–	++	6	–
165563	Bruceantin	141	230	178	133	143	21	*	*	*	–(–)	49	*
166100	Prospidine	114	159	183	145	185	37	*	–	*	–	5	–
169780	L-ICRF	172	229	142	213	177	33	*	*	*	–	10	–
172112	Spirohydantoin mustard	142	>290	263	149	286	25	–	–	–	++(–)	4	–
182896	AZQ	269	238	170	121	325	17	*	+	*	++	11	–

NSC No.	Compound	P-388	L1210	B16 melanoma	Lewis lung	Colon 26	Colon 38	CD8F1	CX-1	CX-2	CX-5	MX-1	LX-1
208734	Aclacinomycin A	NT	236	148	NT	123	R	11	*	*	—	—	—
218321	2'-Deoxycoformycin	105	118	NT	NT	NT	NT	NT	—	*	—	—	—
219733	Diacridinyl hexanediamine	143	180	206	125	215	70	47	+	*	—	+	—(+)
224131	PALA	122	140	199	266	229	21	1	—	—	—	—	—
234714	Aphidicolin	122	155	176	126	175	65	R	—	*	*	*	—
246131	AD-32	>521	>560	288	118	241	6	3	—	*	*	—	—
249992	AMSA	185	216	243	125	130	25	3	*	—	—	—	—
259272	Ara-A-5'-Phosphate	134	NT	131	126	120	R	R	—	(−)	*	(−)	—(−)
259968	Bouvardin	129	188	152	119	133	44	80	(−)	*	—	(−)	—
264880	Dihydro-5-azacytidine	228	227	125	120	>303	40	35	+	*	**	+(−)	—(−)
279836	Dihydroxy anthracenedione	274	>450	>506	276		23	29	—	**	*	(−)	—
288411	Indenoquinoline carboxylic acid	141	172	169	NT	NT	62	R	—	*	—	—	—
289642	Macromycin	182	218	265	116	227	R	R	—	*	*	—	+
526417	Quinomycin A	126	205	189	111	104	123	67	—	*	—	—	—

Murine tumors survival time models, activity considered significant:

P-388 T/C ≥ 120%

Leukemia L1210; B16 melanoma T/C ≥ 125%

Lewis lung carcinoma T/C ≥ 140%

Colon carcinoma 26 T/C ≥ 130%

Tumor inhibition models:

Colon carcinoma 38; CD8F1 mammary tumor T/C ≤ 42%

T/C = Ratio of treated survival time to control survival time × 100

NT = Not tested

R = Activity being confirmed

Human tumor xenografts:

CX-1, CX-2, CX-5, MX-1, LX-1

++ Tumor regression T/C < 1

+ Retardation of tumor weight T/C ≤ 42%

— Inactive T/C ≥ 42%

* Not evaluated

** Test results inconclusive

( ) Results of later test

T/C Ratio of treated tumor weight to control tumor weight × 100.

activity against MX-1; PCNU with activity against CX-5; 2,5-piperazinedione with activity against MX-1; AT-125 with activity against MX-1; and AZQ with activity against MX-1. The predictability value, of course, of the new screen with respect to these compounds must await clinical trial.

In summary, certain generalizations may already be made based on the available data. The primary generalization that appears to be emerging is that high broad-spectrum activity in a variety of experimental test systems prospectively increases the possibility for prediction for clinical activity for at least one and possibly more or even a broad spectrum of human tumors. If this generalization remains valid it would result in an increase in the number of true positive compounds, a decrease in the number of false positives and false negatives, and possibly an accurate designation of true negatives.

It is suggested that it is possible to predict for selection of drugs that will have activity against tumors of different organ systems or specific histologic types. This was more evident with the prediction for breast tumor than for colon tumor or lung tumor.

It may be important to focus on the drugs that have definitive activity in the xenograft systems, particularly since these tumors may be somewhat more naturally resistant to therapy with many of the drugs.

As an adjunct to the screening panel it may be advisable to employ a small battery of human tumors of the same histologic type, i.e., a series of colon tumors, a series of lung tumors, a series of breast tumors.

Alternatively, instead of employing a whole series of tumors of the same histologic type there could be judicious choice of one virtually resistant and one relatively sensitive tumor for each histologic type. This may increase the possibility for discovering new compounds of interest.

Firm conclusions concerning these generalizations that are emerging await additional clinical investigations of the new compounds selected by the screening panel.

References

1. Cain BF, Atwell CJ (1974) The experimental antitumor properties of three congeners of the acridylmethanesulphonanilide (AMSA) series. Eur J Cancer 10: 539−549
2. Collins KD, Stark GR (1971) Aspartate transcarbamylase interaction with the transition state analog, *N*-(phosphonacetyl)-L-aspartate. J Biol Chem 246: 6599−6605
3. Detre SI, Davies AJS, Connors TA (1975) New models for cancer chemotherapy. Cancer Chemother Rep (Part 2) 5: 133−143
4. Goldin A, Schepartz SA, Venditti JM, Devita VT, Jr (1979) Historical development and current strategy of the National Cancer Institute drug development program. In: De Vita VT, Busch H (eds) Methods in cancer research, vol XVI. Academic Press, New York London, pp 165−245
5. Goldin A, Serpick AA, Mantel N (1966) A commentary. Experimental screening procedures and clinical predictability value. Cancer Chemother Rep 50: 173−218
6. Goldin A, Venditti JM (1978) Retrospective and prospective approaches to screening and to comparative evaluation of analogs in the USA. In: Umezawa H, Carter SK, Goldin A, Kuretani K, Mathe G, Schurai Y, Tsukagoshi S (eds) Advances in cancer chemotherapy. Japan Science Society Press, University Park Press, Tokyo Baltimore, pp 179−200
7. Goldin A, Venditti JM, Muggia FM, Rozencweig M, Devita VT jr (to be published) New animal models in cancer chemotherapy. Proc Int Union Against Cancer

8. Johnson RK, Houchens DP (1979) The use of human tumor xenografts for selection of new agents against tumors with poor response to established drugs. In: Muggia F, Rozencweig M (eds) Lung cancer: Progress in therapeutic research. Raven Press, New York, pp 37–44

9. Johnson RK, Inouye T, Goldin A, Stark GR (1976) Antitumor activity of N-(phosphon-acetyl)-L-aspartic acid; a transition-state inhibitor of aspartate transcarbamylase. Cancer Res 36: 2720–2725

10. Johnson RK, Swyryd EA, Stark GR (1978) Effects of N-(phosphonacetyl)-L-aspartate on murine tumors and normal tissues in vivo and in vitro and the relationship of sensitivity to rate of proliferation and level of aspartate transcarbamylase. Cancer Res 38: 371–378

11. Livingston RB, Venditti JM, Cooney DA, Carter SK (1970) Glutamine antagonists in cancer chemotherapy. In: Garattini S, Goldin A, Hawking F, Kopin IJ (eds) Advances in pharmacology and chemotherapy, vol VIII. Academic Press New York, pp 57–120

12. Mitchley BCV, Clarke SA, Connors TA (1975) Hexamethylmelamine-induced regression of human lung tumors growing in immune deprived mice. Cancer Res 35: 1099–1102

13. Osieka R, Houchens DP, Goldin A, Johnson RK (1977) Chemotherapy of human colon cancer xenografts in athymic nude mice. Cancer 40: 2640–2650

14. Ovejera AA, Houchens DP, Barker AD (1978) Chemotherapy of human tumor xenografts in genetically athymic mice. Ann Clin Lab Sci 8: 50–56

15. Sofina ZP, Goldin A, Belousova AK (to be published) Analysis of experimental data and correlations with the clinic. In: Goldin A, Kline I, Sofina ZP, Syrkin AB (eds) Experimental evaluation of antitumor drugs in the USA and USSR and clinical correlations. USA-USSR Monograph, Washington, DC – US-Govt Print Office

16. Venditti JM, Goldin A, Miller I, Rozencweig M (1978) Experimental models for antitumor testing in current use by the National Cancer Institute USA: Statistical analysis and methods for selecting agents for clinical trials. In: Carter SK, Goldin A, Kuretani K, Mathé G, Sakurai Y, Tsukagoshi S, Umezawa H (eds) Advances in cancer chemotherapy. Japan Science Society Press, University Park Press, Tokyo Baltimore, pp 201–219

17. Wasserman TH, Comis RL, Goldsmith M, Handelsman H, Penta, JS, Slavik M, Soper WT, Carter SK (1975) Tabular analysis of the clinical chemotherapy of solid tumors. Cancer Chemother Rep (Part 3) 6: 399–419

Selected Anticancer Drugs in Phase I Trials in the United States (1979–1980)

F. M. Muggia, J. S. Penta, R. Catane, M. S. Jensen-Akula, and L. M. Charles, Jr.

Cancer Therapy Evaluation Programm, Division of Cancer Treatment, National Cancer Institute, USA – Bethesda, MD 20205

Introduction

Since 1975 the antitumor activity of new agents introduced by the Division of Cancer Treatment (DCT) has been detected or confirmed in animal screening systems consisting of a panel of six spontaneous allografted murine tumors, and three human tumor xenografts [25]. A plan of clinical development has been formulated which includes, as a minimum requirement, testing all new agents in a clinical panel that matches in disease orientation those preclinical screening systems [50]. Accordingly, Phase II studies with every drug are expected to be completed in patients with breast, colon, and lung carcinomas, malignant melanoma, acute leukemia, and lymphoma. It is hoped that such a plan will obviate incomplete clinical evaluations which were all too prevalent in the past [64].

Such a restructuring of the drug development program of the National Cancer Institute reflects trends favoring utilization of systems other than murine leukemias in the hope of identifying new types of chemical entities. In addition, increased attention to natural products and to agents intellectually selected on the basis of unique biologic or biochemical concepts has diversified the input into this panel [48]. Studies in the panel have also triggered renewed interest in older compounds that had received inadequate clinical testing [54]. Finally, a number of drugs introduced for evaluation represent analogs bearing a variable relationship to previously tested compounds [47, 56]. Rationales for analog development are becoming increasingly better delineated, and this area represents a fertile field of investigation requiring a team approach [48].

The current review will confine itself to drugs in or soon to be in Phase I clinical trial during 1979. Phosphonacetyl-L-aspartate (PALA) has been an example of a drug evoking special interest because of its rational synthesis, specific biochemical action, and unique spectrum. However, it will not be covered here because it was subject to extensive prior review [57]. Instead, we have chosen drugs that illustrate other features of drug development or have already yielded some noteworthy findings. For convenience we have subdivided our review into three major categories: (1) drugs that represent new chemical structures (see below for chemical correspondence, of these well-known abbreviated designations): *m-AMSA, 2'-deoxycoformycin, and AT-125;* (2) drugs that have been rediscovered recently for clinical evaluation: *DON, methyl-GBG, and thymidine;* and (3) drugs that have been derived from other known anticancer agents and thus constitute second generation compounds: *pentamethyl-*

melamine and AZO. Our focus shall be on those features that either identified their antitumor potential or led to a renewal of interest. The plan of development of individual drugs will be outlined, and preliminary clinical findings will be summarized, whenever available.

New Chemical Structures (Fig. 1)

4'-(9-acridinylamino)methanesulfon-M-anisidide (*m*-AMSA; methane sulfonamide, *N*-[4-(9-acridimylamino)3-methoxyphenyl]; NSC 249992).

m-AMSA is one of various acridine derivatives synthesized by Cain and Atwell [4]. The preclinical antitumor spectrum, biochemical and biologic effects, pharmacologic disposition in rodents after parenteral and oral administration, and toxicology studies have been previously reviewed [57]. The results of the initial Phase I clinical studies in solid tumors were published within one year of their onset [39, 63]. Table 1 summarizes the findings of these and subsequent studies and provides an indication of the dose schedules that were explored. The major toxic effect observed was moderate to severe leukopenia; mild thrombocytopenia and superficial phlebitis were also observed but otherwise the drug was well tolerated. Because of these acceptable

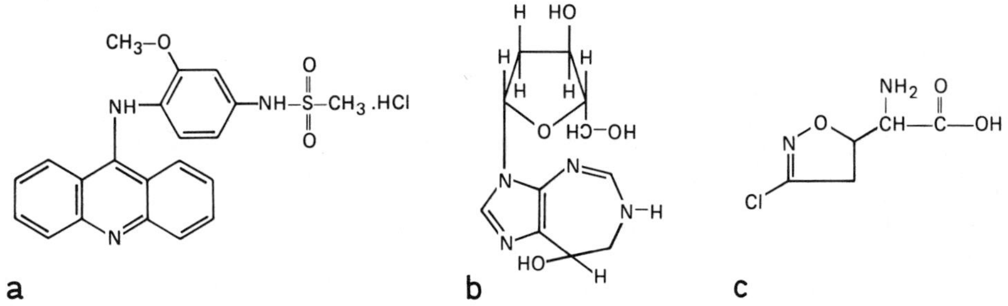

Fig. 1a–c. New chemical structures: **a** The DNA intercalating agent *m*-AMSA (4'-(9-acridinylamino) methane-sulfon-gmm-anisidide NSC-141549). **b** The adenosine deaminase inhibitor 2'-doxycoformycin (pentostatin)(d'dcF; Pentostatin, NSC 218321). **c** The glutamine antagonist AT-125 (5-isoxazoleacetic acid, α-amino-3-chloro-4,5-dihydro

Table 1. Phase I studies with AMSA

Institution (reference)	Disease	Maximal tolerated dose (MTD)
Mt. Sinai [26]		90 mg/m²/week
M. D. Anderson [38, 39]	Solid tumors	40 mg/m²/day × 3 q 3 weeks
	Acute leukemia	90 mg/m²/day × 5 q 3 weeks
NCI [63]		120 mg/m² q 4 weeks
BCRP [60]	Solid tumors	120 mg/m² q 2 weeks
	Acute leukemia	250 mg/m² q 3 weeks
Memorial Sloan-Kettering		90 mg/m²/week

toxicologic properties, coupled with occasional therapeutic responses observed, m-AMSA is currently undergoing extensive Phase II testing in the clinical panel [50]. Studies are being carried out in lung, colon, and breast cancers and malignant melanoma and lymphoma, as well as other tumors which are not part of the clinical panel.

Of special interest are studies being carried out in acute leukemia [49]. During the Phase I studies at Anderson MD and at the Baltimore Cancer Research Program (BCRP), NCI, doses were escalated in patients with acute leukemia in an effort to achieve marrow aplasia. The Anderson MD Hospital study utilized a 3–10 day daily schedule to total doses of 240–750 mg/m^2, which is more than five times the tolerable dose for solid tumors [38]. These observations have been confirmed by other investigators [26]. Similarly, at BCRP the single dose administered was escalated to 240 mg/m^2 [60]. Complete remissions were observed primarily in the repetitive daily schedules. At these higher doses, additional toxicities became manifest and included convulsions (3 of 25 patients at Anderson MD). Hepatotoxicity, nausea, and vomiting also became more prominent at the higher doses. The tolerance of leukemic patients to much higher doses of AMSA may be related to the nearly pure myelotoxic effects of the drug, or it could reflect the phenomenon of greater tolerance to anticancer drugs in the presence of leukemia described with deazuridine [49] and possibly other anticancer drugs. An experimental counterpart to this finding has been recently described [27] and suggests that explanations must be sought for this greater tolerance in the presence of leukemia, other than the simple fact that more aggressive regimens are employed in these patients in an effort to achieve hypoplasia of the replaced bone marrow.

Preliminary information from Phase II trials indicate activity for m-AMSA in leukemia and lymphoma, and possibly in breast cancer and melanoma. It is likely, therefore, that m-AMSA will be incorporated in drug combinations in these disease. Special consideration must be given to possible cross-resistance with adriamycin in some of these studies.

2'Deoxycoformycin (2'dCF)

Adenosine deaminase (ADA) catalyzes the deamination of adenosine and is an important enzyme system required for the function and viability of lymphocytes. ADA has been reported to be deficient in lymphocytes of patients with severe combined immunodeficiency [16, 24, 53]. Studies with inhibitors of ADA such as 2'dCF or erythro-9-(2-hydroxy-3-noryl)adenine (EHNA) indicate that these drugs induce lymphocytotoxicity which occurs as a result of sensitivity of lymphocytes to deoxyadenosine (AdR) metabolic products, particularly dATP [33]. Preclinical studies have confirmed the immunosuppressive and lympholytic effects of 2'dCF [7]. Interest in its antitumor properties was aroused by its ability also to inhibit the deamination of the purine nucleoside analog 9-β-D-arabinofuranosyladenine (ara-A) [37]. This latter compound is known for its selective antiviral activity [23, 51] as well as its antitumor activity in certain transplantable murine tumors [69]. Potentiation of the effect of ara-A by 2'dCF has been established in the P388 and L1210 leukemias and in the Ridgway Osteogenic Sarcoma murine systems. This potentiation is most apparent in the latter system [59]. The combination of ara-A and 2'dCF is also effective in L1210/ara-C and P388/ara-resistant sublines, although the former exhibits only partial sensitivity [59].

Interest in 2'dCF has been further stimulated by preliminary phase I clinical and pharmacologic studies [62]. Antileukemic activity with 2'dCF was demonstrable [33, 62]. As expected, the major toxic effect was related to profound lymphopenia: the peripheral lymphocyte count fell by more than 95% at the highest dose level (0.25 mg/kg daily × 5) in all eight patients so treated, with recovery occurring by day 11–18 [62]. Severe uric acid nephropathy occurred in one patient. Pharmacologic studies indicate persistence of $2 \times 10^{-8}\ M$ plasma levels by 24 h with 32% of the drug recovered in the urine. Of seven patients with acute lymphoblastic leukemia in the Phase I study, one complete remission was obtained, and two other patients exhibited improvement in their leukemic picture. Thrombocytopenia was also seen but was relatively mild.

Current efforts are directed toward additional studies of 2'dCF alone in leukemia. Laboratory studies correlating results with ADA levels in lymphocytes and the extent of inhibition achieved are planned. The sensitivity to 2'dCF of various lymphocyte subpopulations remains to be delineated [11]. In addition, there is interest in studying the combination of 2'dCF and ara-A clinically, and toxicology is ongoing to determine effects of the combination in dogs. It is likely that immunosuppressive effects of 2'dCF, as well as the potentiation of the antiviral effects of ara-A, will also be exploited. Finally laboratory studies indicate that 2'dCF also enhances the biologic activity of cordycepin (3'deoxyadenosine) and other adenosine analogs [31]. Clearly, 2'dCF offers exciting opportunities for exploring consequences of manipulating intracellular nucleoside metabolism, and for important laboratory and clinical correlations.

AT-125 (α-amino-3-chloro-2-isoxazoline-5-acetic acid; NSC 163501)

AT-125 is an amino acid antibiotic isolated from fermentation broths of *Streptomyces sviceus*. This drug has been found to be an inhibitor of glutamine utilization by L-asparagine, a property it shares with other glutamine antagonists such as DON (6-diazo-5-oxo-L-norleucine) [13]. Toxicity studies indicate its greater sensitivity for female mice, and particularly for younger animals [52]. Similar results have been observed with the antitumor antimetabolite 3-deazauridine [2]. These observations may have in common the fact that cytidine triphosphate synthetase, which is the primary target of 3-deazauridine inhibition, is a glutamine-dependent amidotransferase also inhibited by AT-125 [46, 52].

The spectrum of antitumor activity of AT-125 [28] is shown in Table 2 in comparison with another glutamine antagonist, DON. Following IP injection against L1210 leukemia, AT-125 was effective on all schedules tested and showed some superiority when given on an intermittent schedule every 3 h on days 1, 5, and 9. Activity against L1210 leukemia was also observed following oral and SC administration of AT-125. An approximate 80% inhibition of tumor growth was obtained against the SC implanted CD8F1 mammary tumor, and AT-125 also caused marginal increase of 47% in the life span of mice inoculated IV with the Lewis lung carcinoma. Only marginal activity was observed against the IC implanted L1210 and P388 leukemias, and there was no activity against the IC implanted murine ependymoblastoma. These data suggest that the penetration of AT-125 and/or metabolites into the CNS is minimal. Against three human tumor xenografts, AT-125 produced 3 of 4 minimal regressions in the MX-1 mammary and 2 of 4 minimal regressions in the LX-1 lung, but was not active in the CX-2 colon.

Table 2. Antitumor activity of glutamine antagonists: DON and AT-125[a]

System	DON	AT-125
Murine tumors		
IP L1210 leukemia	81% ILS ++	123% ILS ++
IP P388 leukemia	118% ILS ++	150% ILS ++
SC CD8F1 mammary	83% TWI +	80% TWI +
IV Lewis lung	–	47% ILS +
IP Colon 26	70% ILS ++	–
SC Colon 38	91% TWI ++	–
Human tumor xenografts		
SC LX-1 lung	96% TWI ++	+
SC MX-1 mammary	94% TWI ++	+
SC CX-2 colon	95% TWI ++	–

[a] Activity score: ++, meets DN2 activity criteria (see Appendix 1); +, reproducible activity; –, not active

Preclinical toxicology studies with AT-125 were performed in beagle dogs, rhesus monkeys, CD8F1 mice, guinea pigs, and rabbits. Clinical manifestations of drug toxicity were mainly limited to gastrointestinal disturbances. Dogs, monkeys, and guinea pigs experienced diarrhea and prostation; in dogs and monkeys, bloody stools were also observed. Dogs and monkeys displayed CNS toxicity such as convulsions of tremors, disorientation, and lethargy.

Hematologic toxicity (thrombocytopenia, lymphocytopenia) was observed in both dogs and monkeys. Alopecia was observed only in monkeys and guinea pigs, and rash in monkeys. No local tissue reaction was induced in guinea pigs and rabbits.

The quantitative toxicity of AT-125 is given in Table 3. In dogs, multiple doses resulted in a nearly 13-fold decrease in the tolerable cumulative dose. However, when dogs were treated with AT-125 on a dose schedule of 7.8 mg/m^2 daily × 5, with a 9-day rest period, for a total of three treatments (cumulative dose of 117 mg/m^2) there was no lethality. This dose is greater than the cumulative dose of 80 mg/m^2 which produced lethality on the daily × 5 and daily × 10 schedules. Furthermore, a single dose of 500 mg/m^2 weekly × 6 weeks given to dogs produced lethality at the cumulative dose of 3 000 mg/m^2, which is a threefold increase over the single dose of 1 000 mg/m^2 which producted lethality. The differential toxicity according to sex is also shown. This phenomenon and the greater tolerance of AT-125 in young males has been extensively studied in mice [52]. Although AT-125 shares many characteristics in common with DON, several differences exist such as in the antitumor spectrum and the type of glutamine sensitive reactions it inhibits [30]. Phase I clinical trial will be initiated late in 1979.

Rediscovered Anticancer Drugs (Fig. 2)

6-diazo-5-oxo-L-norleucine (DON; NSC 7365)

DON is an antibiotic isolated from a *Streptomyces* discovered in 1953 simultaneously with azaserine because of its antitumor activity against Sarcoma 180. It was soon

Table 3. Quantitative toxicity of AT-125

Species	Dose definition[a]	Drug schedule mg/m^2	Cumulative dose mg/m^2
Dog	LD	1,000 × 1	1,000
	TDH	500 × 1	500
	TDL	125 × 1	125
	HNTD	62.5 × 1	62.5
Dog	LD	15.6 × 5	78
	THD	7.8 × 5	39
	TDL	2.0 × 5	10
	HNTD	1.0 × 5	5
Dog	LD	7.8 × 10	78
	TDH	4.0 × 10	40
	TDL	1.0 × 10	10
	HNTD	0.5 × 10	5
Monkey	LD	31.7 × 5	158
	TDH	15.8 × 5	79
	TDL	4.0 × 5	20
	HNTD	1.9 × 5	9.5
Mouse (male)	LD$_{90}$	2,228 × 5	11,140
	LD$_{50}$	939 × 5	4,695
	LD$_{10}$	396 × 5	1,980
Mouse (female)	LD$_{90}$	639 × 5	3,195
	LD$_{50}$	313 × 5	1,565
	LD$_{10}$	154 × 5	770

[a] LD, lethal dose; TDH, toxic dose high; TDL, toxic dose low; HNTD, highest nontoxic dose

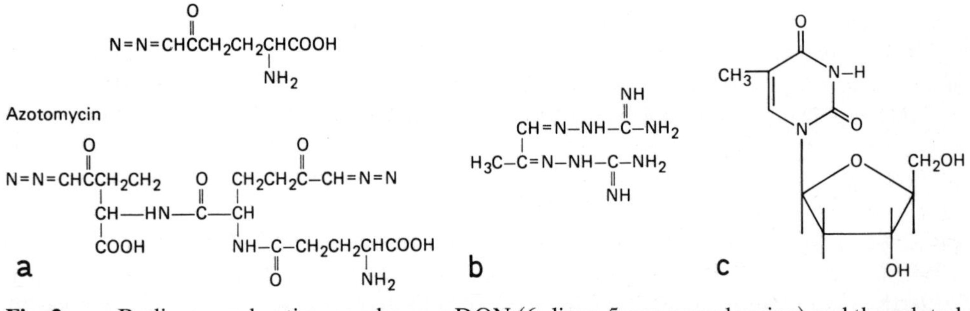

Fig. 2a–c. Rediscovered anticancer drugs: **a** DON (6-diazo-5-oxo-L-norleucine) and the related drug azotomycin. **b** Methylglyoxal bis-guanylhydrazone (Methyl-GAG, NSC 32946). **c** Thymidine (TdR)

identified as a glutamine antagonist because its potency was dramatically reduced in the presence of arginine and glutamine. L-glutamine plays an important role in the biosynthesis of proteins and nucleic acids; although it is a nonessential amino acid, some tissues are dependent on exogenous glutamine and are unable to synthesize it. Notably, various neoplastic tissues showed low L-glutamine, synthetase activity [20].

None of the glutamine antagonists, however, became established in clinical practice [43]. A few exceptional results were reported: DON was markedly effective against choriocarcinoma [42], and azotomycin showed some activity in colon cancer [66]. Azotomycin also produced by *Streptomyces* (Fig. 2) is actually a molecule formed by the condensation of two DON and one glutamine acid. It is rapidly converted to DON in vivo [55] and is inactive unless hydrolyzed [3].

Further clinical trials of a combination of azotomycin and 5-Fluorouracil (5-FU) in colon cancer yielded a relatively high response rate, 10 of 22 patients responding (45%) [65]. Because of those encouraging preliminary results and the lack of active chemotherapeutic agents in colon cancer, we shought to reevaluate the glutamine antagonists clinically.

The effects of azotomycin and DON on human tumor xenografts in nude mice were recently studied. Remarkable activity in these xenografts with a high therapeutic ratio was shown for both drugs [5]. DON, which is more readily available, was therefore selected for trial. Clinical data from the 1 950s indicated that DON had only moderate therapeutic activity [6], but it had been given only in low, daily, oral doses, which caused dose-limiting mucositis [44]. Recently, a new Phase I study was activated in Sloan-Kettering Memorial Hospital, in which the intermittent, IV administration of high doses of DON was investigated. Other dose schedules, such as single dose every 3 weeks or daily for 3 or 5 days, will also be explored in Phase I before going on to Phase II trials.

Methyl-GBG (Methyl-glyoxal bis-Guanylhydrazone; Methyl-GAG; NSC 32946)

Methyl-GBG is a substituted guanylhydrazone compound (see Fig. 2) synthesized in 1958 and found to be active against mouse L1210 leukemia [22]. Many years later, its mechanism of action was linked to its potent inhibition of 5-adenosylmethionine decarboxylase which catalyzes synthesis of spermidine and spermine [14]. This inhibition occurs at drug concentrations much lower than those utilized to inhibit protein synthesis or mitochondrial respiration in earlier experiments. Polyamines have been demonstrated to interact at a number of different intracellular levels. However, a major role of spermidine appears to be in the initiation of DNA synthesis, possibly through stabilization of the DNA polymerase-helix complex [10]. Recent research has demonstrated that polyamines are excreted in excess amounts in patients with cancer and that the pattern of polyamine excretion may vary directly with response to therapy [19].

A series of trials initially demonstrated significant activity in human acute leukemia (154 patients − 53 CR, 34%) [41]. The drug was generally administered daily until response or toxicity, and toxicity was prohibitive, including severe mucositis, myelosuppression, hepatic and renal damage, and hypoglycemia (occasionally fatal). Although very limited experience was obtained in solid tumors, Falkson reported five partial remissions in 21 patients with esophageal cancer. The daily dose schedule used was again associated with serious drug toxicity [21]. Delayed urinary excretion ot intact drug may explain the toxicity of daily schedules; only 60% of an administered IV dose is excreted in the urine and less than 20% in the feces, over a 3 week period (Davidson 1965, cit. by [15]).

A broad Phase II trial by the Eastern Drug Evaluation Program and the Eastern Cooperative Oncology Group (ECOG) using a weekly or biweekly intramuscular schedules of 6–10 mg/kg per week demonstrated responses in a number of tumors (breast 2 of 8, colon 2 of 15, esophagus 2 of 3, lymphoma 4 of 7) with somewhat improved therapeutic index [61]. Nevertheless, no new studies with Methyl-GBG were initiated for several years.

More recently, Dr. William Knight (San Antonio), in a Southwest Oncology Group Phase I–II pilot study, has reevaluated the drug using a weekly IV dose schedule. In a poor risk population (average ECOG scale performance status 2.6, mostly pretreated patients with solid tumors), he observed no toxicity at 500–700 mg/m^2 weekly in 34 of 47 patients (74%). Toxicity, when encountered, consisted mainly of mucositis (11 of 47, 23%, only one life threatening). The incidence of weight loss, malaise, vasculitis, neuromyopathy, balanitis, and ileus was estimated to be less than 10%. Myelosuppression is minimal or absent at the dose utilized [32].

Notably, this study not only continues to provide strong hints of antitumor activity but also indicates that tolerable dose schedules may be devised. Of 47 patients evaluable for response, three complete responders (one transitional cell bladder, one clear cell, primary unknown, and one acute myeloid leukemia) and two partial responders (one adenocarcinoma of colon, one squamous esophagus) were reported. Two of the patients with complete responses had underlying renal impairment and thus suggests responsiveness may increase as higher doses are used.

Because of these results, we are obtaining information on the full spectrum of preclinical antitumor activity, including the newer xenograft models. Phase I trials in several new schedules followed by complete evaluation of the clinical panel in Phase II studies are planned. Studies of polyamine metabolism and drug pharmacology, in addition, may add new dimensions to these clinical investigations.

Thymidine (TdR; NSC 21548)

Clinical trials with TdR as an antitumor agent were begun in January 1979. Interest in utilizing TdR clinically was sparked by laboratory observations by Lee, Giovanella, and Stehlin [35], and subsequently by pharmacologic studies done by one of the investigators on himself in collaboration with Zaharko [70]. The observation that millimolar (mM) levels were achievable and sustained during TdR infusion for 24 h prompted the initiation of Phase II efficacy trials. These were instituted to mimic the experimental circumstances demonstrating effectiveness of TdR on a variety of human tumor xenografts [34, 36].

Interest in TdR's action on neoplastic cells is not new. In addition to its use as a radioactive marker when incorporated ino DNA of dividing cells, the agent has been used as a cell synchronizing agent in tissue culture. This latter action has been attributed to the inhibition of DNA which follows the feedback inhibition from high TTP levels. Restoration of DNA synthesis of ribonucleotide reductase can be achieved by administration of deoxycytidylate triphosphate (dCTP) which is depleted as a result of this inhibitory activity. Possible therapeutic use of TdR was postulated by Beltz and co-workers (1972) [1]. Increased susceptibility of neoplastic cells to TdR in tissue culture had been demonstrated by several investigators. Giovanella was further encouraged by the greater sensitivity of transformed or neoplastic tissues than their normal counterparts. In a series of experiments designed to provide high doses of TdR for long periods of time, he and his co-workers were able to first confirm in vivo inhibition of tumor growth and then actually regression of human tumors growing in human tumor xenografts [34, 36]. Millimolar concentrations and several courses were required to produce regression. Curiously, complete regression often followed a sudden increase in tumor size, and upon TdR withdrawal. These experiments have only partially been confirmed by Howell, who noted some activity against human melanoma growing in these mice [29].

To achieve millimolar levels in humans, doses must be administered in large fluid volumes (more than 5 liters of TdR in hypotonic saline) delivering 75 g/m^2 per day. TdR is rapidly degraded to thymine, but with the amounts administered, saturation of the phosphorylase system takes place causing a slower rate of degradation of TdR and the feasibility of sustained millimolar concentrations. Large amounts of both TdR and thymine are, of course, excreted in the urine. Thymine, being less soluble, may crystallize in the urine upon refrigeration [8].

The clinical effects of TdR in high doses are becoming better delineated. Leukopenia and thrombocytopenia result from 0−4 days after 5-day infusions of the drug and are reversible in a few days [8]. Severe leukopenia has been recorded but is rare. Commonly seen are a number of other symptoms of moderate severity, including headaches, which may be attributed in part to fluid overload and isotonic volume expansion. On the other hand, central nervous symptoms such as somnolence, memory impairment, and visual illusions are not well explained, Nausea, vomiting, anorexia, and diarrhea also occur in over two-thirds of patients.

Antitumor activity manifested by clearing of circulating blasts has been readily demonstrable in leukemic patients. However, no complete remissions have been reported and blasts rapidly return following termination of the infusion [8, 67]. This latter phenomenon may be an indication of synchronization. In a variety of solid tumors, primarily colon cancer and melanomas, activity has not been striking although some transient objective regressions have been noted [8, 67]. The lack of disease progression which has been reported is difficult to interpret. Plans are proceeding to continue Phase II clinical studies in a minimum clinical panel of tumors.

Preceding and concurrently with these studies, efforts have been initiated seeking to improve the therapeutic effectiveness of 5-FU or methotrexate when given in combination with TdR. More recently, interest in TdR plus ara-C combinations has also been awakened. The rationale for these combinations has been recently reviewed [45] and lies beyond the scope of this report. It is noteworthy, however, that the rediscovery of Tdr's therapeutic potential alone or in combination is related to our ability to monitor pharmacologic levels of these nucleosides, analogs, and related antimetabolites. Elucidation of the tumor selectivity of drugs such as 5-FU, MTX, and ara-C may result from these manipulations.

Second Generation Anticancer Drugs (Fig. 3)

Pentamethylmelamine (PMM; NSC 118742)

PMM is a monodemethylated derivative of hexamethylmelamine (HMM, NSC 13875, see Fig. 3). Since HMM is sparingly soluble in aqueous solutions, it must be administered orally despite its dose-limiting gastrointestinal toxicity. It is metabolized in man by extensive *N*-demethylation and proceeds through PMM as the first intermediate in the process. PMM has 23.7 times the solubility in water of HMM [12] and was thus developed as a suitable alternative for parenteral administration. The mechanism of action of these compounds is unknown. Although they exhibit a spectrum of toxicity and activity similar to many alkylators, both compounds were inactive in the *p*-nitrobenzyl pyridine chemical test of alkylating activity [68], and HMM has demonstrated activity in patients whose tumors are resistant to alkylating agents [40]. They display equivalent activity in animal antitumor screens, i.e., minimal activity against a wide variety of rodent tumors [9] but moderate activity against the human MX-1 and MX-2 breast xenografts [9] and a human lung tumor xenograft (P246) [12]. Animal toxicology studies with PMM demonstrated significant acute central nervous system stimulation, including seizures and sudden death, which was dose-rate dependent, i.e., rapid injection could produce stimulation even at relatively low dose levels [9]. Other toxic effects included damage to the integumentary (injection site), lymphatic, renal, and reproductive (male) systems with equivocal involvement of the cardiovascular, respiratory, and gastrointestinal symptoms.

The parent HMM has demonstrated activity in a wide variety of tumors including lymphoma, bronchogenic carcinoma and breast, cervical, and ovarian cancer, but the studies were hampered by its gastrointestinal intolerance [40]. PMM is now undergoing active Phase I studies in a daily (for 5–10 days), intermittent (weekly and

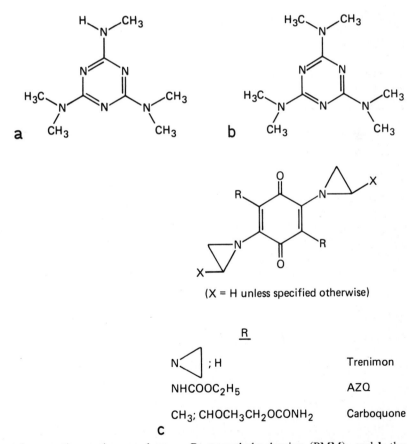

(X = H unless specified otherwise)

	R	
N△ ; H		Trenimon
NHCOOC$_2$H$_5$		AZQ
CH$_3$; CHOCH$_3$CH$_2$OCONH$_2$		Carboquone

c

Fig. 3a–c. Second generation anticancer drugs: **a** Pentamethylmelamine (PMM), and **b** the parent compound hexamethylmelamine (HMM), and **c** AZQ and related aziridinylbenzoquinones

Table 4. Antitumor activity of AZQ

System	Drug route	Activity[a]
Murine tumors		
IP L1210 leukemia	IP	120% ILS[b] ++
IP P388 leukemia	IP	138% ILS ++
IP B16 melanoma	IP	70% ILS ++
IP Colon 26	IP	> 225% ILS ++
IC L1210 leukemia	IP	84% ILS ++
IC Ependymoblastoma	IP	> 349% ILS ++
IC P388 leukemia	IP	60% ILS +
SC CDF$_1$ mammary	IP	89% TWI[c] +
SC Colon 38	IP	83% TWI +
IV Lewis lung	IP	−
IC B16 melanoma	IP	−
Human tumor xenografts		
S.R.C.[d] MX-1 mammary		++
S.R.C. LX-1 lung		−
S.R.C. CX-1 colon		−

[a] Activity: ++, meets decision network 2A activity criteria; +, reproducible activity; −, not active
[b] %ILS, percent increase in life span
[c] %TWI, percent tumor weight inhibition
[d] Subrenal capsule assay

ever 3−4 weeks) and continuous infusion schedule. The drug is given over at least one hour to minimize the potential for acute neurotoxic reactions seen in animal studies, and to date no such reactions have been observed. Sporadic thrombocytopenia, which was not clearly dose related, and gastrointestinal disturbances appear to be the only reproducible toxicities to date. The availability of a parenteral form related to HMM should allow a more interpretable result of efficacy in Phase II studies and its relationship to dose-rate. Similar observations concerning neurotoxicity will also be crucial with regard to the ultimate potential of these drugs beyond a period of induction. The relationship of neurotoxicity and efficacy to pyridoxine administration must also be reassessed.

Aziridinylbenzoquinone (AZQ; 1,4-Cyclohexadiene-1,4-dicarbamic acid, 2,5-bis(1-aziridinyl)-3,6-dioxo-, diethyl ester; NSC 182986)

AZQ is an aziridinyl quinone. Antitumor agents which contain the quinone moiety include mitomycin C, adiramycin, daunomycin, streptonigrin, lapachol, and porfiromycin [18]. More closely related are the aziridinylbenzoquinones which include triethyleniminebenzoquinone (Trenomon) and carboquone [58]. Aziridinylbenzoquinones have been known to posses physicochemical properties which are associated with penetration of CNS, and many of these compounds have been found to be effective against the IC implanted L1210 leukemia. A comparison of more than 30 aziridinylbenzoquinones in IC and IP implanted murine tumor systems showed AZQ

Table 5. Toxic dose levels of AZQ in dogs and mice

Species	Defined dose[a]	Daily dose mg/m^2	Cumulative dose mg/m^2
Dog	LD	25×1	25
	TDH	12.5×1	12.5
	TDL	3.2×1	3.2
	HNTD	1.6×1	1.6
Dog	LD	6.2×5	31
	TDH	3.2×5	16
	TDL	1.6×5	8
	HNTD	0.8×5	4
Mice	LD_{90}	32.4×1	32.4
	LD_{50}	30×1	30
	LD_{10}	25.8×1	25.8

[a] LD, lethal dose; TDH, toxic dose high; TDL, toxic dose low; HNTD, highest nontoxic dose

to be the superior compound; and also because of its favorable water solubility, AZQ was developed for clinical trials [17].

The antitumor activity of this drug against murine tumors and human tumor xenografts is summarized in Table 4. In the IC implanted ependymoblastoma, there was a greater than 349% increase in life span (% ILS) when AZQ aas administered on a QD × 5 schedule. Although less effective in the IC implanted leukemias, AZQ showed a greater than 50% ILS on a QD × 9 schedule. There was no activity against the IC implanted B16 melanoma. However, AZQ showed a 70% ILS against IP B16 melanoma on the QD × 9 schedule and, in addition, showed activity against the solid tumors colon 26, colon 38, and CD8F mammary tumor. Against the IP implanted L1210 leukemia, AZQ was effective on every schedule which was tested, and there was some superiority for the QD × 9 and day 1, 5, 9 schedules. It shows some activity against the MX-1 human mammary tumor xenograft.

Preclinical toxicology studies indicate that major clinical manifestations of drug toxicity involve the gastrointestinal system. Clinical signs of emesis and/or hematemesis and bloody stolls were observed in dogs. Both dogs and monkeys exhibited hematologic toxicity with the major change being dose-related, reversible leukopenia.

The quantitative toxicity of AZQ in dogs and mice is summarized in Table 5. A daily dose of 6.2 mg/m^2 was lethal when given in a five or ten daily dose schedule whereas a single dose of 25 mg/m^2 was lethal. Rest intervals had no ameliorating effect on toxicity. Phase I clinical trials will probably proceed at starting doses of 1.0 mg/m^2 single dose or 0.5 mg/m^2 daily × 5 days, which correspond to one-third of toxic dose low (TDL) values.

Summary

In summary, Phase I trials in 1979 include some drugs representing totally new structures, new schedules of old compounds undergoing reevaluation, and second

Appendix 1. DCT tumor panel screening protocol

Tumor model	Site of tumor transplant	Treatment route-schedule	Parameter	Activity criteria	Decision network criteria[a]
Mouse tumors					
Leukemia L1210	IP	IP-qd, d 1–9	ILS (%)[b]	25	50
B16 Melanoma	IP	IP-qd, d 1–9	ILS (%)	25	50
CD8Fl Mammary	SC	IP-q7d × 5	TWI (%)[c]	58	90
Lewis lung	IV	IP-qd, d 1–9	ILS (%)	40	50
Colon 38	SC	IP-q7d × 2	TWI (%)	58	90
Human tumor xenografts					
Colon – CX-1, 5	SC	IP-q4d × 3			
Mammary – MX-1	SC	or	TWI (%)	58	90
Lung – LX-1	SC	IP-q7d × 4			
Prescreen					
Leukemia P388	IP	IP-qd, d 1–9	ILS (%)	20	75

[a] DN$_2$ is decision point to proceed with further formulation, scale-up and toxicologic studies to pass it requires having established antitumor activity with above criteria
[b] ILS, Increase in life span
[c] TWI, Tumor weight inhibition

generation compounds. The rational development of analogs based on structure-activity relationships and on overcoming pharmacologic or toxicologic problems of parent compounds requires much future emphasis; two such examples (pentamethylmelamine and AZQ) are cited here. For all drugs, a plan of clinical development should ensure a more thorough initial evaluation as well as validation of concepts and systems that have prompted their introduction into the clinic. Establishment of clinical usefulness for the new structures, and particularly for three compounds herein reintroduced after a long period of oblivion, would constitute tangible proof of methodological and technocological advances that have taken place in the development and clinical evaluation of anticancer drugs.

References

1. Beltz RE, Jolley WB, Waters RN, Hinshaw DB (1972) Growth inhibitors rapidly inactivated by the host as potential antineoplastic agents in intra-arterial infusion chemotherapy. Oncology 26: 121–133
2. Bloch A, Dutschman G, Grindey G, Simpson CL (1974) Prevention by testosterone of the intestinal toxicity caused by the antitumor agent 3-deazauridine. Cancer Res 34: 1299–1303
3. Brockman RW, Pittillo RF, Shaddix S, Hill DL (1970) Mode of action of azotomycin. Antimicrob Agents Chemother 1969: 56–62
4. Cain BF, Atwell GJ (1974) The experimental antitumor properties of three congeners of the acridylmethanesulphonanilide (AMSA) series. Eur J Cancer 10: 539–549
5. Catane R, Ovejera AA, Houchens DP, von Hoff DD, Davis HL jr, Wolpert MK, Rozencweig M, Muggia FM (1978) Rationale for further clinical trials with 6-diazo-5-oxo-L-norleucine (DON). Proc Am Assoc Cancer Res Proc Am Soc Clin Oncol 19: 317
6. Catane R, von Hoff DD, Glaubiger DL, Muggia FM (to be published) Azaserine, DON and azotomycin: Three diazo analogs of L-glutamine with clinical antitumor activity. Cancer Treat Rep
7. Chassin MM, Chirigos MA, Johns DG, Adamson RH (1977) Adenosine deaminase inhibition for immunosuppression (Letter to the editor). N Engl J Med 296: 1232
8. Chiuten DF, Wiernik PH, Zaharko DS, Edwards L (1979) Phase I–II trial and clinical pharmacology of continuously infused high-dose thymidine. Proc Am Assoc Cancer Res Proc Am Soc Clin Oncol 20: 76
9. Clinical Brochure (1978) Pentamethylmelamine (NSC-118742), Investigational Drug Branch, Cancer Therapy Evaluation program, Division of Cancer Treatment
10. Cohen S (1971) Organic cations in the structure and function of the nucleic acids. In: Englewood C (ed) Introduction to the polyamines. Prentice-Hall, New Jersey, pp 111–146
11. Coleman MS, Greenwood MF, Hutton JJ, Holland P, Lampkin B, Krill C, Kastelic JE (1978) Adenosine deaminase, terminal deoxynucleotidyl transferase (TdT), and cell surface markers in childhood acute leukemia. Blood 52: 1125–1131
12. Connors TA, Cumber AJ, Ross WCJ, Clarke SA, Mitchley BCV (1977) Regression of human lung tumor xenografts induced by water-soluble analogs of hexamethylmelamine (letter). Cancer Treat Rep 61: 927–928
13. Cooney DA, Jayaram HN, Ryan JA, Bono VH (1974) Inhibition of L-asparaginase synthetase by a new amino acid antibiotic with antitumor activity: L(αS, 5S)-α-amino-3-chloro-4,5-dihydro-5-isoxazoleacetic acid (NSC-163501). Cancer Chemother Rep 58: 793–802

14. Corti A, Dave C, Williams-Ashman HG, Mihich E, Schenone A (1974) Specific inhibition of the enzymatic decarboxylation of S-adenosylmethionine by methylglyoxal bis (guanyl-hydrazone) and related substances. Biochem J 139: 351−357

15. Oliverio V, Zubrod CG (1965) Clinical pharmacology of the effective antitumor drugs. Ann Rev Pharmacol Toxicol 5: 351

16. Dissing J, Knudsen B (1972) Adenosine-deaminase deficiency and combined immuno-deficiency syndrome. Lancet II: 1316

17. Driscoll JS, Dudeck L, Congleton G, Geran RI (1979) Potential CNS antitumor agents. VI: aziridinylbenzoquinones III. J Pharm Sci 68: 185−188

18. Driscoll JS, Hazard GF, Wood HB jr, Goldin A (1974) Structure − antitumor activity relationships among guinone derivatives. Cancer Chemother Rep 4: 1−362

19. Durie BGM, Salmon SE, Russell DH (1977) Polyamines as markers of response and disease activity in cancer chemotherapy. Cancer Res 37: 214−221

20. El-Asmar FA, Greenberg DM (1966) Studies of the mechanism of inhibition of tumor growth by the enzyme glutaminase. Cancer Res 26: 116−122

21. Falkson G (1971) Methyl GAG (NSC 32946) in the treatment of esophagus cancer. Cancer Chemother Rep 55: 209−212

22. Freedlander BL, French FA (1958) Carcinostatin action of polycarbonyl compounds and their derivatives. II. Glyoxal bis (guanylhydrazone) and derivatives. Cancer Res 18: 360−363

23. Furth JJ, Cohen SS (1967) Inhibition of mammalian DNA polymerase by the 5'-triphosphate of 9-β-D-arabinofuranosyladenine. Cancer Res 27: 1528−1533

24. Giblett ER, Anderson JE, Cohen F, Pallara B, Meawissen H Adenosine-deaminase deficiency in two patients with severely impaired cellular immunity. Lancet 2: 1067−1069

25. Goldin A, Venditti JM, Muggia FM, Rozencweig M, de Vita VT (1979) New animal models for anticancer agents. In: Fox BW (ed) Advances in medical oncology, research and education. Proceedings of the XIIth International Cancer Congress, Buenos Aires, vol 5. Pergamon Press, Oxford New York, pp 113−122

26. Goldsmith MA, Bhardwaj S, Ohnuma T, Greenspan EM, Holland JF (1979) Phase I study of m-AMSA in patients with solid tumors and leukemias. Proc Am Assoc Cancer Res Proc Am Soc Clin Oncol 20: 344

27. Hagenbeek A (1977) Master's thesis, Erasmus University, Rotterdam

28. Houchens DP, Ovejera A, Sheridan M, Johnson RK, Bogden AE, Neil GL (1979) Therapy for mouse tumors and human tumor xenografts with the antitumor antibiotic AT-125. Cancer Treat Rep 63: 473−476

29. Howell SB, Jenkins R (1979) Evaluation of thymidine as a chemotherapeutic agent against human tumor xenografts in nude mice. Proc. Am Assoc Cancer Res 20: 259

30. Jayaram HN, Cooney DA, Ryan JA, Neil G, Dion RL, Bono VH (1975) L-[αS,5S]-α-ami-no-3-chloro-4,5-dihydro-5-isoxazoleacetic acid (NSC-163501): A new amino acid antibiotic with the properties of an antagonist of L-glutamine. Cancer Chemother Rep 59: 481−491

31. Johns DG, Adamson RH (1976) Enhancement of the biological activity of cordycepin (3'-deoxyadenosine) by the adenosine deaminase inhibitor 2'-deoxycoformycin. Biochem Pharmacol 25: 1441−1444

32. Knight WA, Livingston RB, Fabian C, Costanzi J (1979) Methyl-glyoxyl bis-guanylhy-drazone in advanced human malignancy. Proc Am Assoc Cancer Res Proc Am Soc Clin Oncol 20: 319

33. Koller C, Grever M, Mitchell B (1979) Treatment of acute lymphoblastic leukemia with the adenosine deaminase inhibitor 2'-deocycoformycin. Proc Am Assoc Cancer Res Proc Am Soc Clin Oncol 20: 382

34. Lee SS, Giovanella BC, Stehlin JS (1977) Effect of excess thymidine on the growth of human melanoma cells transplanted in thymus deficient nude mice. Cancer Lett 3: 209−214

35. Lee SS, Giovanella BC, Stehlin JS (1977) Selective lethal effect of thymidine on human mouse tumor cells. Physiologist 92: 401–405
36. Lee SS, Giovanella BC, Stehlin JS, Brunn JC (1979) Further studies on the long-term effects of high-dose thymidine infusion on human tumors heterotransplanted in nude mice. Proc Am Assoc Cancer Res Proc Am Soc Clin Oncol 20: 234
37. Le Page GA, Worth LS, Kimball AP (1976) Enhancement of the antitumor activity of arabinofuranosyladenine by 2'-deoxycoformycin. Cancer Res 36: 1481–1485
38. Legha SS, Bodey GP, Keating MJ, Blumenschein GR, Hortobagyi GN, Buzdar AU, McCredie K, Freireich EJ (1979) Early clinical evaluation of acridinyl-amino methane-sulfon-*m*-anisidide (AMSA) in patients with advanced breast cancer and acute leukemia. Proc Am Assoc Cancer Res 20: 416
39. Legha SS, Gutterman JV, Hall SW, Benjamin RS, Burgess MA, Valdivieso M, Bodey GP (1978) Phase I clinical investigation of 4'-(9-acridinylamino)-methanesulfon-*m*-anisidide (NSC-249992), a new acridine derivative. Cancer Res 38: 3712–3716
40. Legha SS, Slavik M, Carter SK (1976) Hexamethylmelamine – An evaluation of its role in the therapy of cancer. Cancer 38: 27–35
41. Levin RH, Henderson E, Karon M, Freireich EJ (1965) Treatment of acute leukemia with methylglyoxyl-bis-guanylhydrazone (methyl GAG). Clin Pharmacol Ther 6: 31–42
42. Li MC (1961) Management of choriocarcinoma and related tumors of uterus and testis. Med Clin North Am 45: 661–676
43. Livingston RB, Venditti M, Cooney DA, Carter SK (1970) Glutamine antagonists in chemotherapy. Adv Pharmacol Chemother 8: 57–120
44. Magill GB, Myers WPL, Reilly HC, Putnam RC, Magill JW, Sykes MP, Escher GC, Karnofsky DA, Burchenal JH (1957) Pharmacological and initial therapeutic observations on 6-diazo-5-oxo-L-norleucine (DON) in human neoplastic disease. Cancer 10: 1138–1150
45. Martin DS, Stolfi RL, Sawyer RC, Nayak R, Spiegelman S, Young CW, Woodcock T (to be published) An overview of thymidine. Cancer
46. McPartland RP, Wang MC, Bloch A, Weinfeld H (1974) Cytidine 5'-triphosphate synthetase as a target for inhibition by the antitumor agent 3-deazauridine. Cancer Res 34: 3107–3111
47. Muggia FM (1978) Clinical evaluation of new antitumor antibiotics. Recent Results Cancer Res 63: 288–297
48. Muggia FM, Bono VH, de Vita VT jr (1978) New anticancer drugs. Antibiot Chemother 23: 42–49
49. Muggia FM, Chiuten D, von Hoff DD, Rozencweig M, Wiernik P (1979) New drugs against human leukemia. In: Crouthner DG (ed) Advances in mediacl oncology, research and education. Proceedings of the XIIth International Cancer Congress, vol 7. Pergamon Press, Buenos Aires, Oxford New York, pp 55–62
50. Muggia FM, Rozencweig M, Chiuten D, Jensen-Akula M, Charles L, Kubota T, Bono V (to be published) Phase II trials: Use of a clinical tumor panel and overview of current resources and studies. Cancer Treat Rep
51. Müller WEG, Zahn RB, Bittingmaier K, Falke D Inhibitions of herpesvirus DNA synthesis by 9-β-D-arabinofuranosyladenine in cellular and cell-free systems. Ann NY Acad Sci 284: 34–48
52. Neil GL, Berger AE, McPartland RP, Grindey GB, Bloch A (1979) Biochemical and pharmacological effects of the fermentation-derived antitumor agent (αS,5S)-α-ami-no-3-chloro-4,5-dihydro-5-isoxazoleacetic acid (AT-125). Cancer Res 39: 852–856
53. Ochs HD, Young JE, Giblett ER, Chen SH, Scott CR, Wedgwood RJ (1973) Adenosine-deaminase deficiency and severe combined immunodeficiency syndrome. Lancet 1: 1393
54. Ovejera AA, Houchens DP, Barker AD (1977) Chemotherapeutic sensitivity to anticancer drugs of human tumor xenografts in athymic mice. Curr Chemother 2: 1144–1146

55. Pittillo RF, Woolley C, Brockman RW, Ho DH (1971) Azotomycin (NSC-156654): Biologic fate in mice and man. Cancer Chemother Rep 55: 47–52

56. Rozencweig M, de Sloover C, von Hoff DD, Tagnon H, Muggia FM (to be published) Anthracycline derivatives in new drug development programs: Proceedings of the NCI-EORTC Symposium on Anthracycline Derivatives. Cancer Treat Rep

57. Rozencweig M, von Hoff DD, Cysyk RL, Muggia FM (to be published) AMSA and PALA: Two new agents in cancer chemotherapy. Clin Chemother Pharmacol

58. Saito T, Himori T (1978) Clinical evaluation of a new anticancer alkylating agent, carboquone (NSC-134679). In: Current chemotherapy, Proceedings of the 10th International Congress of Chemotherapy, vol II, pp 1235–1238

59. Schabel FM (1979) Test systems for evaluating the antitumor activity of nucleoside analogues. In: Walker RT, DeClercq E, Eckstein F (eds) Nucleoside analogues: Chemistry, biology, and medical applications. Plenum Press, New York, pp 363–394

60. Schneider R, Sklaroff R, Ochoa M jr, Young C (1979) Phase I trial of AMSA [4'-(9-acrindylamino)-methane-sulfon-m-anisidide]. Proc Am Assoc Cancer Res Proc Am Soc Clin Oncol 20: 114

61. Shnider BI, Colsky J, Jones R, Carbone PP (1974) Effectiveness of methyl-GAG (NSC 32946) administered intramuscularly. Cancer Chemother Rep 58: 689–695

62. Smyth JF, Chassin MM, Harrap KR, Adamson RH, Johns DG (1979) 2'-deoxycoformycin (DCF): Phase I trial and clinical pharmacology. Proc Am Assoc Cancer Res Proc Am Soc Clin Oncol 20: 47

63. Von Hoff DD, Howser D, Gromley P, Bender RA, Glaubiger D, Levine AS, Young RC (1978) Phase I study of methanesulfonamide, N-4-(9-acridinylamino)-3-methoxyphenyl-(m-AMSA) using a single dose schedule. Cancer Treat Rep 62: 1421–1426

64. Von Hoff DD, Rozencweig M, Soper WT, Helman LJ, Penta JS, Davis HL, Muggia FM (1977) Whatever happened to NSC? Cancer Treat Rep 62: 759–768

65. Weiss AJ, Mastrangelo MJ (1970) Phase I study of a combination of azotomycin and 5FU in malignant disease. Cancer Chemother Rep 54: 109–111

66. Weiss AJ, Ramirez G, Grage T, Strawitz J, Goldman L, Downing V (1968) Phase II study of azotomycin. Cancer Chemother Rep 52: 611–614

67. Woodcock T, Damin L, O'Hehir M, Hansen H, Andreeff M, Young C (1979) Early clinical and pharmacokinetic evaluation of thymidine therapy in patients with advanced cancer. Proc. Am Assoc Cancer Res Proc Am Soc Clin Oncol 20: 114

68. Worzalla JF, Johnson BM, Ramirez G, Bryan GT (1973) N-demethylation of the antineoplastic agent hexamethylmelamine by rats and man. Cancer Res 33: 2810–2815

69. York JL, Le Page GA (1966) A proposed mechanism for the action of 9-β-D-arabino-furanosyladenine as an inhibitor of the growth of some ascites tumors cells. Can J Biochem 44: 19–26

70. Zaharko DS, Bolten BJ, Giovanella BC, Stehlin JS (1979) Thymidine and thymine measurements in biological fluids: mouse, monkey, and man. Proc Am Assoc Cancer Res Proc Am Soc Clin Oncol 20: 62

Fundamental Studies on Bestatin: A Small Molecular Microbial Product Enhancing Immune Responses

H. Umezawa

Institute of Microbial Chemistry, 14–23, Kamiosaki 3-Chome, Shinagawa-ku, J – Tokyo 141

The author initiated the screening study of enzyme inhibitors produced by microorganisms in 1965, and found about 50 new microbial products. These small molecular enzyme inhibitors have various bioactivities, but no significant antimicrobial activity. The finding of these inhibitors indicates that microorganisms in nature have acquired the ability to produce various compounds that have no obvious function in the growth of microbial cells and that have widely varied chemical structures [12, 14]. Therefore, if an exact screening method can be established, it is reasonable to search for small molecular microbial products which can modulate immune responses.

In this paper, the author will review the studies on the discovery and development of bestatin.

Discovery of Small Molecular Microbial Immunomodulators

The administration of a very small dose of coriolin group antibiotics and their active derivatives (Fig. 1) which inhibited Na^+-K^+-ATPase [9] increased the number of antibody-forming cells in mouse spleen [7]. Diketocoriolin B, one of the derivatives, at 0.1 ng/ml also increased the number of antibody-forming cells in cultured mouse spleen lymphocytes and was suggested to act on B cells. Glycopeptides such as lectins bind to the surface of immune cells, cause mitogenesis, and enhance immune responses. Therefore, the author thought that the action of coriolins and diketo-coriolin B to increase the number of antibody-forming cells might be due to their binding to Na^+-K^+-ATPase on the membrane of cells involved in immune reactions. The author also thought that small molecular compounds that bound to the surface of immune cells might modulate immune responses, and he searched for inhibitors of enzymes on the surface of immune cells.

We found that aminopeptidases which hydrolyzed N-terminal peptide bonds were located not only in cells but also on the cell surface of all kinds of animal cells including macrophages and lymphocytes, but they were not released extracellularly [2]. We also found that alkaline phosphatase and esterase were located on the cellular surface.

On the other hand, during this study on enzymes located on the surface of animal cells, we [16] found bestatin (Fig. 2) which inhibited aminopeptidase B (prepared from rat liver) and leucine aminopeptidase (prepared from hog kidney).

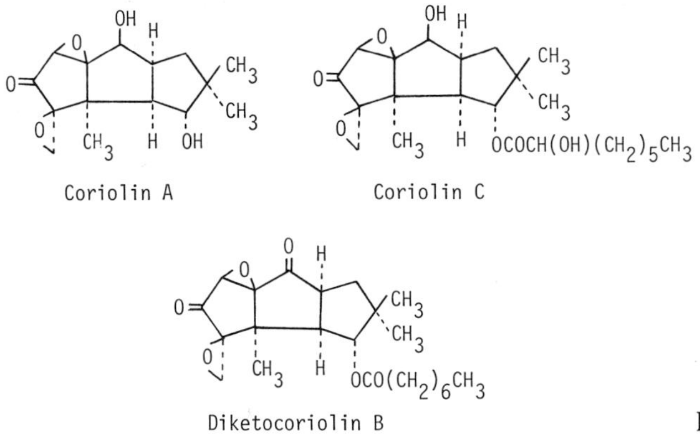

Coriolin A   Coriolin C

Diketocoriolin B   **Fig. 1.** Coriolins

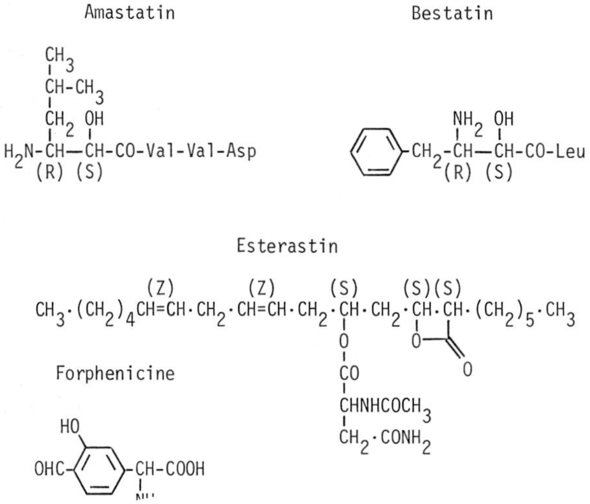

Amastatin   Bestatin

$$CH_3$$
$$CH-CH_3$$
$$CH_2 \; OH$$
$$H_2N-CH-CH-CO-Val-Val-Asp$$
$$\quad (R) \; (S)$$

$$-CH_2-CH-CH-CO-Leu$$
$$\qquad NH_2 \; OH$$
$$\qquad (R) \; (S)$$

Esterastin

$$CH_3 \cdot (CH_2)_4 CH=CH \cdot CH_2 \cdot CH=CH \cdot CH_2 \cdot CH \cdot CH_2 \cdot CH \cdot CH \cdot (CH_2)_5 \cdot CH_3$$
$$\quad (Z) \qquad (Z) \qquad (S) \qquad (S)(S)$$

Forphenicine
$$CO$$
$$CHNHCOCH_3$$
$$CH_2 \cdot CONH_2$$

$$OHC-\bigcirc-CH-COOH$$
$$HO$$

Fig. 2. Amastatin, bestatin, forphenicine, and esterastin

Bestatin was a strong inhibitor of these enzymes and the type of the inhibition was competitive with the substrates. The binding of bestatin to rat macrophages, lymphocytes, and mouse spleen cells was shown by the inhibition of aminopeptidase activities of these cells and by experiments using ^{3}H-bestatin. As will later be described in detail, bestatin enhanced delayed-type hypersensitivity to sheep red blood cells. In the screening of an inhibitor of aminopeptidase A which hydrolyzed the N-terminal glutamyl and aspartyl bond, we [3] found a tetrapeptide which we named amastatin (Fig. 2). It inhibited aminopeptidase A (prepared from human serum) and leucine aminopeptidase (prepared from hog kidney). The type of inhibition was competitive with the substrates. Amastatin also inhibited not only the action of aminopeptidase A and leucine aminopeptidase of human B-type leukemic cells, but also inhibited the aminopeptidase B of the cell lines, suggesting the binding of amastatin to these cells. Intraperitoneal injection of 10 or 100 μg of amastatin at the time of immunization increased the number of sheep red blood cell antibody-forming cells 2.5–3.5 times. In the screening of inhibitors against chicken intestine alkaline phosphatase, we found a new amino acid which we [4] named forphenicine (Fig. 2). It inhibited chicken intestine alkaline phosphatase very strongly, and the type of inhibition was

Table 1. Km and Ki of amastatin, bestatin, forphenicine and esterastin and the types of their inhibition

Inhibitors	Enzymes	Substrates	Km $(\times 10^{-4}\,M)$	Ki $(\times 10^{-8}\,M)$	Type of inhibition
Amastatin	AP-A[a]	L-Glutamic acid NA[b]	1.0	15	Competitive
	Leu-AP	L-Leucine NA	37	160	Competitive
Bestatin	AP-B	L-Arginine NA	1.0	6.0	Competitive
	Leu-AP	L-Leucine NA	5.8	2.0	Competitive
Forphenicine	Alkaline phosphatase	PNPP[c]	4.6	16.4	Uncompetitive
Esterastin	Esterase	PNPA[d]	4.0	0.016	Competitive

[a] Aminopeptidase A
[b] L-Glutamic acid β-naphthylamide
[c] p-Nitrophenyl phosphate
[d] p-Nitrophenyl acetate

uncompetitive with the substrate (p-nitrophenyl phosphate). Forphenicine inhibited only very weakly alkaline phosphatases from other sources. The binding of forphenicine to animal cells including lymphocytes was shown by using its labeled analog. The intraperitoneal administration of forphenicine enhanced delayed-type hypersensitivity to sheep red blood cells and increased the number of antibody-forming cells.

An inhibitor of esterase which we named esterastin (Fig. 2) was also found in *Streptomyces* [15]. It was a very strong inhibitor and the type of the inhibition was competitive with the substrate (p-nitrophenyl acetate). Intraperitoneal injection of 62 µg/mouse or more suppressed both delayed-type hypersensitivity to sheep red blood cells and antibody-formation.

Table 1 shows Ki values of bestatin against aminopeptidase B (rat liver) and leucine aminopeptidase (hog kidney), amastatin against aminopeptidase A (human serum) and leucine aminopeptidase (hog kidney), forphenicine against chicken intestine alkaline phosphatase, and esterastin against esterase (hog pancreas). Ki value of esterastin is in the order of $10^{-10}M$ and extremely small compared with Ki values of others. It is not yet certain whether the enhancement or the suppression of immune responses is due to the binding strength or to the difference in receptors.

Among the immunomodulators thus found, forphenicine and bestatin exhibited a strong inhibition against slowly growing subcutaneous tumors of Gardner lymphosarcoma and IMC carcinoma. But forphenicine was not effective by oral administration. Bestatin exhibited its action by its oral administration and therefore we studied bestatin most in detail.

Actions of Bestatin in Enhancing Immune Responses and in the Treatment of Cancer

In a footpad test, bestatin enhances delayed-type hypersensitivity to sheep red blood cells or oxazolone. The reaction elicited by the injection of an antigen in young mice is much stronger than that in old mice. The strength of the reaction is also dependent on mouse strains. The test using CDF_1 male mice older than 10 weeks can show the action of bestatin to enhance delayed-type hypersensitivity to sheep red blood cells. As shown in Table 2, 0.1, 1.0, 10, 100 µg of bestatin given orally or intraperitoneally at the time of the immunization enhances delayed-type hypersensitivity [17]. If mice are sensitized to sheep red blood cells and the reaction is elicited by human red blood cells, or vice versa, bestatin shows no effect.

Oral, intraperitoneal, or intravenous administration of bestatin at the time of sensitization enhances delayed-type hypersensitivity to sheep red blood cells, but the administration at the time of the elicitation of the reaction does not. A large dose such as 1 000 µg/mouse of bestatin increases the number of antibody-forming cells but does not enhance delayed-type hypersensitivity significantly. Oral, intravenous, and intraperitoneal administration of bestatin shows the same action, but subcutaneous injection does not.

Bestatin (Fig. 2) has three asymmetric carbon atom and all stereoisomers were synthesized. Then, the S configuration of the α-carbon atom of the 3-amino-2-hydroxy-4-phenylbutanoyl moiety was shown to be the absolute requirement for inhibition of aminopeptidase B and leucine aminopeptidase [10]. All isomers containing R configuration of this carbon atom shows much weaker inhibition of these enzymes than the others containing S configuration. The isomers which inhibit aminopeptidase B strongly enhance delayed-type hypersensitivity in almost the same degree as bestatin. It suggests that the enhancement of delayed-type hypersensitivity is due to the binding of bestatin to aminopeptidases of cells involved in immune responses.

The delayed-type hypersensitivity reduced by cyclophosphamide can be recovered by the oral administration of 10 µg or 1 000 µg/mouse of bestatin: 6 mg of cyclophosphamide was intravenously given on day 0; bestatin was given daily on days 1−5; immunization by the streaking of 5% oxazolone ethanol solution was given on the shaved skin in the abdomen on day 6; the reaction was elicited by streaking the oxazolone ethanol solution on a footpad on day 8; the thickness of the edema of the footpad was measured on day 10: the edema of the normal control, 0.68 ± 0.09 mm; those given cyclophosphamide, 0.20 ± 0.09 mm; those given cyclophosphamide and 1 000 µg of bestatin/day, 0.89 ± 0.07 mm; those given cyclophosphamide and 10 µg of bestatin/day, 0.88 ± 0.06 mm [6].

Bestatin treatment also recovered the delayed-type hypersensitivity reduced by the inoculation of Ehrlich carcinoma cells to CDF_1 mice: 10^6 carcinoma cells were inoculated intraperitoneally on day 0; 5% oxazolone ethanol solution was streaked on the shaved skin on day 4; 0.1, 10, or 1 000 µg/mouse of bestatin was given orally once at the time of the immunization; the reaction was elicited by streaking the oxazolone ethanol solution on a footpad on day 6; the thickness of the edema of the footpad was measured on day 8; the normal control 0.68 ± 0.09 mm; those to which the carcinoma cells were inoculated, 0.21 ± 0.13 mm; those bearing carcinoma and given 0.1 µg, 10 µg, or 1 000 µg of bestatin, $0.78 \pm 0.15, 0.70 \pm 0.11, 0.73 \pm 0.17$ mm respectively. The result indicates that the reduced immune response to oxazolone in mice 4 days after the inoculation of 10^6 Ehrlich carcinoma cells can be recovered by bestatin to the normal value. But this bestatin treatment does not influence the survival days of mice bearing Ehrlich carcinoma [6].

The mitogenic effect of bestatin on mouse lymphocytes was tested in the following three culture conditions: 1) mouse (CDF_1) spleen cells (1.5×10^7) were cultured in

Table 2. Effect of bestatin on delayed-type hypersensitivity[a] to sheep red blood cells (SRBC) in mice of 4, 8, or 14 weeks

μg/mouse	Age of mice[b] 4 weeks		8 weeks		14 weeks	
	Increase of footpad thickness[d]	T/C%	Increase of footpad thickness[d]	T/C%	Increase of footpad thickness[d]	T/C%
0	8.6 ± 0.2		8.1 ± 0.9		8.1 ± 1.5	
0.1	8.0 ± 0.5	93	9.9 ± 0.7	122	13.1 ± 0.8	162
1.0	9.6 ± 1.5	112	10.5 ± 0.8	130	14.0 ± 0.7	173
10.0	9.0 ± 1.9	105	12.5 ± 1.0	154	13.8 ± 0.8	170
100.0	8.3 ± 2.0	97	10.4 ± 0.8	128	9.9 ± 1.0	159
1000.0	7.6 ± 1.5	88	9.3 ± 0.7	115	12.9 ± 0.5	122

[a] 10^8 SRBC were injected into a footpad, 4 days thereafter the reaction was elicited by injection of same number of SRCB and the thickness of edema was measured 24 h thereafter bestatin was given orally at the time of the immunization
[b] CDF$_1$ (Balb/c × DBA/2) male mice
[c] Oral administration at the time of immunization
[d] Increase of footpad thickness (× 0.1 mm, ± S.E.)

1 ml of RPMI 1640 medium containing fetal calf serum at 20% for 2 h; 2) the spleen cells were cultured in the same medium with anti-θ-serum and complement for 2 h; and 3) after 1 and 2 h culture adherent cells were removed repeatedly. Each of these groups 1−3 was thereafter cultured with or without 1.0 μg of bestatin for 24 h; the supernatant cells of each group were collected, washed, and subjected to Ficoll-Paque sedimentation; 0.2 ml of 1.5×10^6 cells of each group was cultured in the same medium described above for 3 days and ^{3}H-thymidine incorporation was tested. The results are shown in Table 3. Bestatin increased the incorporation of ^{3}H-thymidine into lymphocytes, when bestatin was cultured with mouse spleen cells for 24 h and lymphocytes were collected and cultured. This bestatin effect was eliminated by the destruction of T cells or by the removal of macrophages. This indicates that macrophages and T cells are involved in the action of bestatin to cause mitogenesis of lymphocytes. But is should be noticed that fetal calf serum which must be antigenic to mouse immune cells was present in the culture medium.

Table 3. Mitogenic effect of bestatin (BS) on mouse lymphocytes

Spleen cells from normal CDF_1 mice
|
a)[a] No treatment
b)[a] Treatment with anti-θ-serum and C' or
c)[a] Collection of nonadherent cells
|
Cultured with or without bestatin[b] for 24 h in 5% CO_2
|
Nonadherent cells (lymphocytes) were subjected to Ficoll-Paque sedimentation
|
Cultured for 3 days (lymphocytes culture)[a]
|
^{3}H-Thymidine incorporation test

Treated with	Addition to precultures	c.p.m./culture[c]	BS/none
Experiment 1			
None	None	17 975	1.54
	BS	27 620	
Anti-θ-serum and C'	None	19 457	0.93
	BS	18 122	
Macrophage-depleted	None	15 208	0.99
	BS	15 136	
Experiment 2			
None	None	15 132	1.94
	BS	29 370	
Anti-θ-serum and C'	None	14 715	0.85
	BS	12 534	

[a] RPMI 1640 medium containing 20% of fetal calf serum
[b] Bestatin: 1 μg/15×10^6 spleen cells
[c] Mean c.p.m. of triplicate cultures

Very low concentrations (0.001–0.1 µg/ml) of bestatin modulate the differentiation of bone marrow stem cells. About 5×10^6 cells can be obtained from a femoral bone marrow of mouse by injecting 1.0 ml of αMEM medium into the marrow of this bone and pushing out the cells. A portion of the cells (7.5×10^4) thus obtained was cultured for 10 days under 10% CO_2 at 37° C with the colony-stimulating factor (0.1 ml of mouse serum obtained 5 h after the injection of 5 µg of endotoxin) and with or without bestatin. Agar was added at 0.3%. If the colony stimulating factor is not added, there is no growth of any colonies. As shown in Fig. 3, bestatin added to the medium at 0.001, 0.01, or 0.1 µg/ml increased the number of colonies of granulocytes. The oral administration of bestatin also increased the number of the colonies. After 2 days starvation (only the drinking water was given), the number of cells obtained from the femoral bone marrow decreased to about a half of the control without starvation. The number of colonies which were observed under the same experimental condition described above was less than a half of the control without starvation treatment. Bestatin added to the medium at 0.01 µg/ml recovered the number of colonies to that of the control without starvation [6].

Bestatin shows therapeutic effect on Gardner lymphosarcoma and IMC carcinoma that grows slowly and on which the tumor growth can be examined for more than 30 days after the inoculation. In this condition, it inhibited the growth of Gardner lymphosarcoma as follows: 0.5 or 5 mg bestatin/kg was orally given for 5 days during day 1 to day 5 of the inoculation of 10^5 cells, the weight of the tumor was measured on day 31 of the inoculation and 59%–77% inhibition was observed. IMC carcinoma is a mouse carcinoma which appeared spontaneously in CDF_1 mouse in the author's laboratory and has been successively transferred through this mouse strain. The effect of bestatin on IMC carcinoma is shown in Table 4. In case 1, 10, or 100 µg bestatin/mouse is given daily orally for 5 days. The treatment started 8 or 14 days after the inoculation of the tumor cells exhibited a stronger inhibition than the treatment started 1 day after the inoculation [6].

The oral administration of 10 or 100 µg bestatin/mouse twice a week for 20 weeks showed a suppressive effect on the induction of squamous cell carcinoma in mouse skin by methylcholanthrene (streaked twice a week for 10 weeks) [6].

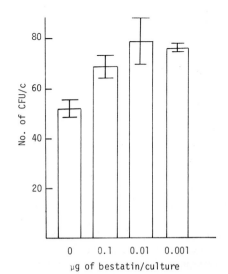

Fig. 3. Effect of varied concentrations of bestatin on colony formation of mouse bone marrow cells stimulated by LPS-induced colony-stimulating factor (CSF) in culture

Tsuruo et al. [11], Cancer Institute, Tokyo, observed an effect of bestatin in preventing the lymph node metastasis of P388 leukemia.

Kawamata [8], Institute of Microbial Diseases of the University of Osaka, has found that the growth of one of the human uterus carcinoma strains in nude mice causes a strong cachexia. He observed that intraperitoneal injection of 500 μg of bestatin on days 1–6 of the inoculation suppressed the growth of the tumor slightly and exhibited a marked effect in preventing cachexia.

As described above, bestatin enhances immune responses in mice and can show a suppressive effect on some slowly growing solid tumors in mice. Bestatin had an extremely low toxicity and seemed to be an immune response-enhancing agent worth clinical study. But before confirmation by the clinical study it was not certain whether the human immune system would produce a response to bestatin or not.

We tested the mitogenetic effect of bestatin on human peripheral white cells. Human buffy coat cells (2×10^7) were collected from 20 ml of healthy human blood and 5×10^6 cells were cultured with 1.0 μg bestatin in 1 ml of RPMI 1640 medium containing fetal calf serum at 20% overnight and nonadherent cells collected were subjected to Ficoll-Paque sedimentation. viable lymphocytes (0.2 ml of 1.5×10^6 cells) thus collected were cultured in the same medium containing fetal calf serum at 20% for 3 days and ^{3}H-thymidine incorporation was tested. Then, as shown in Table 5, ^{3}H-thymidine incorporation was increased 2.3 or 2.9 times by culturing the mixture of human lymphocytes and macrophages with bestatin in a medium containing fetal calf

Table 4. Effect of bestatin on IMC-carcinoma

Bestatin μg/mouse/day	Treatment days and % inhibition mean (range)			
	− 7 to − 1	1 to 5	8 to 12	14 to 18
1	–	43.1 (52−27)	48.7 (89−0)	55.0 (76−3)
10	–	41.7 (75−26)	82.0 (89−76)	71.0 (84−58)
100	42.3 (91−0)	36.3 (63−0)	71.6 (82−61)	71.3 (81−62)

Table 5. Mitogenic activity of bestatin on human lymphocytes

Buffy coat cells from	Addition to preculture	Lymphocytes culture	
		c.p.m./culture[a]	Ratio
H. I.	None	2 060	1.00
	Bestatin[b]	4 802	2.33
T. S.	None	990	1.00
	Bestatin[b]	2 905	2.93

[a] Results in 3 days cultures
[b] Bestatin 1 μg to 5×10^6 cells in 1 ml

serum. However, according to Blomgren et al. (1979), Radiation Institute of Royal Karolinska Institute, bestatin does not show the mitogenic effect, if the cells are cultured in a medium containing human serum instead of fetal calf serum. These observations suggest that the presence of antigen might be necessary for the mitogenic action of bestatin.

Clinical studies in the last two years in Japan have shown that daily oral administration of 30 mg of bestatin increases T cell percent. This has been confirmed also by Blomgren et al. [5]. Furthermore, Blomgren et al. [5] found that bestatin enhanced NK-cell activity. Preincubation of healthy human lymphocytes with bestatin at 0.001, 0.1, or 10.0 µg/ml for 20 h increased the cytotoxic index. Natural killer (NK) cell activity in cancer patients increased after 2 weeks or more bestatin treatment. NK-cell activity increase during bestatin administration was also confirmed by Aoike et al. (1), Medical School of Kyoto Furitsu University.

Various oral daily doses such as 30, 60, 100, 200, 400, 700, and 900 mg of bestatin have been studied by Japanese doctors, who found that daily doses of 200 mg or more caused the decrease of T cell percent. Thus, the optimum daily dose in increasing T cell percent has been suggested to be in the range of between about 30 and 100 mg/patient. As will be reviewed by Oka in this book, in the clinical study, daily oral administration of 30 mg has shown interesting therapeutic effects.

An immunostimulator may be not able to exhibit its action strongly enough to compete with the action of a big tumor in decreasing cell immunity, but even in this case, the action of an immunostimulator may exhibit its action in young patients who can recover immune responses, or in metastatic lymph nodes where cancer cells are surrounded by immune cells. There may be two types of immunotherapy depending on the positive or negative antigenicity of tumors. Immunostimulators may enhance the host defense, for instance, as shown by the enhancement of NK-cell activity. In the case of a tumor which contains a masked antigen, if this antigen is released, an immunostimulator may show a rapid and strong action in destroying the tumor. Although there remain many unknown mechanisms in cancer immunology, it is possible that the immunotherapy combined to surgery, radiation, and chemotherapy will increase the rate of cure from cancer.

Bestatin given orally is very well absorbed and excreted into urine. A gas mass spectroscopic method which can determine ng amount of bestatin has been developed. By this method, bestatin concentrations in blood and urine after its oral administration has been measured.

As shown by an example in Fig. 4, during daily administration of 30 mg, the lowest concentration of bestatin just before the oral administration was about 50 times lower than the highest concentration about 1 or 2 h after the administration. The maximum concentration in blood was $1-2$ µg/ml and a fairly high concentration of $0.2-0.5$ µg/ml was maintained for more than 3 h. A small amount of bestatin orally given is oxidized to p-hydroxybestatin and about $0.005-0.5$ µg/ml of this metabolite is found in blood (Fig. 4). More than 85% of bestatin is excreted into urine and $1\%-15\%$ was metabolized to p-hydroxybestatin.

p-Hydroxybestatin has about five times stronger activity than bestatin in inhibiting aminopeptidase B. As shown in Table 6, 1, 10, or 100 µg p-hydroxybestatin/mouse orally given at the time of immunization enhanced delayed-type hypersensitivity to sheep red blood cells in footpad test. It is noteworthy that the oral administration of 0.1, 1, 10, or 100 µg/mouse given at the time of the elicitation of the reaction also enhanced delayed-type hypersensitivity. As already described, bestatin given at the

	Intact concentration of bestatin (ng/ml)	Metabolite concentration of p-OH-bestatin (ng/ml)
0 h	86.0	trace
1 h	1 533.0	trace
2 h	12 213.0	174.05
4 h	4 832.5	489.40
6 h	2 424.5	399.40
8 h	905.0	205.30

——○——   ‒ ‒●‒ ‒

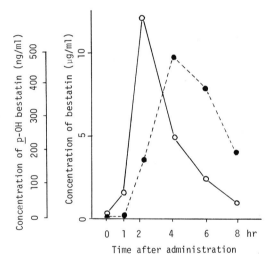

Fig. 4. Blood level of bestatin and *p*-hydroxybestatin after the oral administration of 300 mg

Table 6. Effect of *p*-hydroxybestatin (HBS) on delayed-type hypersensitivity to sheep red blood cells (SRBC) (footpad test)

On day 0	On day 4	Thickness of edema on day 5
10^8 SRBC	10^8 SRBC	7.4 ± 1.1
10^8 SRBC + HBC, 100 µg, p.o.	10^8 SRBC	9.1 ± 0.9
10^8 SRBC + HBC, 10 µg, p.o.	10^8 SRBC	10.1 ± 1.2
10^8 SRBC + HBC, 1 µg, p.o.	10^8 SRBC	10.6 ± 0.7
10^8 SRBC + HBC, 0.1 µg, p.o.	10^8 SRBC	8.0 ± 1.1
10^8 SRCB[a]	10^8 SRBC + HBS, 100 µg, p.o.	9.9 ± 0.4
10^8 SRCB[a]	10^8 SRBC + HBS, 10 µg, p.o.	12.2 ± 1.3
10^8 SRCB[a]	10^8 SRBC + HBS, 1 µg, p.o.	13.9 ± 1.4
10^8 SRCB[a]	10^8 SRBC + HBS, 0.1 µg, p.o.	11.3 ± 1.4

[a] CDF_1 mice, female, 11 weeks

Table 7. Effect of hydroxybestatin on delayed-type hypersensitivity to oxazolone

Immunization with or without bestatin	Thickness of edema in footpad[a] (HBS) ($\times$ 0.1 mm)	
	24 h[b]	48 h[b]
Streak of 5% oxazolone ethanol on the shaved skin in the abdomen	3.0 ± 1.05	5.6 ± 1.1
+ HBS, 1000 µg, p.o.	6.9 ± 1.5	6.8 ± 1.1
+ HBS, 100 µg, p.o.	6.0 ± 1.3	7.0 ± 1.0
+ HBS, 10 µg, p.o.	3.5 ± 0.9	6.7 ± 1.6

[a] Oxazolone ethanol solution was streaked on a footpad 48 h after the immunization
[b] 24 h or 48 h after the elicitation of the reaction

Table 8. Effect of hydroxybestatin on the number of antibody-forming cells against sheep red blood cells (SRBC)

Immunization	PFC/spleen
10^8 SRBC	$482\,000 \pm 36\,200$
10^8 SRBC + HBS 1000 µg, IP	$829\,600 \pm 32\,100$
10^8 SRBC + HBS 100 µg, IP	$1\,044\,000 \pm 120\,890$
10^8 SRBC + HBS 10 µg, IP	$832\,000 \pm 28\,700$
10^8 SRBC + HBS 1 µg, IP	$703\,000 \pm 32\,900$
10^8 SRBC + HBS 0.1 µg, IP	$565\,000 \pm 22\,940$

time of the elicitation of the reaction did not enhance delayed-type hypersensitivity to sheep red blood cells.

p-Hydroxybestatin showed a stronger enhancement of the hypersensitivity to oxazolone than bestatin when p-hydroxybestatin (10, 100, or 1 000 µg) was given orally at the time of the immunization. The enhancement of the hypersensitivity by 100 or 1 000 µg/mouse was shown already 24 h after the second streaking of oxazolone (Table 7). Thus, the reaction occurred more rapidly in the case of p-hydroxybestatin than in bestatin.

A hundred or 1 000 µg p-hydroxybestatin given orally at the same time with intravenous injection of 10^8 sheep red blood cells to 10-week-old CDF_1 male mice increased the number of antibody-forming cells in the spleen. As shown in Table 8, intraperitoneal injection of 1, 10, 100, or 1 000 µg of p-hydroxybestatin to 6-week-old ddY/S female mice increased more markedly the number of antibody-forming cells in the spleen than in CDF_1 mice. As described above, p-hydroxybestatin is an active metabolite of bestatin and the effect of p-hydroxybestatin may be involved in the effect of bestatin given orally.

As shown by the study of bestatin, small molecular immune-enhancing agents will be useful in the treatment of cancer. Such compounds may also be useful in the treatment of infections resistant to present chemotherapy. Although the effect of bestatin on bacterial infection has not yet been studied enough in detail, in a preliminary

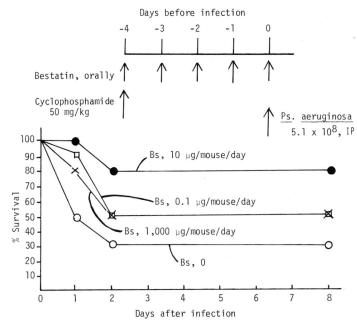

Fig. 5. Effect of bestatin (Bs) on Pseudomonas aeruginosa infection in mice treated with cyclophosphamide

experiment it has been shown that the administration of bestatin to mice treated with cyclophosphamide before a light infection of *Pseudomonas aeruginosa* can exhibit a preventive effect: in the condition where 70% of mice died in 3 days after the infection, 70% survived in the group given 10 μg of bestatin, 50% in two groups given 0.1 μg or 1 000 μg (Fig. 5). Small molecular immunostimulators will be studied in both purposes for treatments of cancer and resistant infections.

Conclusion

As shown by the author's study, even small molecular compounds that bind to the surface of immune cells modulate immune responses. The compounds with such an activity can be found by the screening of microbial products. Small molecular compounds are not antigenic in general and such compounds which enhance or decrease immune responses will be not only useful in the treatment of cancer but also tools in the analysis of mechanisms of immune responses. Bestatin, which enhanced immune responses of mice, has shown favorable effects in the treatment of human cancer.

References

1. Aoike A (1980) Effect of bestatin on natural killer activity. Small molecular immuno-modulators of microbial origin – fundamental and clinical studies of bestatin. Japan Scientific Societies Press, Tokyo
2. Aoyagi T, Suda H, Nagai M, Ogawa K, Suzuki J, Takeuchi T, Umezawa H (1976) Aminopeptidase activities on the surface of mammalian cells. Biochim Biophys Acta 452: 131−143

3. Aoyagi T, Tobe H, Kojima F, Hamada M, Takeuchi T, Umezawa H (1978) Amastatin, an inhibitor of aminopeptidase A produced by actinomycetes. J Antibiot (Tokyo) 31: 636−638
4. Aoyagi T, Yamamoto T, Kojiri K, Kojima F, Hamada M, Takeuchi T, Umezawa H (1978) Forphenicine, an inhibitor of alkaline phosphatase produced by actinomycetes. J Antibiot (Tokyo) 31: 244−246
5. Blomgren H, Strender LE, Edsmyr F (1979) Studies on the immunostimulatory effect of bestatin in vitro and in vivo. Bestatin Conference, March 10, Tokyo
6. Ishizuka M, Aoyagi T, Takeuchi T, Umezawa H (1979) Further study of effect of bestatin on immune responses. Bestatin Conference, March 10, Tokyo
7. Ishizuka M, Iinuma H, Takeuchi T, Umezawa H (1972) Effect of diketocoriolin B on antibody-formation. J Antibiot (Tokyo) 25: 320
8. Kawamata J (1979) Effect of bestatin on cachexia caused by human uterus carcinoma inoculated to nude mice. Bestatin Conference, March 10, Tokyo
9. Kunimoto T, Umezawa H (1973) Kinetic studies on the inhibition of (Na^+-K^+)-ATPase by diketocoriolin B on antibody-formation. Biochim Biophys Acta 318: 78−90
10. Suda H, Aoyagi T, Takeuchi T, Umezawa H (1976) Inhibition of aminopeptidase B and leucine aminopeptidase by bestatin and its stereoisomers. Arch Biochem Biophys 177: 196−200
11. Tsuruo T, Kataoka T, Tsukagoshi S, Sakurai K (1979) Effect of bestatin on lymph-node metastasis of P388. Bestatin Conference, March 10, Tokyo
12. Umezawa H (1972) Enzyme inhibitors of microbial origin. University of Tokyo Press, Tokyo
13. Umezawa H (1976) Structures and activities of protease inhibitors of microbial origin. Methods Enzymol 45: 678−695
14. Umezawa H (1977) Recent advances in bioactive microbial secondary metabolites. Jpn J Antibiot [Suppl] 30: 138−163
15. Umezawa H, Aoyagi T, Hazato T, Uotani K, Kojima F, Hamada M, Takeuchi T (1978) Esterastin, an inhibitor of esterase, produced by actinomycetes. J Antibiot (Tokyo) 31: 639−641
16. Umezawa H, Aoyagi T, Suda H, Hamada M, Takeuchi T (1976) Bestatin, an inhibitor of aminopeptidase B, produced by actinomycetes. J Antibiot (Tokyo) 29: 97−99
17. Umezawa H, Ishizuka M, Aoyagi T, Takeuchi T (1976) Enhancement of delayed-type hypersensitivity by bestatin, an inhibitor of aminopeptidase B and leucine aminopeptidase. J Antibiot (Tokyo) 29: 857−859

A Review of Clinical Studies on Bestatin, 1976–1978

S. Oka

Institute of Microbial Chemistry, 14–23, Kamiosaki 3-Chome,
Shinagawa-ku, J – Tokyo 141

As Professor Umezawa et al. found bestatin inhibits aminopeptidase B and leucine aminopeptidase, binds to the surface of animal cells including macrophages and lymphocytes, enhances delayed-type hypersensitivity, and exhibits antitumor effect on slowly growing experimental solid tumors. Moreover, bestatin treatment enhances the therapeutic effect of chemotherapeutic agents such as bleomycin and adriamycin on experimental animal tumors. Bestatin has extremely low toxicity by both parenteral and oral administration. Bestatin is a small molecular compound and does not have any antigenicity.

Pilot studies on the clinical use of bestatin were initiated in November 1976 by Dr. Ichikawa and his colleagues. They found that bestatin had no clinical toxicity; and that the frequency of T lymphocytes, identified by sheep erythrocyte rosette formation, was found to increase after bestatin medication, when used on immunosuppressive patients. Moreover patients with residual lesions left by chemotherapy and/or radiotherapy, showed a favorable response to bestatin alone.

On the basis of these findings, the Cooperative Group Study on bestatin, consisting of investigators of 16 institutions throughout Japan, was organized, and Phase I studies were started in August 1978.

Members of the Cooperative Group Study were: Dr. Wada and Dr. Kumamoto, Sapporo Medical College, Sapporo; Dr. Tsuji, Hokkaido University, Sapporo Medical College, Sapporo; Dr. Knno, Tohoku University, Sendai; Dr. Ideka, Saitama Medical School, Saitama; Dr. Isono, Chiba University, Chiba; Dr. Majima, Chiba Cancer Center, Chiba; Dr. Hirokawa, National Tachikawa Hospital, Tachikawa; Dr. Wada and Dr. Niijima, University of Tokyo, Tokyo; Dr. Isurugi, National Medical Center Hospital, Tokyo; Dr. Taketa, Tokyo Medical College, Tokyo; Dr. Abe, Keio University, Tokyo; Dr. Furue, Teikyo University, Tokyo; Dr. Arimori and Dr. Miyake, Tokai University, Isehara; Dr. Oshima, Kyoto University, Kyoto; Dr. Orita and Dr. Kimura, Okayama University, Okayama, and Dr. Kuramoto, Hiroshima University, Hiroshima.

The present review is concerned with the findings of the pilot studies as well as those of phase I studies now underway.

Clinical Study

Toxicity

Five healthy adult volunteers were each given oral doses of 30, 100, and 200 mg bestatin. These tests revealed no subjective toxicity.

Laboratory examinations of these adults carried out 24 h after administration of the drug showed no apparent pathologic findings in complete blood counts, hepatic enzymes, BUN and serum electrolytes, except those of leukocytes. However, there tended to be a decrease in the number of leukocytes and lymphocytes after administration of bestatin at a high dose of 200 mg. These findings provided indications in establishing an optimal dose level for clinical use.

About 80 patients who had entered the pilot studies were given a daily dose of 30 mg bestatin during a period of 3 months in most instances and some patients received bestatin for longer than 12 months. None of these patients had subjective toxicity, and routine laboratory examinations showed no pathologic findings during or after bestatin medication. Therefore, bestatin at clinical dose level was confirmed as having no toxicity.

Absorption and Excretion

Bestatin was administered orally to each of five healthy volunteers in doses of 30, 100, and 300 mg, and the serum concentration of bestatin and its metabolite, p-hydroxybestatin, were measured by gas chromatography-mass spectrography. The highest mean serum concentrations of bestatin showed about 2 μg/ml, 2.5 μg/ml, or 8 μg/ml 30–180 min after administration of 30, 100, or 300 mg bestatin respectively, and they rapidly decreased and disappeared from the blood within 24 h. p-Hydroxybestatin was also detected in the blood, but in lower concentrations. This indicated that there was no distinct dose dependency in relation to the obtained serum concentration. About 80% of bestatin, including p-hydroxybestatin, was excreted in the urine within 24 h.

These findings were useful in establishing an optimal dose of bestatin for immunochemotherapy, and in determining the necessary interval between repeated administrations of bestatin.

Phase I Studies of Bestatin

The Phase I studies were designed to determine an immunologically active optimal dose and an optimal dose schedule for bestatin. A dose of 10, 30, or 60 mg or more per day was administered, once, twice, or every day per week, and then stopped to find the effect of bestatin on the immunocompetent lymphocytes. Parameters used were: the number and frequency of T cells and B cells; tests of NK activity, K activity, suppressor T cells, and blastogenesis of lymphocytes with PHA, Con A, or PWA were also carried out, where possible. Skin tests with PPD, candida, and varidase were also studied in patients who had received 4 weeks to 3 months administration of bestatin.

However, the test methods in these examinations varied among the laboratories which participated in this trial. Therefore, in the present paper the evaluation of these findings made in accordance with the individual judgments of investigators.

Changes in the peripheral blood lymphocyte populations after bestatin administration were studied by Dr. Konno and Dr. Kumano, Tohoku University, in four cases of lung cancer patients. Lymphoid cells were isolated from the heparinized venous blood (by centrifugation on Ficol-Paque) on days 1, 3, and 8 after a 30 mg dose of bestatin, and subjected to rosette tests in a microtest plate, as proposed by Kondo et al. The indicator cells used were: (1) neuraminidase-treated sheep RBC (E) for identifying T lymphocytes, (2) ox RBC sensitized with rabbit anti ox RBC IgG (EA) for cells possessing Fc-receptors for IgG, and (3) trypsin-treated sheep RBC sensitized with rabbit anti-SRBC IgM reacted with human serum as a source of complement (EAC) for those possessing complement receptors or B lymphocytes. Usually 300−400 cells were scored to assess the frequency of each cell population. Percentage of T and B lymphocytes were calculated according to the following formula (corrections for contaminating monocytes and granulocytis cells)

$$T\ (\%) = E \times \frac{E + C}{E + (C - P)} \tag{1}$$

$$B\ (\%) = C - P) \times \frac{E + C}{E + (C - P)}, \tag{2}$$

where E: E-rosette forming cells (%), C: EAC-rosette forming cells (%), and P: peroxidase positive cells (%). $E + C = 100 \pm 4$.

An increment of T lymphocyte population was found on day 1 and day 3, except in one case, and then seemed to return to the values scored before bestatin administration (Table 1).

The findings suggested that bestatin could be given twice or 3 times a week instead of a daily administration.

Responses of these lymphocyte preparations to PHA and Con A were also studied. Two-tenths of a milliliter of peripheral blood lymphocytes (1×10^6 cells/ml in RPMI 1640 containing 20% heat inactivated FCS) in each well of a microtest plate were cultured in the presence or absence of optimally diluted PHA or Con A, for 72 h at 37° C in a humidified atmosphere of 5% CO_2 in air. Incorporation of ^{3}H-thymidine (0.04 μCi/well) into DNA during the last 24 h of incubation was measured in a liquid scintillation counter.

Blastogenesis of lymphocytes with PHA or Con A showed no definite tendency to increase or decrease in the four patients with lung cancer (Table 2).

The relation between bestatin doses and T lymphocyte population was studied by Dr. Majima, Chiba Cancer Center Hospital. A dose of 10, 30, 100, 300, and 900 mg bestatin was administered to patients with cancer. The optimum bestatin dosages required for maximal E rosette formation was found to exist in the dose range from 30−100 mg, and E rosette formation was inhibited at higher doses than 100 mg. On the other hand, an enhancement of blastogenesis of lymphocytes with PMA was found to have no strong correlation with the dose level.

Dr. Aoike, Kyoto Municipal University of Medicine, studied the effect of bestatin on NK activity in patients with gastric cancer by measuring ^{51}Cr release from labeled target Namalwa cells, cultivated in cytotoxic assay system. ^{51}Cr release was 2% in one patient and 9% in another before bestatin administration, but increased to 12% and 38%, respectively, after administration of 60 mg/bestatin per day for 5 days. Therefore, an enhancement of NK activity was found in cancer patients with bestatin medication.

Table 1. Changes in the peripheral blood lymphocyte populations after bestatin administration in lung cancer patients

Case No.	Before		Day 1		Day 3		Day 8	
	T(%)	B(%)	T(%)	B(%)	T(%)	B(%)	T(%)	B(%)
I (S. S., 65, M)	75.7	18.5	85.7	12.5	96.4	16.8	67.3	31.2
II (T. H., 58, M)	66.9	28.0	82.7	11.9	83.5	14.3	72.2	21.8
III (S. O., 70, M)	70.9	14.5	71.4	17.1	N.D.[a]	N.D.	87.6	14.5
IV (N. Y., 55, M)	78.1	20.8	67.5	29.8	N.D.	N.D.	68.2	36.7

Bestatin: 30 mg × 1, p.o., on day-0
[a] ND, not determined

Table 2. Changes in mitogen responses of the peripheral blood lymphocytes after bestatin administration in lung cancer patients

Case No.	Before		Day 1		Day 3		Day 8	
	PHA	Con A	PHA	Con A	PHA	Con A	PHA	Con A
I (S. S., 65, M)	43.5	5.6	18.9	4.0	52.0	8.7	19.5	2.4
II (T. H., 58, M)	19.9	5.8	3.8	N.D.[a]	10.9	1.6	15.0	2.6
III (S. O., 70, M)	10.4	3.5	41.8	4.2	N.D.	N.D.	58.5	3.1
IV (N. Y., 55, M)	8.5	6.0	23.5	3.0	N.D.	N.D.	32.3	2.8

Each value represents stimulation index

$$S.I. = \frac{cpm \text{ with mitogen}}{cpm \text{ without mitogen}}$$

Bestatin: 30 mg × 1, p.o., on day-0
[a] ND, not determined

Findings of the Pilot Study

Findings in Cancer Patients Treated with Bestatin Alone. A 68-year-old patient with penile cancer had residual lesions with histologically positive cancer cells after treatment with bleomycin and irradiation. He was given a daily dose of 30 mg bestatin alone by Dr. Hirokawa, Tachikawa National Hospital. Eight months later, biopsied specimens from the site of headed lesions revealed no cancer cells. The patient showed no signs of relapse during 20 months of bestatin medication. The number of lymphocytes and T cells were about 800 cells and 450 cells/ml before bestatin treatment, but they increased to around 3 000 cells and 2 000 cells/ml respectively during bestatin medication.

An 82-year-old female with breast cancer was treated by Dr. Majima, Chiba Cancer Center Hospital, with FT-207 and cytoxan for 13 months, but showed no response. As she had accidental traumatic fracture of the right femur, chemotherapy was discontinued, and 30 mg bestatin alone was given daily.

Two months later, a 45 × 65 mm sized breast tumor had shrunk to a 5 × 14 mm sized tumor. This response was observed for 5 weeks, and then the tumor gradually grew large again in spite of 100 mg bestatin administration. A definite increase in the number of lymphocytes and T cells was found after bestatin medication.

A 44-year-old patient with breast cancer underwent mastectomy in 1972, but between 1973 and 1976, she showed metastasis successively in the left subclavicular lymph nodes, the anterior chest wall, the right IV-V ribs, the right axillary lymph nodes, and the spinous process of VI-VIII ribs. During this period, she received bilateral oophorectomies, irradiation, and anticancer chemotherapy. However, in July 1978, a 38×31 mm sized tumor mass developed in the left anterior chest wall and simultaneously paralysis of both legs, which remained in spite of anticancer chemotherapy with steroid hormone. At this time, she was given a daily dose of 30 mg bestatin by Dr. Fujii, Tokyo University. Two months later, the tumor completely disappeared and the paralysis of both legs improved to a certain degree. She is under observation.

Two patients with skin cancer after surgery received bestatin in order to prevent recurrence of the imperceptible disease. One patient had no relapse for 6 months and another for 16 months after bestatin administration.

The frequency of T rosettes so far as examined remained within normal range or increased after treatment, but skin reaction to PPD showed no distinct change.

Findings in Stage I and Stage II Cancer Patients Treated with Bestatin in Combination with Anticancer Agents (Table 3). Synergistic antitumor activity was found in a combination of bestatin with pepleomycin in four patients with stage I squamous skin carcinoma, since the total dosage required to achieve regression of the tumors was found to be less than that of pepleomycin treatment alone, as reported by Dr. Ikeda, Saitama University. These stage I patients received bestatin alone after surgery. They had no recurrence during about 12 months of observation.

Three patients having stage II skin cancer and one patient having stage II malignant melanoma who were treated with anticancer agents and bestatin underwent surgical procedure, and afterwards were given bestatin in combination with anticancer agents in order to prevent recurrence of the imperceptible disease. They had no relapse during $7-17$ months of observation.

The number of circulating lymphocytes was found to increase after treatment in five patients, but it remained within normal range in eight patients, while it decreased in one patient as far as examined. The frequency of T rosettes showed no distinct change in patients with stage I to II cancer. Blastogenesis of lymphocytes with PHA and skin reaction to PPD showed no obvious change before or after treatment.

Findings in Stage III and Stage IV Cancer Patients Treated with Bestatin in Combination with Anticancer Agents (Table 4). Forty-four advanced cancer patients, with metastases in most instances, were treated with bestatin in combination with anticancer agents. They included five patients with kidney cancer, five with bladder cancer, one with ureteral cancer, two with testicular cancer, one with ovarian tumor, two with skin cancer, ten with stomach cancer, three with lung cancer, and five with malignant lymphoma.

Of these 44 patients, 38 patients survived throughout observation. One patient with renal cancer and lung metastases, one patient with testicular tumor, and one patient with bladder tumor survived longer than 12 months, suggesting a favorable modification in anticancer chemotherapy by the administration of bestatin.

Table 3. Findings in stage I and II cancer patients treated with bestatin combined with anticancer agents

Disease	Stage	No. of cases	M	F	Average age	Chemotherapy	Post-therapy	n.c. Ly	%T	PHA	PPD	Duration of follow-up (months)
Skin carcer	I											
Squamous cell cancer		4	3	1	52	PEP	Op. → Bs	↗ 2, n.c. 5	7	4	7	No recurrence (12)
Sarcoma		2	2	0	49	FT-207		↘				
Adenocarcinoma		2	1	2	66							
Malignant melanoma	I	3	2	1	64	DTIC, MeCCNU, VCR	Op. → Bs	↗ 1, n.c. 1, ↘ 1	3	3	2	No recurrence (12)
Malignant lymphoma	I	1	0	1	17	PEP	CTX, 6MP × Bs	↗ 1, n.c., ↘	1			No recurrence (13)
Skin cancer	II											
Squamous cell cancer		1	0	1	9	Op, FT-207		↗ 1, n.c. 2, ↘	2	2	1	No recurrence (7)
Adenocarcinoma		2	2	0	75		Bs	↘				
Malignant melanoma	II	1	1	0	52	Op, PEP, DTIC, VCR	Bs	↗ 1, n.c., ↘	1		1	No recurrence (17)

Bs, bestatin; PEP, pepleomycin; Op., surgical operation; n.c., no change; ↗ = increased and within normal range; ↘ = decreased below normal range

Table 4. Findings in stage III and IV cancer patients treated with bestatin combined with anticancer agents

Disease (metastasis)	No. of cases	Sex M	Sex F	Average age	Bestatin treatment combined with	Parameters n.c.	Ly	T	PHA PPD (S.I.)	Alive under observation (months)	Died (months)
Kidney cancer (Lung) (Bone)	5	5	0	56	FAMT[a] BLM Radiation	↗ n.c. ↘	2 2 1	3 1 1	1 1 1	(7), (4), (3), (3)	(7)
(Lung) 1, (brain) 1, (pancreas) 1	4			58	FAMT					(14), (3), (3)	(2)
Bladder cancer (Lymphnodes) 1, (no metastasis) 4	5	5	0	67		↗ n.c. ↘	3 2	1 4	4	(15), (8), (7), (6)	
Ureter cancer	1	1	0	72	BLM Hormone	n.c. ↗	1 1	1 1		(11)	
Testicular cancer	2	2	0	38	VAB[b]	↗ n.c. ↘	2	1 1	5	(8), (2)	(4)
(Lung) 3, (retroperitoneum) 1, (no metastasis) 2	6	6	0	42	FOBEM[c]					(12), (8), (5) (4), (2)	(4)
Ovary cancer	1	0	1	64	5FU, MMC					(2)	
Skin cancer Squamous cell cancer Adenocarcinoma	2	1	1	52	PEP[d], MMC, FT-207 [60]Co	↗ n.c. ↘	2 2	2			(6),(3)

Melanoma (Systemic metastases 4, no metastasis) 1	5	4	1	36	DTC CCNU VCR	↗ n.c. ↘	1 2 2	1 1		2 3	(1), (1), (1)
Stomach cancer	10	5	5	63	FT-207	↗ n.c. ↘	2 6 2	4 2 4	5 4 1	2 6 2	2(4), 4(3), 4(2)
Lung cancer	3	2	1	59	Ca, CTX FT-207						(8), (3), (3)

[a] FAMT (5FU, cyclophosphamide, mitomycin, toyomycin)
[b] VAB (vinblastine, actinomycin D, bleomycin)
[c] FOBEM (5FU, vincristine, bleomycin, cyclophosphamide, mitomycin C)
[d] PEP (pepleomycin)

The eight patients who died did so at an average of 4 months after the beginning of bestatin treatment; three patients with stage III or IV malignant melanoma died within 1 month and one patient with stage IV renal tumor and bone metastases died within 2 months after bestatin administration. Therefore, bestatin was unlikely to restore immunity in extremely immunodepressed patients.

Leukocyte counts increased in 10 (33%) of 30 patients, the frequency of T rosettes in 10 (37%) of 27 patients, and blastogenesis of lymphocytes with PHA in 11 (45%) of 22 patients, so far studied. These findings are under investigation in relation to responses of patients to immunochemotherapy. The choice of anticancer agents best combined with bestatin is being studied in advanced cancer patients.

Bestatin Treatment Combined with Radiotherapy. Dr. Isono, Chiba University, used bestatin in combination with bleomycin and radiotherapy for preoperative treatment of six patients with esophageal cancer.

He found roentgenographic defects of the esophagus markedly reduced in size 10−14 days after this preoperative treatment. Most of the resected specimens showed a degeneration of more than two-thirds of cancer lesions, and the cancer lesions in one patient were found to be changed into scars. As he had never seen any such findings before in this kind of preoperative treatment, he assumed that these findings were due to a possible synergistic antitumor effect between bestatin and radiotherapy.

Dr. Majima, Chiba Cancer Center Hospital, treated virchow lymph node metastasis in stomach cancer with bestatin in combination with irradiation. A 47-year-old male with 30×40 mm virchow nodes received MCCNU, FT-207, FD-1, and 5-FU alternately for 20 months, but the tumor grew to 90×160 mm. Therefore, all medication was discontinued and 30 mg bestatin was administered daily. After 4 weeks irradiation in addition to bestatin, medication was given to the metastatic lymph nodes up to a total tumor dose of 3 800 rad. After 3 weeks, the metastatic lesion began to shrink and completely disappeared 5 weeks after this treatment.

A 68-year-old female having a 12×20 mm sized virchow node metastasis received FT-207 and MMC for one year, but with no response. A daily dose of 30 mg bestatin was given, combined with cobalt irradiation (6 000 tumor dose in 6 weeks). The virchow node completely disappeared.

Dr. Majima emphasises that adenocarcinoma of the stomach is basically radio-resistant, so bestatin in addition to irradiation must be a definite factor in complete remission of virchow's metastasis.

Summary

1) Bestatin has no clinical toxicity.
2) The frequency of T cells was found to increase after bestatin medication in immunodepressive cancer patients, except in extremely immunodepressive ones.

   Furthermore, NK activity was also found to be enhanced. Dr. Blomgren reported at the 2nd Meeting of the Cooperative Group Study on Bestatin, held in February 1979 in Tokyo, that NK activity increased after bestatin treatment in patients with advanced metastatic solid tumor which failed to respond to conventional therapy. Therefore, bestatin was confirmed as enhancing the activity of cells involved in immunity.

3) The pilot studies of bestatin showed that bestatin alone produced a beneficial effect against residual cancer lesions left by chemotherapy, surgery, and radiotherapy. Bestatin in combination with anticancer agents was useful for cancer lesions which are refractory to conventional methods of treatment in some instances.
However, the most suitable choice of anticancer agents to be combined with bestatin remains to be investigated.

4) Bestatin in combination with radiotherapy showed a favorable response against virchow metastatic lymph nodes. Preoperative treatment, with bestatin combined with chemotherapy and radiotherapy, was found to be very effective against cancer of the esophagus.

5) An optimal dose of bestatin was thought to exist in a dose ranging from 10—100 mg, and could be administered daily, twice, or three times a week, although no definite conclusion was reached. Therefore, studies are being carried out to establish an optimal dose schedule for immunochemotherapy or immunorestoration.

References

1. Aoyagi T, Suda H, Nagai M, Ogawa K, Suzuki J, Takeuchi T, Umezawa H (1976) Aminopeptidase activities on the surface of mammalian cells. Biochim Biophys Acta 452:131—143
2. Kondo T, Watanabe N, Tachibana T (1978) Rapid and simple assay in microtest plate for enumeration of human T and B lymphocyte populations (in Japanese). Igaku No Ayumi 107:312—314
3. Tachibana T, Yoshida A (1974) Determination of human T and B lymphocyte populations in microtest plate (an improved method). In: Japanese Society for Immunology (eds) Experimental methods in immunology A (in Japanese), pp 907—914
4. Umezawa H (1977) Recent advances in bioactive microbial secondary metabolites. Jpn J Antibiot 30:138—163.
5. Umezawa H, Aoyagi T, Suda H, Hamada M, Takeuchi T (1976) Bestatin, an inhibitor of aminopeptidase B, produced by actinomycetes. J Antibiot (Tokyo) 29:97—99
6. Umezawa H, Ishizuka M, Aoyagi T, Takeuchi I (1976) Enhancement of delayed-type hypersensivity by bestatin, an inhibitor of aminopeptidase B and leucine aminopeptidase. J Antibiot (Tokyo) 29:857—859

Phase I–II Study
of N^4-Behenoyl-1-β-D-Arabinofuranosylcytosine

K. Kimura, K. Yamada, Y. Uzuka, T. Maekawa, F. Takaku,
M. Shimoyama, M. Ogawa, I. Amaki, S. Osamura, M. Ito,
Y. Sakai, M. Oguro, K. Hattori, A. Hoshino, Y. Hirota,
K. Ohta, T. Nakamura, T. Masaoka, I. Kimura,
and M. Ichimaru*

1st Department of Internal Medicine Nagoya, University School of Medicine 65 Tsurumaicho, Showa-ku, J – Nagoya

1-β-D-Arabinofuranosylcytosine (ara-C) [7] is the mainstay of the treatment of acute myelogenous leukemia in adults [6]. It has, however, several drawbacks in that it has an extremely short half-life [11] and is very schedule-specific [17], which makes it less than ideal for clinical use. For this reason, attempts have been made to find other derivatives that might act as masked precursors, have long half-lives as well as less schedule dependency, give less toxicity, and perhaps achieve better clinical results [8, 10, 12, 13].

Aoshima, Sakurai, et al. [1] found that a series of newly synthesized N^4-acyl derivatives of ara-C with longer chains of fatty acids in their acyl groups exhibited a high level of antitumor activity against the mouse leukemia L-1210. One of those compounds, N^4-behenoyl-1-β-D-arabinofuranosylcytosine (BH-AC; Fig. 1) [2] was found to possess such features as a high level of antitumor activity and therapeutic index among ara-C analogs, schedule independence, resistance to cytidine deaminase, and long-lasting effect.

Preclinical and clinical pharmacologic studies [20] showed that BH-AC had a longer plasma half-time than ara-C and was converted to ara-C in vivo. The process appeared to be sufficiently slow to permit the maintenance of maximally effective ara-C levels when BH-AC was given once each day.

N^4–Behenoyl(1–β–D–arabinofuranosyl)cytosine   **Fig. 1**

*   We gratefully acknowledge the support of Asahi Chemical Industry in supplying the BH-AC used in these study, and Dr. Y. Sakurai and his group in supplying the experimental data on which these studies were based

The present report describes the results of phase I-II study of BH-AC conducted by a cooperative study group in Japan.

Patients and Methods

Phase I Study

Patients with documented metastatic malignancies and leukemias for whom there was no proven effective therapy and patients who were no longer responsive to effective therapy were considered eligible to receive BH-AC. No patient had received chemotherapy or radiotherapy within 3 weeks of receiving the drug. All patients had a complete history and physical examination with documentation of measurable disease (if present). Blood examinations including hemoglobin, hematocrit, WBC count and differential, platelet count, and renal and liver function profiles were obtained prior to treatment. Blood counts were taken twice weekly during the study.

Two schedules of drug administration were employed: (1) a single dose of BH-AC was given IV at day 1 only with dose ranges of 1.5−9.0 mg/kg; (2) daily consecutive doses of the drug was given IV for 3−21 days with dose ranges of 2.0−10.0 mg/kg. Dosage modifications were usually not made in individual patients.

Phase II Study

All adults with acute leukemia who were previously untreated were eligible for inclusion in the study regardless of morphological type, clinical status, elevation of leukocyte, degree of bleeding, or other considerations. The drug was administered by IV infusion lasting 3 h per day with dosages ranging from 3.5−8.0 mg/kg daily for 5−21 days. The drug was discontinued when a hypoplastic marrow resulted, and of further progression of leukopenia and/or production of marrow hypocellularity had not occured, the starting dose was resumed. Dosages were usually not modified in individual patients. The aim throughout was to continue drug administration during the induction phase to the point of the maximum tolerable amount, and thus a hypoplastic marrow or complete remission resulted. Throughout the studies, supportive therapy, including leukocyte and platelet transfusions, was used where indicated and feasible.

Responses were evaluated by the criteria of the Japan Hematological Society [14]. In the results to be discussed, only complete remission (CR) is considered significant. Marrow and/or peripheral blood remission in the presence of progression or persistence of disease elsewhere, i.e., node involvement, hepatosplenomegaly, etc. are not included among remissions.

Drug Administration

BH-AC was supplied by the Asahi Chemical Industry Co., Ltd. (Tokyo), in a 50 mg vial which contained 350 mg of hydrogenated castor oil polyethylene glycol ether (HCO-60; Nikko Chemical Co., Ltd., Tokyo) as a solvent. Five ml of sterile water were added to the vial, which was placed in boiling water for 5 min. After being cooled, BH-AC was completely dissolved to give a clear solution. The designated dose of BH-AC was added to 500 ml 5% dextrose solution and was administered by IV infusion lasting 3 h per day.

Results

Phase I Study

A total of 126 patients, 75 men and 51 women, were entered in the study. The median age was 51 years, with a range from 11−88 years. Fifty-one patients received a single dose of BH-AC at day 1 only, and 75 received daily consecutive doses.

Toxicity

All patients entered in the study were considered evaluable for immediate side effects, and only those patients with solid tumors who received daily consecutive administration of the drug were analyzed for myelosuppressive toxicity. The incidence of the various side effects of BH-AC relative to the dosage and the schedule are shown in Tables 1 and 2. In the day 1 only schedule nausea occurred in only 4 of 51 patients receiving the drug at daily dosage levels of 3−5 mg/kg, and was associated with vomiting in two patients (Table 1). Salivation and epilation, possibly related to the drug, were observed in one patient each. Forty-two (82%) of 51 patients had no toxic manifestation whatsoever. In the daily consecutive schedule, the most common side effects were nausea and vomiting (Table 2). Nausea occurred in 20 (26%) of 75 patients, and was associated with vomiting in three patients. Anorexia and malaise were observed in nine patients (12%) each. Further effects noticed in a small number of patients, perhaps attributable to the drug, were liver dysfunctions, erythematous rash, and fever.

The myelosuppressive toxicity was analyzed relative to the total WBC and platelet counts (Table 3). Only the myelosuppression related to the first 5 or 10-day courses is tabulated. Minimal myelosuppression was observed in the ten patients receiving five day courses of the drug at 2.0−3.5 mg/kg per day.

Table 1. Incidence of toxic effects of BH-AC at different dosage levels a single dose at day 1 only

	Dose (mg/kg/day)			
	−3.5	3.6−5.0	5.1−7.5	7.6−9.0
No. of patients treated	35	11	4	1
No. with toxic effects (%)				
Nausea	3 (9)	1 (10)	0	0
Vomiting	2 (6)	0	0	0
Anorexia	0	1 (10)	0	0
Salivation	0	1 (10)	0	0
Epilation	1 (3)	0	0	0

At higher dosage levels, the myelosuppresion became increasingly severe, such that all six patients receiving 5.1—9.0 mg/kg per day × 5 days or 3.6—5.0 mg/kg per day 10 days had either severe leukopenia or thrombocytopenia. There was no cumulative myelosuppression with prolonged administration of the drug. Analysis of the time course of the myelosuppression revealed that the median lowest leukocyte count was recorded on day 11, and for platelet, the median lowest count occured on day 12 in the first five-day course of treatment (Table 4).

Phase II Study

A total of 37 patients with acute leukemia in adults, 21 men and 16 women, were entered in the study. The mean age was 51 years, with a range from 15—72 years.

Table 2. Incidence of toxic effects of BH-AC at different dosage levels; daily consecutive doses

	Dose (mg/kg/day)			
	−3.5	3.6—5.0	5.1—7.5	7.6—9.0
No. of patients treated	37	24	9	5
No. with toxic effects (%)				
Nausea	10 (28)	9 (4)	1 (12)	0
Vomiting	1 (3)	2 (9)	0	0
Anorexia	6 (17)	2 (9)	1 (12)	0
Malaise	2 (6)	6 (25)	1 (12)	0
Erythemateous rash	1 (3)	0	0	0
Fever	1 (3)	0	0	0
Hypotension	1 (3)	0	0	0
Anemia	0	2 (9)	0	0
Liver dysfunctions	1 (3)	0	0	0

Table 3. Myelosuppression with BH-AC in patients with solid tumors

Dose (mg/kg/day)	No. of patients	No. of patients with		
		WBC 4 × 10³	Platelets/mm³	
			10 × 10⁴	2 × 10⁴
5-day courses				
2.0—3.5	10	2	1	0
3.6—5.0	4	2	4	2
5.1—9.0	6	4	2	2
10-day courses				
2.0—3.5	6	2	2	0
3.6—5.0	6	4	4	2
5.1—9.0	−	−	−	−

Twenty-six suffered from acute myelogenous leukemia (AML), six from acute monocytic leukemia (AMoL), two from acute promyelocytic leukemia (AMPL), two from acute lymphocytic leukemia (ALL), and one from smoldering type of AML. Table 5 gives an overall summary of the results. Responses with CR were noted with an overall rate of 35%. Of the patients who received BH-AC therapy, 50% of the 26 with AML and 16% of the six with AMoL responded with CR. Distribution of the patients relative to the total doses and total days of drug administration is shown in Table 6. In case of AML, patients receiving a total dose of more than 40 mg/kg for total days of more than ten had a significantly higher rate of CR (50%) than patients receiving smaller doses for fewer days (16%). Complete remissions were obtained at all age levels among adult patients with AML. A median total of 54 mg/kg of the drug, with a range of from 33−160 mg/kg, and a median total of 20 days of treatments, with a range from 10−33 days, were necessary for induction of CR. Complete remissions were obtained 28−60 days after the start of BH-AC, with a median of 35 days (Table 7).

Table 4. Time course of myelosuppression with BH-AC in patients with solid tumors

Dose (mg/kg/day)	Day[a] of (range) − lowest count	
	WBC	Platelet
5-day courses		
2.0−3.5	12 (3−21)	12 (1−14)
3.6−5.0	7 (3−9)	7 (3−13)
5.1−9.0	7 (9−13)	7 (5−13)
	11 (3−21)	12 (1−14)
10-day courses		
2.0−3.5	9 (7−24)	17 (9−21)
3.6−5.0	12 (11−26)	12 (11−13)
5.1−9.0	−	−
	11 (7−24)	13 (11−21)

[a] Median values for both days and counts

Table 5. Response of adults with acute leukemia to BH-AC therapy

DX	Total No. Rxed	CR	PR	F	Per cent CR
AML	26	13	7	6	50.0
AMoL	6	1	3	2	16.7
AMpL	2	−	1	1	−
Smold. AL	1	−	−	1	−
ALL	2	−	2	−	−
Total	37	14	13	10	35.1

The incidence and degree of drug toxicity were measured, the predominant effects being those related to marrow depression (Table 8). Leukocyte and platelet depressions were prominent, and transfusions of those two fractionated cells were frequently performed. The gastrointestinal effects were significantly less frequent than those reported by others using daily infusions lasting for 3 h per day. Liver dysfunctions were noted in two of 37 patients, but these were moderate in degree and reversible.

Table 6. Number of patients with AML relative to total doses and days of BH-AC therapy

Dx	Total doses (mg/kg)	Day of treatment			
		5–9	10–14	15–20	20–
AML	− 40	4 (0)	3 (1)	–	–
	41–100	2 (1)	6 (4)	–	–
	101–120	–	3 (2)	2 (1)	2 (1)
	121–	–	–	3 (3)	1 (0)
	Total	6 (1)	12 (7)	5 (4)	3 (1)

( ) CR

Table 7. Median total days and doses of BH-AC therapy in cases obtained CR

Total days (range) Rxed	Total doses administered (mg/kg/d)	Days reaching to CR
20 (10–33)	54 (33–160)	35 (28–60)

Table 8. Toxic effects of 3 h daily infusion of BH-AC in adults with acute leukemia

	%
Fall to WBC 1.0–3.0 ($\times$ 10^3/mm^3)	55
< 1.0	33
Fall to platelet < 30	55
Marrow hypocellularity < 30	48
Gastrointestinal tract:	
N and V	17
Anorexia	6
Eruptions	6
Hepatic dysfunctions	6
Total no. patients	37

Discussion

Both preclinical and clinical pharmacologic studies [20] showed that BH-AC had the longest plasma half-time among ara-C analogs. It was found that BH-AC was converted to ara-C in vivo, which was subsequently inactivated to ara-U by deamination in the usual way. However, conversion of BH-AC to ara-C is not instantaneous, and the process appeared to be sufficiently slow to permit the maintenance of maximally effective ara-C levels when BH-AC was given once each day, and therefore, BH-AC may serve as an in vivo reservoir of ara-C. Thus, BH-AC appeared to be a prime candidate for clinical trials of phase I-II study, which was conducted by a cooperative study group.

Three-hour infusion instead of rapid injection was employed in both phase I and II study because of the presence of the solvent HCO-60 in the drug preparation, which was reported to show hypotensive and histamine-releasing effects in dogs [18]. A recommended maximum dosage of HCO-60 for clinical use is 350 mg/day for IV, and therefore a single dose of BH-AC had to be limited to certain extent.

The immediate side effects following administration of BH-AC included nausea and vomiting, malaise, etc. Gastrointestinal toxicity was comparably less in incidence and severity than that observed with ara-C [3], and was not dose-limiting. As with the other side effects, epilation, salivation, fever, and itchy eruption occurred in sporadic incidences. No syncopal episode associated with postural hypotension or parotid pain was observed [4].

The major dose-limiting toxic effect observed was myelosuppression. At dosage levels of 5.1−9.0 mg/kg per day × 5 days, all patients had myelosuppression. The median lowest count of leukocytes and of platelets occurred at 11 days and 12 days, respectively. As with ara-C, there was no evidence that prolonged administration of BH-AC resulted in cumulative marrow toxicity.

In phase II study, significant responses were noted in AML patients, and complete remissions were obtained at all ages among adults. The dosage regimen used was infusion lasting 3 h per day, with the drug continued to the point of marrow depression where possible. Responses were noted, with an overall rate of 35% CR. Of the 26 patients with AML, there were 13 CR. The results are superior to those which have been reported for ara-C with the various dose regimens [3, 5, 6].

As was expected, the therapeutic effectiveness of BH-AC was found to be primarily time-dependent, i.e., dependent on the total length of treatment (thereby related to the total dose administered), and less dependent on the daily dose given, although a dosage of 4−5 mg/kg/per day seemed optimal for induction therapy of acute leukemia.

Combination chemotherapy studies with ara-C in acute leukemia have shown very positive results [9, 15, 19]. In solid tumors, a combination of ara-C, mitomycin C, and 5-FU was reported to have considerable efficacy against gastrointestinal adenocarcinoma [16]. In both cases, BH-AC is expected to be a promising alternative to ara-C because of its therapeutic potentiation.

Its minimal toxicity and the established therapeutic effectiveness over ara-C indicate that BH-AC deserves further clinical trials, particularly for phase III study in acute leukemia as well as in solid tumors, and such studies are now underway.

Summary

A phase I-II study of N^4-behenoyl-1-β-D-arabinofuranosyl-cytosine (BH-AC) was conducted by a cooperative study group. In phase I study, a total of 126 patients, 64 of whom had metastatic solid tumors and 62 of whom had leukemia, were administered BH-AC in a single IV dose at day 1 only or in daily IV doses for 3 to 21 days, with dose ranges of 1.5—10.0 mg/kg. Side effects included nausea and vomiting, which were significantly less in incidence and severity than those observed with ara-C. Myelosuppressive toxicity became severe with doses 3.6—5.0 mg/kg per day $\times$ 10 days.

In phase II study, a total of 37 adult patients with acute leukemia were entered in the study. Responses were noted, with an overall rate of 35% complete remission. Of th 26 patients with AML, there were 13 CR. The recommended schedule of treatment for BH-AC, based on our data, is daily infusion of 4—5 mg/kg over 3 h for approximately 3 weeks. The results with BH-AC in patients with acute leukemia are superior to those which have been reported for ara-C.

References

1. Aoshima M, Tsukagoshi Y, Sakurai Y, Ishida T, Kobayashi H (1976) Antitumor activities of newly synthesized N^4-behenoyl-1-β-D-arabinofuranosylcytosine. Cancer Res 36: 2726—2732
2. Aoshima M, Tsukagoshi S, Sakurai Y, Oh-Ishi J, Ishida T, Kobayashi H (1977) N^4-behenoyl-1-β-D-arabinofuranosylcytosine, as a potential new antitumor agent. Cancer Res 37: 2481—2486
3. Bodey GP, Freiereich EJ, Monto RW, Hewlet JS (1969) Cytosine arabinoside therapy for acute leukemia in adults. Cancer Chemother Rep 53: 59—66
4. Burgess MA, Bodey GP, Minow RA, Gottlieb JA (1977) Phase I-II evaluation of cyclocytidine. Cancer Treat Rep 61: 437—443
5. Ellison RR, Holland JF, Silver RT, Boiron M (1966) Cytosine arabinoside: A new drug for induction of remission in acute leukemia. Abstract, 9th Internat. Cancer Congr, p 645
6. Ellison RR, Holland JF, Weil M, Jacquillat C, Boiron M, Bernard J, Sawitsky A, Rosner F, Gussoff B, Silver RT, Karanas A, Cuttner J, Spurr CL, Hayes DM, Blom J, Leone LA, Haurani F, Kyle R, Hutchison JL, Forcier RJ, Moon JH
7. Evans JS, Musser EA, Bostwick JL, Mengel GD (1964) The effect of 1-β-D-arabinofuranosylcytosine hydrochloride on murine neoplasms. Cancer Res 24: 1285—1293
8. Fox JJ, Falco EA, Wempen D, Pomeroy MD, Dowling MD, Burchenal JH (1972) Oral and parenteral activity of 2,2'-anhydro-1-β-D-arabinofuranosyl-5-fluorocytosine (AAFC) against both intraperitoneally and intracerebrally inoculated mouse leukemia. Cancer Res 32: 2269—2272
9. Gee TS, Yu K-P, Clarkson BD (1969) Treatment of adults acute leukemia with arabinosylcytosine and thioguanine. Cancer 23: 1019—1032
10. Gray GD, Nichol FR, Michalson MM (1972) Immunosuppressive antiviral and antitumor activities of cytarabine derivatives. Biochem Pharmacol 27: 466—475
11. Ho DHW, Freireich EJ (1971) Clinical pharmacology of 1-β-D-arabinofuranosylcytosine. Clin Pharmacol Ther 12: 944—954
12. Ho DHW, Rodriguez V, Loo T, Bodey GP, Freireich EJ (1974) Clinical pharmacology of O^2, 2'-cyclocytidine. Clin Pharmacol Ther 17: 66—72
13. Hoshi A, Kanazawa F, Kuretani K (1972) Antitumor activity of cyclocytidine in a variety of tumors. Gann 63: 353—360

14. Kimura K (1965) Chemotherapy of acute leukemia with special reference to criteria for evaluation of therapeutic effect. In: Advances in chemotherapy of acute leukemia. A seminar on chemotherapy of acute leukemia under the U.S.-Japan Cooperative Science Program. Sept. 27–28. Bethesda MD, USA, pp 21–23. Published by The Editorial Committee for the Symposium on Recent Advances in Acute Leukemia, Nagoya, Japan.

15. Ohno R, Hirano M, Koie K, Kamiya T, Nishiwaki H, Ishiguro J, Yamada K, Uetani T, Sako F, Imamura K (1975) Daunorubicin, cytosine arabinoside, 6-mercaptopurine and prednisolone (DCMP) combination chemotherapy for acute myelogenous leukemia in adults. Cancer 36: 1945–1949

16. Ota K, Kurita S (1972) Combination therapy with mitomycin C (NSC-26980), 5-fluorouracil (NSC-19893), and cytosine arabinoside (NSC-63878) for advanced cancer in man. Cancer Chemother Rep 56: 373–385

17. Skipper HE, Schabel FM, Wilcox WS (1964) Experimental evaluation of potential anticancer agents. XIII. On the criteria and kinetics associated with "curability" of experimental leukemia. Cancer Chemother Rep 35: 1–111

18. Tajima T, Shoji T, General pharmacological effects of menaquinone-4 (in Japanese). Pharmacometrics 5: 489–504

19. Whitecar JP jr, Bodey GP, Freireich EJ (1972) Cyclophosphamide (NSC-26271), vincristine (NSC-67574), cytosine arabinoside (NSC-63878), and prednisolone (NSC-10023) (COAP) combination chemotherapy for acute leukemia in adults. Cancer Chemother Rep 56: 543–550

20. Yamada K, Kawashima K, Kato Y, Morishima Y, Tanimoto M, Ohno, R (1980) Pharmacological and clinical studies of N^4-behenoyl-1-β-D-arabinofuranosylcytosine. In: Carter SK, Sakurai Y (eds) Recent Results in Cancer Research, vol 70. Springer, Berlin Heidelberg, pp 219–229

Gastric Cancer

The FAM Regimen for Gastric Cancer: A Progress Report*

P. S. Schein, J. S. Macdonald, P. V. Woolley, F. P. Smith, D. F. Hoth, M. Boiron, C. Gisselbrecht, R. Brunet, and C. Lagarde

Vincent T. Lombardi Cancer Research Center, Georgetown University School of Medicine, USA – Washington, DC 20007

The FAM regimen for upper gastrointestinal cancer was developed during 1974. It incorporated three anticancer drugs which had demonstrated independent activity against gastric cancer: 5-fluorouracil, adriamycin [2], and mitomycin-C [3]. In an attempt to insure adequate patient tolerance and allow for chronic administration, an intermittent schedule was designed (Table 1). In particular, mitomycin-C was to be administered only once every 2 months because of its then appreciated delayed and cumulative bone marrow toxicity. We have recently reported the criteria for entry into this study, including the strict requirement for followable disease criteria for patient response, as well as the initial response rates and survival curves [1]. This progress report describes the updated results in the treatment of 62 patients with advanced and measurable gastric cancer.

The patient population consists of 38 men and 24 women, with a median age of 62 years (range 28–83). The median Eastern Cooperative Oncology Group (ECOG) performance status (PS) was 2, asymptomatic but in bed less than 50% of the time, with a range of 0–4. The primary tumor had been resected in only 28 of the 62 cases. The principal site of followable disease was as follows: palpable abdominal mass, 50%; hepatic metastases, 36%; palpable lymphadenopathy, 6%; osseous metastases, 8%.

Table 1. FAM combination chemotherapy

Drug	Dose	Method of administration	Day 1	8	28	35	56	
5-Fluorouracil	600 mg/m^2	IV	X	X	X	X	R	
							E	C
Adriamycin	30 mg/m^2	IV	X		X		P	Y
							E	C
Mitomycin-C	10 mg/m^2	IV	X				A	L
							T	E

* This study was supported by NIH-NCI NOI-CM 67110. This work has been convected, in part, under the French-American Agreement in Cancer Research

Twenty-six patients (42%) have achieved a partial response. The median duration of response is 9 months with a range of 2−20 months. The influence of known prognostic variables for response were analyzed. In regard to performance status, 46% of 41 patients with PS 0−2 achieved an objective response, but 31% of cases with PS 3−4 still benefited from treatment. The sites of principal followable disease made an apparent contribution to the outcome; 50% of patients with malignant hepatomegaly responded, compared to 32% with abdominal masses and 20% with osseous metastasis. All four patients with followable lymphadenopathy achieved a partial remission. An interesting result was obtained from the analysis of tumor differentiation: 68% of patients with poorly differentiated tumors demonstrated a partial response compared to only 32% with well or moderately differentiated histology. The potential importance of age or sex were also analyzed; the median age of responders and nonresponders did not differ (64 years versus 63 years), whereas women fared slightly better than men, 50% response versus 32%.

The survival of this patient group is presented in Fig. 1. The median survival of the entire group is 6 months. The median survival of responding patients is 13 months (range 5−37 months) which is significantly longer than the 4-month median (range 0.5−8 months) for the nonresponders.

The toxicity of the FAM regimen was, in general, well tolerated. There was remarkably little serious acute gastrointestinal regimen as one commonly encounters with combinations containing a chloroethylnitrosourea. Myelosuppression was at an acceptable level, only 10% of patients demonstrating a white blood cell count below $1\,500/mm^3$ or platelet count less than $30\,000/mm^3$ during their entire period of treatment. After a full year of treatment patients were still able to take 75% of the original projected doses based upon measurements of body surface area. No adriamycin cardiac toxicity was encountered, as might be expected in view of the relatively low cumulated dose, $360\,mg/m^2$, during the first year of treatment.

The response rate found in this pilot study has now been confirmed in a large controlled trial conducted by the Southwest Oncology Group [4]. At the present time the FAM regimen represents a useful treatment option for the patient with either advanced or locally unresectable gastric cancer. Surgical adjuvant trials with this

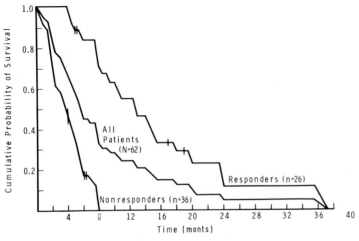

Fig. 1. Survival after initiation of FAM chemotherapy

combination have now been initiated or are being planned by several cooperative groups.

References

1. MacDonald JS, Woolley PV, Smythe T, Ueno W, Hoth D, Schein PS (to be published) 5-Fluorouracil, adriamycin, and mitomycin-C (FAM) combination chemotherapy in the treatment of advanced gastric cancer. Cancer
2. Moertel CG (1976) Chemotherapy of gastrointestinal cancer. Clin Gastroenterol 5: 777
3. Moore GE, Bross IDJ, Ausman R, Nadler S, Jones R, Slack N, Rimm AA (1968) Efficacy of mitomycin-C in 346 patients with advanced cancer. Cancer Chemother Rep 52: 641
4. Panettiere FJ, Heibrun L (1979) Experiences with two treatment schedules in the combination chemotherapy of advanced gastric carcinoma. In: Carter S, Crooke S (eds) Mitomycin-C: Current status and new developments. Academic Press, New York San Francisco London

Adjuvant Studies in Gastric Cancer in the United States

G. A. Higgins

Veterans Administration Medical Center, 50 Irving Street N.W.
USA – Washington, DC 20422

For reasons yet unknown, there has been a steady decrease in the rate of gastric cancer in the United States for the past four decades. Despite this providential decline, however, the estimated 1979 incidence of 23 000 new cases and 14 000 deaths continues to place gastric malignancy high on the list of formidable problems facing American oncologists. The World Health Statistics Manual shows a highly variable worldwide incidence rate, the most prevalent areas of gastric cancer being geographically widely separated countries such as Japan, Chile, Costa Rica, and Hungary. Among the 44 countries from which statistics have been compiled, the United States ranks No. 40 in males and No. 43 in females; and with few exceptions, the incidence in males is considerably higher than in females in the countries surveyed. The overall adjusted 5-year survival rates in the United States remain distressingly low, being 12% in males and 13% in females. However, in those patients with localized disease and hence favorable for surgical resection, the adjusted survival rates are approximately 40% [7]. Unfortunately the symptoms of gastric cancer are nonspecific and all too often appear late in the course of the disease, with only 18% of patients having a localized stage of disease at the time of diagnosis. Even when all obvious malignancy has been removed following surgical resection, appearance of recurrent or persistent disease remains a frequent and discouraging problem. This presentation will be concerned with a review of the clinical trials conducted in the United States in which other modalities of therapy have been combined with surgery in an attempt to prolong and augment the postoperative survival rate.

Completed Trials

When the large cooperative group studies were instituted in the late 1950s, two adjuvant surgical groups, one composed of University Hospitals [1] and a second composed of Veterans Administration Hospitals [9], designed and instituted protocols to study the effects of the administration of chemotherapy at the time of the operation and in the immediate postoperative period. These trials were based on observations that the peripheral blood of patients with cancer contain cells which closely resemble the neoplastic cells found in the primary tumor and that the number of cells is increased in the peripheral blood and especially in the venous blood draining the tumor area during operative manipulation of the tumor at the time of operation. Also, animal studies had demonstrated that chemotherapeutic agents administered to animals could significantly reduce the implantation and growth of cells in recipient animals. Because of previous animal studies, as well as prior experience with its use in man, thio-TEPA was selected as the experimental drug by both study groups. In the Veterans Administration (VA) group trial, thio-TEPA was administered both intravenously and intraperitoneally at the close of operation and the drug was then administered intravenously on each of the first and second postoperative days. The University group protocol differed slightly in that the dosage of thio-TEPA at the end of surgery was given intravenously and into a portal vein tributary rather than intraperitoneally. In addition, both male and female patients were included in the University study, whereas only male patients were entered into the VA trials. This phase of the study, referred to as the "full dosage scheduling", was discontinued when analysis of the 30-day mortality data suggested an adverse effect of the drug. This adverse effect observed in the VA study was not seen in data accruing in the University study group. Careful study of the postoperative mortality data showed a significant increase in those patients receiving the drug who had also had splenectomy in conjunction with gastrectomy. Subsequent animal studies also showed a decreased tolerance to thio-TEPA following splenectomy [4]. Consequently, a "reduced dosage schedule" was instituted omitting the intravenous dosage of thio-TEPA administered at the close of operation. Over 900 patients were randomized into the various stratifications of these two cooperative trials; however, no benefit in survival could be demonstrated in patients receiving the drug, compared with patients treated by surgery alone [1, 3, 5].

Following termination of entry into these trials, the VA Surgical Adjuvant Group next ran a study using fluorodeoxyuridine as the anticancer drug [6]. Randomization was carried out on the first postoperative day and those patients selected to receive the drug were given intravenous doses on the first, second, and third postoperative days. A second course was then instituted between the 35th and 45th postoperative days. This consisted of five full doses on successive days followed by four half-doses on alternate days, if toxicity permitted. Extensive analysis of survival data of 459 patients entered into this trial showed no demonstrable treatment benefit from the drug in any of the three stratification groups [3, 6]. Following completion of accrual of patients in this protocol, the VA group discontinued study of gastric cancer, partly because the number of patients available for such studies had decreased appreciably.

Ongoing Trials

In 1974 the VA group resumed the study of gastric cancer, using a combination o methyl-CCNU (MeCCNU) and 5-Fluorouracil (5-FU) as the study drugs. Based on surgical findings and study of the resected specimens, patients are stratified into three groups: group A, resection of the primary lesion without microscopic evidence of residual tumor; group B, resection of the primary lesion, but with microscopic evidence of residual disease; and group C, primary lesion not resected. Administration of drugs is begun as soon as the patient's postoperative condition permits, usually between the 7th and 14th postoperative days. The 5-FU is administered intravenously in a daily dosage of 9 mg/kg on 5 successive days with MeCCNU given orally in a dose of 4 mg/kg body wt. on the first day of treatment. At this time, approximately 275 patients have been randomized into this trial but observations on recurrence and survival are too early to permit any statement on drug effect (Fig. 1).

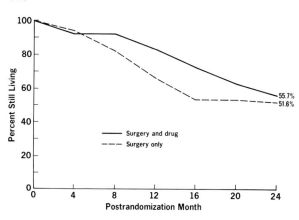

Fig. 1. Survival curves of patients in the Current Veterans Administration Surgical Oncology Group trial comparing surgery alone with a combination of 5-FU and MeCCNU

Currently there are at least five additional clinical trials in progress in the United States, as well as one in Canada and one in Europe, which will be briefly reviewed [9] (Table 1).

The Eastern Cooperative Oncology Group (ECOG) also has a two-arm trial in which MeCCNU and 5-FU are administered to those patients randomized to receive the drug. Patients entered into this trial have undergone a complete en bloc distal subtotal or total resection of all known tumor within 6 weeks prior to study entry. Intravenous 5-FU is given on 5 successive days with MeCCNU administered orally on the first day of treatment. Courses are repeated every 10 weeks until there is evidence of recurrence or for a total of ten courses. No survival or recurrence data are as yet available.

The Southwest Oncology Group (SWOG) has instituted a protocol in patients having potentially curative surgery. The treatment arm of this trial consists of a combination of 5-FU, adriamycin, and mitomycin C, the FAM regimen which has shown promise in patients with advanced disease. The drug is started approximately 4−8 weeks following surgery and is repeated at 8-week intervals for a total of six courses. No data are as yet available.

The Gastro-Intestinal Tumor Study Group (GITSG) is also conducting a two-arm trial in patients undergoing potentially curative resection. In those patients randomized to receive the drug, therapy is instituted when the patient's postoperative condition permits and it consists of intravenous 5-FU on 5 successive days, with MeCCNU to be given orally on day 1. Drug courses are repeated every 5 weeks, but MeCCNU is given only on the first day of alternate courses. Therapy is continued for 2 years or until relapse or prohibitive toxicity. Patients are stratified by extent of resection, tumor type, and location of the primary lesion. Accrual of patients continues in this trial.

At the Mayo Clinic a randomized trial is currently underway to determine whether a combination of 5-FU and supervoltage radiation can improve survival of patients who have poor prognosis and who have operable gastric cancer. Only those patients undergoing potentially curative surgery who have lymph node involvement, diffuse infiltrative, scirrhous lesions, or those with lesions of the cardia are included. In those patients randomized to the treatment arm, therapy is instituted 3−4 weeks following operation. This consists of supervoltage radiotherapy to a total dose of 3 000 rads to the tumor area delivered during a 28-day period with 5-FU administered intravenously on days 1 through day 3 of radiotherapy.

Table 1. Tabulation of adjuvant trials in gastric cancer now in progress in the United States and Canada (from Compilation of Clinical Protocol Summaries, Third Edition, April 1979) [8]. For details of names of groups and treatment regimens, see text

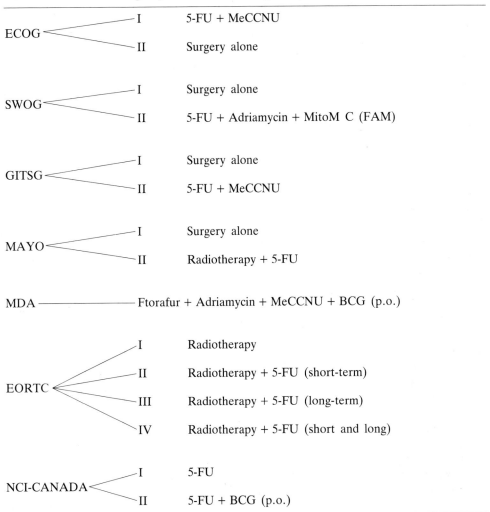

Group	Arm	Regimen
ECOG	I	5-FU + MeCCNU
	II	Surgery alone
SWOG	I	Surgery alone
	II	5-FU + Adriamycin + MitoM C (FAM)
GITSG	I	Surgery alone
	II	5-FU + MeCCNU
MAYO	I	Surgery alone
	II	Radiotherapy + 5-FU
MDA		Ftorafur + Adriamycin + MeCCNU + BCG (p.o.)
EORTC	I	Radiotherapy
	II	Radiotherapy + 5-FU (short-term)
	III	Radiotherapy + 5-FU (long-term)
	IV	Radiotherapy + 5-FU (short and long)
NCI-CANADA	I	5-FU
	II	5-FU + BCG (p.o.)

At the M.D. Anderson Hospital, a nonrandomized study is underway, utilizing patients who have undergone surgery for removal of the tumor within ten weeks of entry and who have no evidence of local or metastatic disease. All patients are given a three-drug combination consisting of ftorafur, adriamycin, and MeCCNU. Courses of drug therapy are continued for 1 year. In addition to chemotherapy these patients are given BCG orally for a period of 2 years.

The National Cancer Institute of Canada [2] has conducted a trial in gastric cancer comparing 5-FU as a single agent with a combination of 5-FU and BCG given orally. The European Organization for Research on the Treatment of Cancer (EORTC) has a four-arm randomized trial in which patients with totally or partially resected localized gastric carcinoma are entered. All patients receive either postoperative radiotherapy alone or radiotherapy combined with a different regimen of 5-FU. In arm I, patients are given a total dosage of 5 550 rads over a period of 6 weeks. In arm II the same dosage of radiotherapy is used and intravenous 5-FU is administered on days 1 through 4 of the first week of radiotherapy. In arm III patients are given the same dosage of radiotherapy followed by intravenous 5-FU to be given every 2 weeks starting approximately 4 weeks after completion of radiotherapy and to be continued for 18 months. Arm IV of the trial calls for the same dosage of radiotherapy plus a combination of short-term chemotherapy as in arm II of the trial followed by the long-term chemotherapy with 5-FU utilized in arm III of the study.

Summary

Early optimism for the chemotherapeutic augmentation of standard surgical treatment of gastric cancer has thus far generally not come to pass. First attempts to destroy circulating cancer cells in small metastatic foci by giving drugs at the completion of operation and in the immediate postoperative period were disappointing.

Numerous large cooperative groups and individual institutions are now studying drugs and drug combinations in various treatment regimens and have introduced the use of radiotherapy and immunotherapy in an effort to improve long-term survival following surgical resection of gastric cancer.

Resurgence of interest in surgical adjuvant studies, and especially recent encouraging results from drug combinations in advanced disease, with the possible augmentation by radiotherapy and immunotherapy, generates optimism that the theoretical potential of this approach to cancer control may soon be realized.

References

1. Dixon WJ, Longmire WP jr, Holden WD (1971) Use of triethylenethiophosphoramide as an adjuvant to the surgical treatment of gastric and colorectal carcinoma: Ten-year follow-up. Ann Surg 173:26
2. Falk RE, Macgregor AB, Ambus H, Landi S, Langer B, Miller AB (1976) The use of adjuvant therapy with BCG combined with chemotherapy in the treatment of gastrointestinal cancer. In: Lamoureux G, Turcotte R, Portelance V (eds) BCG in cancer immunotherapy. Grune & Stratton, New York, pp 217–225
3. Higgins GA (1976) Chemotherapy, adjuvant to surgery, for gastrointestinal cancer. Clin Gastroenterol 5:795–808
4. Higgins GA jr, Flynn T, Gillespie J (1964) Effect of splenectomy on tolerance to thio-TEPA. Arch Surg 88:627–632
5. Serlin O, Keehn RJ, Higgins GA, Harrower HW, Mendeloff GL (1977) Factors related to survival following resection for gastric carcinoma. Analysis of 903 cases. Cancer 40:1318–1329
6. Serlin O, Wolkoff JS, Amadeo JM, Keehn RJ (1969) Use of 5-fluorodeoxyuridine (FUDR) as an adjuvant to the surgical management of carcinoma of the stomach. Cancer 24:223–228
7. Silverberg E (1979) Cancer Statistics, 1979. CA 29:6–21
8. U.S. Dept. Health, Education and Welfare, Public Health Service, National Institutes of Health, National Cancer Institute (1979) Compilation of clinical protocol summaries, 3rd ed. DHEW/NIH 79–1116
9. Va Surgical Adjuvant Cancer Chemotherapy Study Group (1965) Use of thio-TEPA as an adjuvant to the surgical management of carcinoma of the stomach. Cancer 18:291–297

Preliminary Results
of A United States-Japan Cooperative Trial
in Patients with Disseminated Gastric Cancer

M. Friedman, M. Ogawa, J. Hannigan, K. Kimura, Y. Sakurai, and S. K. Carter*

University of California, San Francisco, Cancer Research Institute, 1282M, USA – San Francisco, CA 94143

Introduction

In December 1977 a joint clinical trial for patients with gastric adenocarcinoma was initiated by investigators in the United States and Japan. This cooperative protocol was the first joint clinical effort sponsored by the United States-Japan Scientific Agreement for Cancer Research, as part of the National Cancer Institute.

The reasons for selecting gastric cancer as the disease to be studied were threefold. Firstly, gastric cancer is probably the most sensitive to chemotherapy of all the enteric adenocarcinomas. Secondly, the expertise of the Japanese oncologists in the research and care of gastric cancer patients is well recognized. Finally, similar chemotherapy approaches are used by physicians in both countries.

The institutions participating in the American program are members of the Northern California Oncology Group (NCOG).

Fourteen institutions are participating on the Japanese side. The study has coordinators and study chairmen from both countries.

Study Design and Purposes

There were considerable problems that had to be dealt with in the design and execution of this binational Phase III trial. After much discussion it was concluded that one similar treatment arm would be studied by both nations and that the United States and Japan would each employ an additional unique arm. This design would permit direct comparisons (for the common arm) and indirect comparisons between all three arms. This study protocol is summarized in Table 1. A variety of pretherapeutic stratification variables were deemed to be important and were elucidated in the protocol randomization:

1) Measurable disease
   a) Nonmeasurable
   b) Measurable

* The authors are grateful to Melanie Gribble and Yoko Shimano for their help in preparing this analysis. This study was supported in part by American Cancer Society Clinical Fellowship 4285, Northern and NCI Contrect No. NOI-CM-22054

2) Prior radiation therapy
   a) No prior radiation
   b) Prior radiation
3) Status of primary tumor
   a) Resected
   b) Nonresected
4) Performance status (Karnofsky)[1]
   a) 40%−70%
   b) 80%−100%
5) Weight loss within last months
   a) ≤ 10%
   b) > 10%

The purposes of this joint investigation were projected to be the following:
1) To determine the feasibility of a joint United States-Japan trial.
2) To determine the comparability of patients, disease biology, drug toxicity, and physician practice in the United States and Japan.
3) To determine the response rates, survival, and toxicity of all three treatments.

Table 1. Schema of Japan gastric cancer study

R

A

N: NCOG Arm
BCNU 100 mg/m^2 IV day 1
Adriamycin 40 mg/m^2 IV day 1[a]   repeat
Ftorafur 2 gm/m^2 IV days 1 and 2   q 28 days

N

D

C: Common arm − NCOG
Adriamycin 50 mg/m^2 IV day 1   repeat
5-FU 500 mg/m^2 IV days 1, 2, and 3   q 21 days

O

M

C: Common arm − Japanese
Adriamycin 35−50 mg/m^2 IV day 1[a]   repeat
5-FU 350−500 mg/m^2 IV days 1, 2, and 3   q 21 days

I

Z

J: Japanese arm
Adriamycin 20−30 mg/m^2 IV day 1 q 3 weeks[a]
Mitomycin C 2.7−4 mg/m^2 IV day 1 q week
Ftorafur 267 mg/m^2/po b.i.d. every week
   or

E

33 mg/m^2 rectally day 1 every day

[a] After cumulative dose of adriamycin of 500 mg/m^2, switch to BCNU + 5FU

1 In Japan, patients were stratified according to Karnofsky Performance Status only

Materials and Methods

Data forms, flow sheets, and computer assisted statistical analysis were provided by the NCOG Central Administrative Office. Randomization was performed independently in both countries, and histologic material will be reviewed by pathologists in both nations.

Patients were considered eligible for randomization if they fit the following criteria:

1) Biopsy proven gastric adenocarcinoma.
2) No prior chemotherapy.
3) No significant intrinsic heart disease.
4) Age less than 75 years old.
5) Karnofsky Performance Status (KPS) < 40%.
6) Adequate physiologic status: a) Bilirubin < 3 mg%, b) SGOT < 4 times normal, c) Creatinine < 2 mg%, d) WBC > 4000 cells/mm^3, and e) Platelets > 100 000 cells/mm^3.

Standard criteria for objective response were employed but patients did not need to have measurable disease to be included in this study. Overall survival was identified as the most significant objective parameter measured.

Modification of drug dosage was based on blood counts and liver function tests.

Table 2. Comparability of patients in NCOG-Japan joint gastric cancer study

Stratification variables		United States			Japan		
		Arm C	Arm N	Total	Arm C	Arm J	Total
No. pts. randomized		19	21	40	24	26	50
Age	35	1	1	2	1	2	3
	35−50	6	2	8	3	6	9
	51−65	9	12	21	15	11	26
	65	3	6	9	5	7	12
Sex	Male	13	14	27	15	16	31
	Female	6	7	13	9	10	19
Tumor	T1	1	1	2	2	1	3
	T2	2	0	2	0	2	2
	T3	3	4	7	5	5	10
	T4	10	12	22	9	7	16
	Unkown	3	4	7	8	11	19
	N0	6	1	7	0	0	0
	N1	5	6	11	1	1	2
	N2	0	4	4	3	2	5
	N3	3	4	7	8	6	14
	N4	0	0	0	0	0	0
	Unknown	5	6	11	12	17	29
Metastases	M0	4	7	11	7	2	9
	M1	15	14	29	17	24	41

Results

Sixteen months after the initiation of this study a total of 90 patients had been entered and could be subjected to a preliminary analysis. Evaluation of these patients based on age, sex, and TNM stratification variables are summarized in Table 2. As can be seen, there is excellent comparability between the American and Japanese patients. There appears to be a slight preponderance of T4 lesions in the American group and of N3 cases in the Japanese group.

The distribution of patients according to measurability of disease, prior therapy, Karnofsky performance status, and weight loss were again comparable between the two groups (Table 3).

Table 3. Comparability of stratification variables in NCOG-Japan; joint gastric protocol

Stratification variables		United States			Japan		
		Arm C	Arm N	Total	Arm C	Arm J	Total
No. pts. randomized		19	21	40	24	26	50
Measurable disease	Non-measurable	6	10	16	9	12	21
	Measurable	13	11	24	10	9	19
Prior radiotherapy	Yes	1	1	2	0	0	0
	No	18	20	38	19	22	41
Surgery	Non-resectable	12	14	26	15	16	31
	Resectable	7	7	14	4	6	10
Karnofsky status	40−70	9	8	17	12	12	24
	80−100	10	13	23	12	14	26
Prior weight loss	< 10	12	13	25	9	12	21
	>10	7	8	15	8	9	17

Table 4. Gastrointestinal and cardiac toxicity observed with common arm (adriamycin + 5-FU) in NCOG-Japan joint gastric cancer study

	Karnofsky status 80−100		
	Number evaluated	Number with severe nausea and vomiting	Number with severe cardiac toxicity
Japanese	10	0	0
NCOG	8	1	1
	Karnofsky status 40−70		
Japanese	7	1	0
NCOG	8	3	0

Table 5. Hematologic toxicity observed with common arm (adriamycin + 5-FU) in NCOG-Japan joint gastric cancer study

	Karnofsky 80−100				
	Number evaluated	Number with WBC		Number with platelets	
		≤ 4 000	≤ 2 000	≤ 100 000	≤ 50 000
Japanese	10	10	0	1	0
NCOG	8	7	1	1	1
	Karnofsky 40−70				
	Number evaluated	Number with WBC		Number with platelets	
		≤4 000	≤ 2 000	≤ 100 000	≤ 50 000
Japanese	7	5	0	0	0
NCOG	8	6	6	2	0

Table 6. Severity of toxicity observed with common arm (adriamycin + 5-FU) in NCOG-Japan joint gastric cancer study

Grade	Nausea and vomiting			
	Cycle 1 and 2		Overall	
	U.S. (19)	Japan (24)	U.S.	Japan
1 (least severe)	26%	25%	26%	25%
2	16%	13%	32%	13%
3	10%	0	26%	0
4 (most severe)	0	4%	0	4%

WBC (cell/mm^3)	Toxicity − White blood cells			
	Cycle 1 and 2		Overall	
	U.S. (19)	Japan (24)	U.S.	Japan
3 000−4 000	21%	17%	21%	17%
2 000−3 000	10%	33%	16%	42%
< 2,000	26%	8%	26%	13%

PLT (cells/mm^3)	Toxicity − platelet			
	Cycle 1 and 2		Overall	
	U.S. (19)	Japan (24)	U.S.	Japan
75−100 000	0	4%	5%	17%
50−75 000	0	0	0	0
< 50 000	11%	4%	11%	4%

Table 7. Toxicity observed with japanese unique arm (mitomycin C + adriamycin + ftoratur) in NCOG-Japan joint gastric cancer study

Number evaluated	Karnofsky Status 80–100	
	Number with severe nausea and vomiting	Number with severe cardiac toxicity
11	0	0
	Karnofsky status 40–70	
6	1	0

Number evaluated	Karnofsky status 80–100			
	Number with WBC		Number with platelets	
	≤ 4 000	≤ 2 000	≤ 100 000	≤ 50 000
11	10	3	4	0
	Karnofsky status 40–70			
6	6	0	1	1

Table 8. Toxicity observed with NCOG unique arm (BCNU + adriamycin + ftorafur) in NCOG-Japan joint gastric cancer study

Number evaluated	Karnofsky Status 80–100	
	Number with severe nausea and vomiting	Number with severe cardiac toxicity
9	2	0
	Karnofsky status 40–70	
8	5	0

Number evaluated	Karnofsky status 80–100			
	Number with WBC		Number with platelets	
	≤ 4 000	≤ 2 000	≤ 100 000	≤ 50 000
9	4	1	3	0
	Karnofsky status 40–70			
8	3	1	3	2

Table 9. Time since randomization (weeks)

	ARM J			ARM C (Japan)			ARM C (NCOG)			ARM N		
	No. pat.[a]	No. deaths	Med. surv.	No. pat.[a]	No. deaths	Med. surv.	No. pat.[a]	No. deaths	Med. surv.	No. pat.[a]	No. deaths	Med. surv.
All patients	9	10	30	18	15	22–25[b]	17	9	27	18	12	27
K.P.S. 40–70	6	4	12–14[b]	7	7	22	9	5	10	7	5	16
K.P.S. 80–100	13	6	36	11	8	28	8	4	30	11	7	31
Measurable	8	5	14–16[b]	9	7	22	10	7	23	9	5	16
Nonmeasurable	11	5	36	9	8	26	6	2	40[c]	9	7	27–33

[a] Number of patients evaluable for survival analysis
[b] % not reaching endpoint stayed equal to 50% for these weeks
[c] Median not reached at 40 weeks, 53% at 27 weeks

Overall, there is a satisfactory balance achieved between the patients in both countries for all the stratification groups. Analysis of adherence to protocol-dictated dosages and schedules also revealed that most patients were properly treated.

Toxicity

Evaluation of toxicity was made in three areas − hematologic, gastrointestinal, and cardiac. Analysis was made according to KPS, treatment, and country. For the common arm (Arm C) there was little detectable gastrointestinal or cardiac toxicity (Table 4).
Hematopoietic toxicity was also overly distributed between both nations (Table 5). Overall, the toxicity of this treatment regimen was such that it could be considered well tolerated. The percentage of patients experiencing severe nausea and vomiting or myelosuppression were small (Table 6). The Japanese unique arm of mitomycin C plus adriamycin plus ftorafur was also well tolerated (Table 7). The same can be said for the NCOG unique arm of BCNU plus adriamycin plus ftorafur (Table 8).

Efficacy

The median survival times (in weeks) of patients which can be evaluated at this time can be seen in Table 9. There is no meaningful difference detectable between any of the treatment programs. Patients with poor KPS ratings seemed to have a poorer overall life expectancy (12−22 weeks median survival). On the other hand, patients with good KPS and nonmeasurable disease had a better overall prognosis (26−40+ weeks median survival).

Discussion

This report is a preliminary one which recognizes the need for further patient accession and more detailed data analysis. Nonetheless, there are several conclusions which can be drawn at this time.
First of all, there is significant comparability between the toxicity and efficacy data for the American and Japanese patients on Arm C. The dosages used, toxicity, and median survival are all quite similar. It is reassuring to note this similarity since it engenders more confidence in this joint trial.
In an overall sense, this study has yielded median survivorships which are consistent with other larger American clinical trials for gastric cancer patients. Moertel et al. [1] have reviewed the Gastro-Intestinal Tumor Study Group's and Eastern Cooperative Oncology Group's data on 517 gastric cancer patients. For patients on 12 studies the median duration of survival was between 16 and 34 weeks. Our current data is consistent with this large composite experience. We may assume that in our study the quality of care has not been diluted in our efforts to make this binational trial succeed. There has been excellent overall cooperation between the American and Japanese investigators in this study. All involved with this study are hopeful that future collaborative efforts will prove even more productive.

Reference

1. Moertel CG, O'Connell MJ, Lavin PT (1979) Chemotherapy of gastric carcinoma. Am Assoc Cancer Res 20: 1168

Combined Modality Studies on Small Cell Carcinoma of the Lung – Current Status in Japan

H. Ikegami, T. Horai, and S. Hattori*

Department of Lung Cancer, Research Institute, The Center for Adult Diseases, 1-3-3-Nakamichi, Higashinari-ku, J – Osaka 537

Introduction

Small cell carcinoma of the lung is thought to be one of the most malignant tumors that occur in man. However, modern therapy has resulted in a marked prolongation of survival in patients with small cell carcinoma of the lung [1, 3, 4, 13, 24, 27]. This paper deals with the current status of the multidisciplinary treatment for patients with small cell carcinoma in Japan.

Treatment in the Center for Adult Diseases, Osaka

Seventy-five patients with cytologically and/or histologically confirmed small cell carcinoma of the lung were treated. In single chemotherapy, cyclophosphamide, 20 mg/kg body wt., was given intravenously once a week for 4–6 weeks. In a combination treatment, cyclophosphamide (CTX) (20 mg/kg once a week, IV), vincristine (VCR) (1 mg/person once a week, IV), and 5-fluorouracil (5-FU) (250 mg/person daily IV) were administered for 4 weeks, followed by radiotherapy (β-tron or linear accelerator; 3 000–5 000 rads) and intradermal injections of BCG-CWS or Nocardia-CWS [29, 30].

Response was defined as follows: Complete response (CR) indicates a complete regression of all of the recognizable tumor; partial response (PR) indicates more than 50% decrease in the initial tumor size on the chest X ray film, and nonresponse (NR) indicates less than 50% decrease (tumor size determined by the product of the longest perpendicular diameters). Survival time was calculated from the onset of treatment.

Data on survival of patients with small cell carcinoma according to tumor regression as a result of chemotherapy are shown in Fig. 1. Median survival times for CR, PR, and NR cases were 14.5 months, 10.5 months, and 7.0 months, respectively. It is recognized that the complete responders survived about twice as long as the nonresponders.

* We are grateful to Dr. M. Ohta, Kyushu Cancer Center, and Dr. M. Nishimura, Aichi Cancer Center, for their kind cooperation in this study. Our research was supported by a Grand-in-Aid for Cancer Research [5, 25] from the Japanese Ministry of Health and Welfare

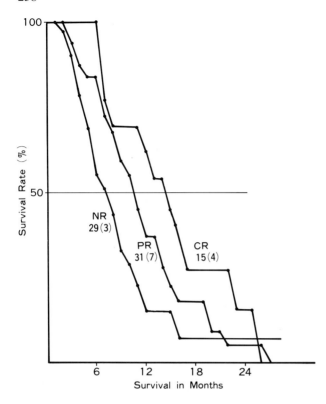

Fig. 1. Survival of patients with small cell carcinoma according to tumor regression by chemotherapy

Table 1. Objective response of small cell carcinoma of the lung to single drugs

Drugs	Percentage responding	Patients treated	References
ACNU	46	28	[5], [14], [22], [25]
Carboquone	43	7	[28]
Ifosfamide	33	12	[15]
Mitomycin C (Dextran sulfate, Urokinase)	50	34	[18]
Cyclophosphamide	51	39	Our result

ACNU, 1-(4-Amino-2-methyl-5-pyrimidinyl) methyl-3-(2-chloroethyl)-3-nitrosourea hydrochloride (NSC-D-245382)

In this institute, the response rate to single chemotherapy using CTX was 51%. This response rate is higher than that to any other single drug commonly used in Japan (Table 1).

The response rate to our polychemotherapy was 61%. The results of polychemotherapy in major Japanese institutes are compared in Table 2.

Survival data in our institute for patients with small cell carcinoma that were treated with chemotherapy alone (CTX), the combination of chemotherapy with radiotherapy (chemoradiotherapy), and chemo-radio-immunotherapy are shown in Fig. 2. Median

Table 2. Objective response of small cell carcinoma of the lung combinations

Drugs	Response		Patients treated	References
	Overall (%)	CR (No.)		
ACNU + CTX + VCR + PROC	81	(7)	26	[6]
CTX + MTX + PROC + VCR	79	(3)	14	[15]
CA + CTX + 5-FU + MMC + TM + VCR	63		8	[20]
CTX + 5-FU + VCR	61	(5)	23	Our result
ADR +Ifosfamide + VCR	50	(1)	10	[15]
CTX + MMC + TESPA + TM	36		11	[20]
CA + 5-FU + MMC	33		9	[20]
BLEO + CTX + 5-FU + MMC + VCR	33	(2)	12	[15]
CA + CQ + 5-FU (or CQ + 5-FU)	26		23	[5]

ADR, adriamycin; BLEO, bleomycin; CA, cytosine arabinoside; CTX, cyclophosphamide; CQ, carboquone; 5-FU, 5-fluorouracil; Ifosfamide, Z4942; MMC, mitomycin C; PROC, procarbazine; TM, chromomycin A_3; TESPA, thio-TEPA; VCR, vincristine

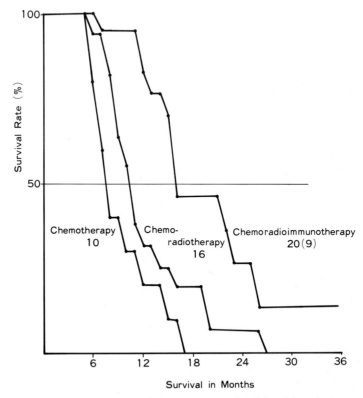

Fig. 2. Survival of patients with small cell carcinoma treated with chemotherapy, chemoradiotherapy, and chemoradioimmunotherapy (cases treated for more than 5 months are compared)

survival times were 7.5 months, 10.2 months, and 15.9 months, respectively. Survival curves in the figure are those only of patients who could be treated for more than 5 months, because treatment for 3 months is necessary to confirm the effect of immunotherapy.

Cooperative Clinical Trials in Three Institutes

Sixty-two patients with small cell carcinoma in three institutes were divided into limited and extensive disease categories. For the screening of metastases, bone marrow aspiration, radioisotopic scanning, radiographic bone survey, and sometimes echography, or computer tomography were performed.

Treatment modalities at the Kyushu Cancer Center were polychemotherapy with VCR (1 mg/person every week, IV), CTX (100 mg/person twice a week, IV), mitomycin C (MMC) (2 mg/person twice a week, IV) and chromomycin A_3 (TM) (0.5 mg/person twice a week, IV) for 4 weeks, followed by intrapleural injections of BCG-CWS or Nocardia-CWS. Treatment modalities at the Aichi Cancer Center were polychemotherapy with MMC (2 mg/person twice a week, IV), CTX (100 mg/person twice a week, IV), TM (0.5 mg/person twice a week, IV) VCR (1 mg/person twice a week, IV), 5-FU (500 mg/person twice a week, IV), and cytosine arabinoside (CA) (20 mg/person twice a week, IV) for 4 weeks, and some patients received subsequent

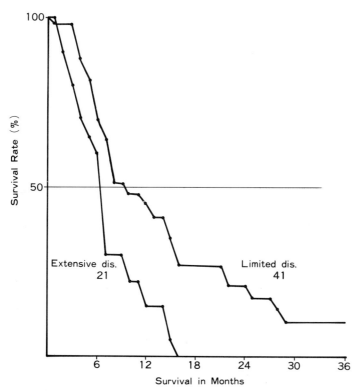

Fig. 3. Survival of patients with small cell carcinoma according to limited or extensive disease categories (cooperative clinical trials in three institutes)

radiotherapy. Treatment modalities at the Center for Adult Diseases, Osaka, were described above.

As shown in Fig. 3, median survival time of limited-disease patients wa 9.0 months and 6.2 months for those with extensive disease. Median survival time of responders was 12.8 months and that of nonresponders was 6.2 months (Fig. 4).

Combination Chemotherapy with Concurrent Small-Dose Radiation Therapy

Treatment with concurrent small-dose irradiation for the purpose of intensifying the effect of chemotherapy has been studied at the Aichi Cancer Center [19] and the Center for Adult Disease, Osaka. Patients were irradiated 100 or 200 rads within 3 h before the IV administrations of anticancer agents once a week for 1−2 months. The total radiation dose was only 800 or 1 600 rads.

The response rate was obviously improved by this method and no side effects were observed. Results are compared with the combination chemotherapy with sequential full-dose radiation therapy in Table 3. As shown in the table, response rates are 52% and 55% in patients treated with chemotherapy alone by CTX and CTX + 5 − FU + VCR, respectively. In the group treated with CTX + 5 − FU + VCR and small-dose radiation therapy, the response rate is improved to 90%. This response rate is comparable to those obtained in the groups treated with chemotherapy and sequential full-dose radiation therapy.

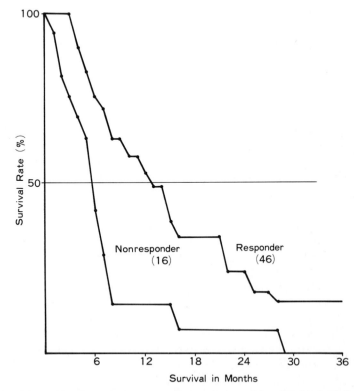

Fig. 4. Survival of patients with small cell carcinoma according to tumor regression by initial chemotherapy (cooperative clinical trials in   three institutes)

Table 3. Response to combination chemotherapy with concurrent radiation therapy

Drugs	Radiation	Response		Patients treated	References
		Overall (%)	CR (%)		
CTX	None	52	4	25	Our result
CTX	sequential full dose	80	24	same patients	Our result
CTX + 5-FU + VCR	None	55	22	18	Our result
CTX + 5-FU + VCR	sequential full dose	94	50	same patients	Our result
CTX + 5-FU + VCR	Concurrent small dose (800 rads)	93	33	15	Our result
CA + CTX + 5-FU + MMC + TM + VCR	Concurrent small dose (1400 rads)	93	50	14	[19]

Cytomorphological Study on the Correlation
with Better Survival of Small Cell Carcinoma Patients

As has been reported by us [8], histologically there was no definitive relation between the subtype of small cell carcinoma and the response to chemotherapy. In spite of numerous efforts with combination chemotherapy for patients with small cell carcinoma, it is undeniable that there is some limit to the effect of the anticancer agents available at present. Therefore, if there is a means of predicting the effect of chemotherapy before the treatment, it will be useful in the selection of treatment modality.

Twenty-six patients who received CTX alone were subjected to the study of cytomorphological characteristics in relation to response to chemotherapy [12]. Cytology materials were obtained directly from the tumor by brushing under bronchoscopy. Immediately after the smearing, specimens were fixed and stained by the ordinary Papanicolaou's method. At least 200 tumor cells in each case were light-microscopically examined. For this kind of cytologic study, the exfoliated cancer cells in the sputum were not useful because of some degenerative changes [10].

Most tumor cells were very well preserved, showing thin nuclear borders and distinct chromatin patterns. The sizes of the nuclei were distributed around 9 μ, with no difference between the good response group and the no-response group. The nuclei were mostly round or oval, with no difference between the good response group and the no-response group.

The tumor cells in the good response group more frequently showed finely granular chromatin evenly distributed throughout the nuclei. The tumor cells in the no-response group predominantly showed deeply stained nuclei with coarsely granular chromatin distributed evenly, or pale nuclei with unevenly distributed chromatin (Fig. 5). This different chromatin pattern will be an indicator to predict the degree of response to CTX.

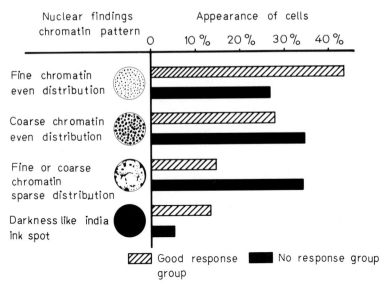

Fig. 5. Cytomorphological studies on the correlation with better survival of small cell carcinoma patients. Tumor cells in the good response group to chemotherapy (cyclophosphamide) more frequently showed a finely granular chromatin pattern, and tumor cells in the no-response group predominantly showed a deeply stained coarse chromatin pattern

Discussion

In this paper, the current status of the multidisciplinary treatment for small cell carcinoma in Japan was described. Sixty-two patients were divided into limited and extensive disease categories. Median survival of limited-disease patients was longer than those with extensive disease. As has been reported by Cohen and others [2], patients with disease confined to one hemithorax, with or without involvement of ipsilateral supraclavicular nodes, have higher response rates and longer survival than patients with more disseminated disease. Therefore, staging of small cell carcinoma will be an important factor influencing response rate to chemotherapy and survival of patient [17]. Hayata [11] reported a good 5-year survival rate for surgically resected intermediate cell type cases in stages I and II. We [9] also reported longer survival in stage I nonresected cases. But the number of stage I nonresected cases in the report is not sufficient for statistical analysis, so that the evaluation of staging of small cell carcinoma remains to be determined.

In our institute, 75 patients were treated with chemotherapy alone, the combination of chemotherapy with radiotherapy (chemo-radiotherapy), and chemoradio-immuno-therapy. Median survival times of CR, PR, and NR were 14.5, 10.5, and 7.0 months, respectively. It was evident that a complete responder had a longer disease-free survival. The response rate to polychemotherapy (CTX + VCR + 5-FU) was better than that to single chemotherapy (CTX). Therefore, combination chemotherapy with or without radiation therapy was more effective than single drug treatment, as described by Minna and others [16].

In recent results of chemotherapy in Japan (Table 2), good response rates were achieved using ACNU + CTX + VCR + PROC (procarbazine) (81%) and MTX +

CTX + PROC + VCR (79%). But in order to obtain a higher response rate than polychemotherapy, combination chemotherapy with concurrent small-dose radiation therapy was performed at the Aichi Cancer Center and at our institute. As reported by Hansen [7] and Ohta [23], the effect of simultaneous combination of chemotherapy and radiotherapy is remarkable. However, indications for the concurrent use of full dosage of both treatments are markedly restricted by its strong side effects.

Attaching great importance to the systemic treatment by chemotherapy, our method seems to be valuable for obtaining faster and stronger local effects than chemotherapy alone.

Concerning the possible mechanism of this intensifying effect, Nishimura [21] described the increase in the permeability of the cell membrane. Sato [26] reported on the effect of irradiation on the cancer cells by the method of cell electrophoresis. Cell electrophoretic mobilities decreased after the irradiation of 100 rads, and its maximum decrease was observed 4 h after the irradiation. Because electrophoretic mobility is mainly dependent upon the charge of the cell surface, it is possible that some changes could be caused in the cell membrane by small-dose irradiation. It may be presumed that the intensifying effect results from the administration of anticancer agents during the instability caused by small-dose irradiation in DNA and the membrane of the cancer cells.

It may become essential, in planning the treatment for individual cases, to predict the degree of response to chemotherapy prior to the initial treatment. Cytomorphological analysis was performed using materials directly obtained by brushing under bronchoscopy before the treatment. Chromatin patterns in the tumor cells of small cell carcinoma varied in individual cases, and there were some differences between responders and nonresponders.

As described in the results, the tumor cells showing abundant coarse chromatin prove to contain a high amount of heterochromatin, while the tumor cells with tightly fine chromatin appear to be rich in euchromatin rather than heterochromatin. Tumor cells with sparse distribution of chromatin probably contain less of the nuclear substances, including chromatin. If active metabolism and rapid cell proliferation are closely related to sensitivity of the cells to anticancer agents, it will be assumed that the sensitive cells must be filled with euchromatin and with less heterochromatin. From these cellular findings we could predict the degree of response to CTX at the time of initial cytologic diagnosis.

Accordingly, seeing these different chromatin patterns of tumor cells, we began two different treatment modalities. For patients for whom we expect a good response, we take the polychemotherapy first, and for those for whom we expect a poor response, we take the combination chemotherapy with concurrent small dose radiation therapy. But this trial is still in progress, and the results will be reported in the future.

Summary

Sixty-two patients with small cell carcinoma in three institutes were carefully divided into limited and extensive disease categories. Median survival time of limited-disease patients was longer than those with extensive disease.

In relation to the survival rate, the degree of response to initial chemotherapy was studied on 75 patients treated in our institute. The complete responders had a significantly better survival rate than the partial responders and nonresponders. Best survival was achieved by multidisciplinary treatment, including polychemotherapy, subsequent radiotherapy, and immunotherapy using BCG-CWS or Nocardia-CWS. Combination chemotherapy with concurrent small-dose radiation therapy for the purpose of intensifying the effect of chemotherapy was introduced. This method significantly improved the response rate without causing any of the side effects associated with radiotherapy.

Cytomorphological studies on the correlation with better survival rates of small cell carcinoma patients were described.

References

1. Abeloff MD, Ettinger DS, Baylin SB, Hazra T (1976) Management of small cell carcinoma of the lung: Therapy, staging, and biochemical markers. Cancer 38: 1394–1401
2. Cohen MH, Fossieck BE Jr, Ihde DC, Bunn PA Jr, Matthews MJ, Shackney SE, Minna JD (1979) Chemotherapy of small cell carcinoma of the lung: Results and concepts. In: Muggia FM, Rozencweig M (eds) Lung cancer-progress in therapeutic research. Progress in cancer research and therapy, vol 11. Raven Press, New York, p 559
3. Eagan RT, Maurer LH, Forcier RJ, Tulloh M (1974) Small cell carcinoma of the lung: Staging, paraneoplastic syndromes, treatment, and survival. Cancer 33: 527–532
4. Edmonson JH, Lagakos SW, Selawry OS, Perlia CP, Bennett JM, Muggia FM, Wampler G, Brodovsky HS, Horton J, Colsky J, Mansour EG, Creech R, Stolbach L, Greenspan EM, Levitt M, Israel L, Ezdinli EZ, Carbone PP (1976) Cyclophosphamide and CCNU in the treatment of inoperable small cell carcinoma and adenocarcinoma of the lung. Cancer Treat Rep 60: 925–932
5. Fukuoka M, Takada M, Tamai S, Hashimoto T, Kusunoki Y, Nagasawa S, Negoro S, Shiota K (1978) Clinical study of ACNU for lung cancer (in Japanese). Cancer Chemother [Suppl] 5: 209–217
6. Fukuoka M, Takada M, Tamai S, Kikui M, Shiota K, Kusunoki Y, Nagasawa S (1978) Combination chemotherapy with cyclophosphamide, vincristine, ACNU and procarbazine (CONP) for small cell carcinoma of the lung. 19th Annual Meeting of the Japan Lung Cancer Society (in Japanese). Lung Cancer [Suppl] 18: 28
7. Hansen HH, Muggia FM, Andrews R, Selawry OS (1972) Intensive combined chemotherapy and radiotherapy in patients with nonresectable bronchogenic carcinoma. Cancer 30: 315–324
8. Hattori S. Ikegami H, Tateishi R, Hayata Y, Ohta M, Yoneyama T, Niitani H, Shimosato Y, Hashimoto K, Hirao F, Nishimura M, Ito M, Murakami K, Saotome K, Sato M, Sawamura K (1978) Multidisciplinary treatment of small cell carcinoma of the lung (in Japanese). Lung Cancer 18: 419–427
9. Hattori S, Matsuda M, Ikegami H, Horai T, Takenaga A (1977) Small cell carcinoma of the lung: Clinical and cytomorphological studies in relation to its response to chemotherapy. Gann 68: 321–331
10. Hattori S, Matsuda M, Nishihara H, Horai T (1971) Early diagnosis of small peripheral lung cancer – Cytologic diagnosis of very fresh cancer cells obtained by the TV-brushing technique. Acta Cytol (Baltimore) 15: 460–467
11. Hayata Y, Funatsu H, Suemasu K, Yoneyama T, Hashimoto K, Doi O, Ohta M (1978) Surgical indications in small cell carcinoma of the lung. Jpn J Clin Oncol 8: 93–100
12. Horai T, Sone H, Takenaga A, Ikegami H, Matsuda M, Hattori (to be published) The effects and resultant cytologic characteristics of oat-cell carcinoma of the lung treated with cyclophosphamide
13. Hornback NB, Einhorn L, Shidnia H, Joe BT, Krause M, Furnas B (1976) Oat cell carcinoma of the lung: Early treatment results of combination radiation therapy and chemotherapy. Cancer 37: 2658–2664

14. Kimura I, Harada H, Ohnoshi T, Urabe Y, Fujii M, Machida K, Murakami N (1978) Clinical trial of 1-(4-amino-2-methyl-5-pyrimidinyl)methal-3-(2-chloroethyl)-3-nitrosoura hydrochloride (ACNU) (in Japanese). Cancer Chemother 5: 767–772

15. Kimura I, Ohnoshi T, Takasugi K, Fujii M, Machida K, Nakata Y, Hayashi K, Kanagawa O, Miyata A, Murakami N, Shirahige Y, Takahashi T (1978) An evaluation of effects of chemotherapy and radiotherapy in small cell carcinoma of the lung (in Japanese) Lung Cancer 18: 231–240

16. Minna JD, Brereton HD, Cohen MH, Ihde DC, Bunn PA, Jr, Shackney SE, Fossieck BE jr, Matthews MJ (1979) The treatment of small cell carcinoma of the lung: Prospects for cure. In: Muggia FM, Rozencweig M (eds) Lung cancer-progress in therapeutic research. Progress in cancer research and therapy. vol 11. Raven Press, New York, p 593

17. Mountain CF, Carr DT, Anderson WAD (1974) A system for the clinical staging of lung cancer. Am J Roentgenol Radium Ther Nucl Med 120: 130–138

18. Niitani H (1978) Treatment with anti-cancer agent in relation to the histologic type of the tumor (in Japanese). Jpn J Chest Dis 37: 337–344

19. Nishimura M (1978) Current status and prospects of non-surgical treatment of lung cancer (in Japanese). J Adult Dis 8: 895–901

20. Nishimura M (1976) Combination chemotherapy for lung cancer (in Japanese). Cancer Chemother 15: 34–40

21. Nishimura M, Kurita S, Ogawa M, Kamei Y, Doi M, Murakami M, Oyama J, Sugiura T, Goto T, Naruto M, Ota K (1977) A new combination therapy for lung cancer. Combining multiple combination chemotherapy with small doses of radiotherapy. Cancer Chemother 4: 1291–1300

22. Ogawa M, Inagaki J, Horikoshi N, Inoue K, Chinen T, Ueoka H, Nagura E, Fujimoto S, Murakami M, Ota K (1978) A clinical study on a new water-soluble nitrosourea derivative (ACNU). Cancer Chemother 5: 585–590

23. Ota K, Nishimura M, Kitagawa T (1971) Simultaneous combination of chemotherapy and irradiation in the treatment of inoperable lung cancer (in Japanese). Jpn J Cancer Clin 17: 269–275

24. Reynolds CRD, O'Dells CS (1978) Combination modality therapy in lung cancer: A survival study showing beneficial results of AMCOF (adriamycin, methotrexate, cyclophosphamide, oncovin and 5-fluorouracil). Cancer 42: 385–389

25. Saijo N, Kawase I, Nishiwaki Y, Suzuki A, Niitani H (1978) Phase II study of ACNU [1-(4-amino-2-methyl-5-pyrimidinyl) methyl-3-(2-chloroethyl)-3-nitrosourea hydrochloride] for primary lung cancer and nodular pulmonary metastases (in Japanese). Cancer Chemother 4: 579–584

26. Sato C (1978) Radiation effects on tumor cell membrane. Cancer Chemother 5: 311–320

27. Selawry OS (1977) Chemotherapy in lung cancer. In: Straus MJ (ed) Lung cancer. Clinical diagnosis and treatment. Grune & Stratton, New York San Francisco London, p 199

28. Suzuki K (1977) Clinical study on esquinone to primary lung cancer (in Japanese). Cancer Chemother 4: 1341–1344

29. Yamamura Y, Azuma I, Taniyama T, Sugimura K, Hirao F, Tokuzen R, Okabe M, Nakahara W, Yasumoto K, Ohta M (1976) Immunotherapy of cancer with cell wall skeleton of mycobacterium bovis-bacillus Calmette-Guerin: Experimental and clinical results. Ann NY Acad Sci 277: 209–227

30. Yamawaki M, Azuma I, Saiki I, Uemiya M, Aoki O, Ennyu K, Yamamura Y (1978) Antitumor activity of squalene-treated cell-wall skeleton of nocardia rubra in mice. Gann 69: 619–626

Small Cell Lung Carcinoma –
Recent Advances and Current Challenges

R. B. Livingston

Division of Oncology, University of Texas Health Science Center,
USA – San Antonio, TX 78284

Therapeutic trials in the early and mid- 1970s led to a number of important questions in the treatment of small cell carcinoma of the lung. This paper will attempt to examine those questions in light of the outcome of subsequent studies, and to consider some concepts that are the subject of current trials.

It has now become apparent that there are two major prognostic factors that influence survival in patients treated for this disease: the patient's functional (performance) status and the clinical extent of disease at the time of presentation (limited versus extensive). The TNM classification and the staging system derived from it are not satisfactory for classification of most patients with small cell carcinoma, since surgery is indicated as a potentially curative maneuver in fewer than 5% of the patients [31]. It now appears that patients with supraclavicular node involvement, even contralateral, and those with superior vena caval syndrome have a prognosis comparable to that of patients with disease that appears "limited" to the hemithorax, at least in terms of survival with combined chemo- and radiotherapy. On the other hand, the presence of clinically detectable pleural effusion, even as the sole clinical evidence of dissemination, appears to place the patient in the same category as other individuals with "extensive" disease [39].

Limited Disease

For patients with limited disease so defined, by 1977 a comparison of results achieved with supervoltage radiation therapy and those of combined radiation and multiple-drug chemotherapy suggested superiority of the latter approach. However, none of these were prospective, controlled comparisons. Thus, an important question was, in the minds of many, unresolved: is combined modality treatment really better than radiation therapy alone? Studies by the ECOG-RTOG (Eastern Cooperative Oncology Group) and the SEG (Southeast Group) cooperative groups in the United States now appear to have answered this question. In the ECOG-RTOG randomized study reported by Creech et al. [8], continuously fractionated radiation to a total dose of 4 500 rads in 5–6 weeks, with or without prophylactic cranial irradiation (PCI) was compared to the same radiation program with the addition of simultaneous cyclophosphamide (CTX) and CCNU. The median duration of response was significantly longer in the combined modality group (5.5 versus 3 months) and the complete response (CR) rate was 38% versus 27%. Neither the difference in CR rate or median survival in the two groups (6 versus 4.5 months) were significantly different. In the SEG randomized study reported by Krauss et al. [22], continuously fractionated radiation to a total dose of 4 500 rads in 5−6 weeks, plus PCI, was compared to the same radiation program with the addition of CTX, adriamycin (ADR) and dacarbazine (DTIC) in the sequence, chemotherapy, radiation therapy, chemotherapy. Both the median duration of response (5.1 versus 2.3 months) and the median survival of responders (9.9 versus 6.6 months) were significantly different in favor of the combined modality approach: the CR rate was 52% versus 33%. Neither the ECOG-RTOG study nor that of the SEG produced survival results in the combined modality treatment group which were as good as the median of 1-year and 2-year survival of 15% reported from earlier, uncontrolled cooperative group efforts by SWOG [28] and CALGB (Cancer and Leukemia Group B) [42]. This is probably related to the fact that the chemotherapy programs utilized in the ECOG-RTOG and SEG randomized trials were suboptimal. Nevertheless, the superiority of the combined approach versus radiotherapy alone was still apparent.

The best CR rate and survival result reported by any group in 1977 (and still the best long-term survival) was that by Johnson et al. from the NCI. The last published analysis of this study [19] revealed a CR rate of 77%, a median survival of 1 year, and 2-year disease-free survival in 14 (39%) of 36 patients with limited disease. Unfortunately, 22% of the patients with limited disease suffered "induction deaths" related to the severe toxicity of chest and whole-brain irradiation plus high-dose, simultaneous ADR, CTX, and VCR chemotherapy. Some additional patients had permanent complications like esophageal stricture that prevented return to a normal life, though they were rendered disease-free. An important question raised by this study is whether one can administer effective, aggressive combination chemotherapy at the same time as radiation to the primary tumor site. The answer appears to be "yes": two subsequent studies have reported that ADR, CTX, and VCR can be administered in this fashion, at somewhat reduced doses [15, 18]. Other studies have reported the combination of CCNU, VCR, CTX, and methotrexate (MTX) [17, 20] and the combination of CTX, ADR adriamycin, cis-platinum, and VP-16 with simultaneous chest irradiation (Eagan 1979, unpublished work). The most striking result yet published is that of Greco et al. [15], in which remission induction chemotherapy and chest plus whole brain irradiation were started together: CTX at 1 000 mg/m^2, ADR at 40 mg/m^2, and VCR at 1 mg/m^2 were given intravenously on the first day of radiotherapy and thereafter every 3 weeks for a total of six cycles. After induction therapy, continued cyclic chemotherapy with the combination of VP-16 (200 mg/m^2) intravenously on days 1 and 8, each month) and hexamethylmelamine (8 mg/kg orally on days 1 through 14 of each month) was administered 3 months. Patients then received MTX "maintenance" chemotherapy, 75 mg/m^2 intramuscularly every 3 weeks, with or without C. parvum immunotherapy. Radiation was given to the primary tumor, mediastinum, and supraclavicular node areas at a total dose of 3 000 rads given in 300-rad daily fractions, as well as PCI on the same schedule in the last 20 patients. Of 32 patients with limited disease treated in this fashion, 29 (91%): had CR 70% of all patients are alive at 1 year of follow-up, with median survival estimated at more than 18 months.

If simultaneous radiation and chemotherapy can produce these results in a pilot study, what of the role today for sequential chemotherapy and radiation ("sandwich" treatment)? Einhorn et al. in another study from a single institution, achieved comparable results with the same three drugs (CTX, ADR, and VCR), followed by a second course of chemotherapy and radiation to the chest and PCI, followed by further sequential chemotherapy and radiation [12]. At 450 mg/m^2 total ADR, dose, maintenance chemotherapy was given consisting of MTX + CTX ± CCNU. Median survival in 19 patients was 18 months, with five patients free of evidence of disease beyond 3 years. It should be noted that the results cited for simultaneous and for sequential combined modality approaches represent the best yet reported: Table 1 summarizes results of a number of other programs as well. At the present time, there is no convincing evidence of superiority for "simultaneous" or for "sequential".

Another serious question in the treatment of limited disease is whether one needs to use radiation therapy to the chest at all. The results of Cohen et al. at the National Cancer Institute suggested that chemotherapy alone might be as or more effective, using high-dose CTX, MTX, and CCNU, alternated after two courses (at 6 weeks) with VCR, ADR, and PROC (CMC-VAP) [7]. A follow-up analysis of this study demonstrated CR in 71% of 19 patients with median survival of 14 months: the CR rate increased from 8 of 19 to 14 of 19 after completion of 2 VAP cycles at 12 weeks [6]. There have now been two prospective, controlled trials reported in which chemotherapy alone was compared to the same chemotherapy plus radiation to the chest. Hansen et al. in a large study, reported no significant difference in response

Table 1. Combined modality programs in limited disease (1979)

Regimen	No. pts.	Cr %	Mst (mo.)	Reference (No.)
Simultaneous programs				
CAV + 3000 rads, 1° + brain	32	91	18+	[15]
CC + 4500 rads, 1° ± brain	77	38	6	[8]
CAV + 3000 rads, 1° + brain	19		9.5	[18]
CMC-V + 3000 rads, 1°	30	30	–	[20]
CMC-V + 4000 rads, 1° only (short course, wide split)	65	–	11	[20]
CAV + XRT (varied), 1° + brain	36	77	12	[19]
Pooled data	259	30–91	6–18+	
Sequential programs				
COMF ⇄ CAV → 3000 rads, 1° + brain → off 2 wks → ± 1500 rads, 1° → chemo	158	–	9	[29]
CAV → 2500 rads, 1° only → CMP	66	24[a]	11	[13]
CAD → 4500 rads, 1° + brain → CAD	37	52	7	[22]
CAV ⇄ DDP + VP 16 → 4500 rads, 1° + brain	17	65[a]	> 12	[33]
CAV → CAV + 1800 rads, 1° + brain → off 3 wks → (CAV) → 1800 rads, 1° + brain	19	–	18	[12]
CAV → V + 3000 rads, 1° + brain → CA 1500 rads, 1° → CA	108	41	12	[28]
Pooled data	405	24–65	7–18	

[a] Assessed prior to XRT

Table 2. Long-term disease-free survival: limited disease

Investigator	Regimen	No. pts > 2 years/total	Reference (No.)
Einhorn et al.	CAV → CAV + XRT (split) → CAV	5/19[a]	[12]
Holoye et al.	CV → XRT (split) → CV	3/16[a]	[14]
Johnson et al.	CAV + XRT	14/36	[19]
Jackson et al.	CAV + XRT	2/12	[18]
Hansen et al.	CMC-V + XRT	12/110	[14]
Eagan et al.	VP-16 ± ADR ± CTX + XRT	5/21	[14]
Kane et al.	CMC-V + XRT	5/19	[20]
Cohen et al.	CMC ⇄ VAP (no XRT)	3/19	[6]
	Total, all regimens	49/252 (19%)	

[a] At risk more than 3 years

duration but statistically superior median survival (14 versus II months) in limited disease patients who received drug treatment alone (CTX, MTX, CCNU, and VCR) [20]. Stevens et al. compared CTX, ADR, and VCR + PCI to the same therapy + chest irradiation, and showed no significant difference in median response duration or median survival [38]. Unfortunately, the radiation therapy in both of these studies was not comparable to that employed in other combined modality programs. Both employed high-dose, short-course fractionation with a wide "split" (3 or 4 weeks) between the first and second halves of the radiation therapy course: this type of regimen is inferior to other dose-time schedules for radiation therapy, in the treatment of nonsmall cell carcinoma (Perez 1979, unpublished work).

A final important question relative to limited disease has to do with the status of patients who are "disease-free" at 2 years: Are they cured? Table 2 summarizes the available information for 252 patients, on a variety of regimens, with minimum follow-up to 2 years. It appears that 15%−20% of patients with limited disease are at risk for long-term disease-free status and possible cure. The two series with the longest follow-up had no relapses between 2 and 3 years, and this pattern appears to be holding in the series from the Southwest Oncology Group as well [39].

Extensive Disease

A somewhat different set of questions have been the subject of intensive investigation over the last 2 years among patients with extensive spread of small cell carcinoma. These were largely generated by the observation which Cohen et al. made of increased CR rates and prolonged survival among patients who received alternating, mutually noncross-resistant regimens on the CMC-VAP program at the National Cancer Institute. The most recently published analysis of this program reveals that, of 42 patients treated, 24% achieved CR at 6 weeks (after two courses of CMC) and an additional 12% by 12 weeks (after two courses of VAP). The overall CR rate was thus 36%, with 24% "disease-free" at 1 year, and median survival of 9.3 months for the entire group [6]. It should be noted that a CR rate almost as high (30%) was reported

Table 3. Intensive combination chemotherapy programs in extensive disease (1979)

Regimen	No. pts.	Resp. %	Cr %	Mst (Mo.)	Reference (No.)
Intensive, repeated single regimen					
CMC-V	73	81		9	[9]
CMC	23	96	30	8.5	[5]
CAV	31			9	[16]
CAV → XRT to 1° → CMP	81	65	10	8	[13]
CAV + HDMTX	19		37		[37]
CAV + MTX (standard dose)	29	72	17	7	[27]
CAV + VP-16	20		45		[40]
CAV + PROC (two series)	50		26	7	(J. Manna, 1979 unpublished work [41])
Pooled data	326		10−45	7−9	
Alternating, sequential regimens					
CMC ⇄ VAP	42	91	24[a] (36)	9.3	[6]
CA + VP-16 ⇄ BOMP	15		20		[1]
CAV ± HDMTX ⇄ VPH	45		24	7+	[16]
VMV ⇄ VAC	26	77	19[a]		(R. Livingston, 1979, unpublished work)
VAB ⇄ CMC-V	12	58	42	7+	[2]
CMC-V ⇄ A + VP-16	73	90		9	[9]
Pooled data	213		19−42	7−9	

[a] Response assessed at 6 weeks

by the same group in a series of 23 patients who received high-dose CMC alone, and that three of these patients had disease-free survival beyond 2 years. Thus, observations from Cohen's own group do not now strongly support the concept that alternating combinations are superior. Table 3 summarizes results of recent trials with alternating sequential combinations and of those with repeated, intensive treatment using a single regimen. Reported CR rates in these trials range from 19%−42% for alternating regimens and from 10%−45% for a single regimen. Available data on median survival suggests that they are comparable, in the range of 7−9 months. It therefore appears that the intentional alteration of mutually noncross-resistant regimens as a general principle is not yet established. CR rates do appear to be increased by more intensive chemotherapy, from 5%−15% up to the range of 15%−35%, and this may translate into a much larger fraction of long-term survivors.

Only two investigational drugs, VP-16 and hexamethylmelamine, have established themselves as definitely active against small-cell disease [24]. Alone, VP-16 may be the best single drug, and it is not cross-resistant with other agents in man. Further exploration of dose, schedule, and combinations with other active drugs is clearly indicated. Other agents currently under investigation in small cell carcinoma include older drugs like MMC, methyl GAG, and vinblastine, and newer compounds such as

AMSA, gallium nitrate, and pentamethylmelamine (the water-soluble derivative of hexamethylmelamine). Little or no activity has been demonstrated, in advanced disease refractory to first-line agents, for 6MP, the nitrosoureas, streptozotocin, or cis-platinum.

Attempts to develop effective "salvage" chemotherapy in resistant or refractory patients have demonstrated activity for VCR and ADR, singly or in combination with PROC [3]. Unfortunately, few patients have achieved useful responses of more than 2−3 months duration, and the addition of hexamethylmelamine to VP-16 is probably no better than VP-16 alone (Kennedy and Livingston 1979, unpublished work).

Immunotherapy

Immunotherapy was explored in small cell carcinoma in a number of studies of the mid- and late-1970s, always in combination with other modalities. Studies with BCG by scarification in the SWOG and by Einhorn et al. demonstrated no benefit to its addition [12, 29]. Jackson et al. compared CTX, ADR, and radiation therapy (XRT) with and without administration of the methanol-extractable residue of BCG (MER). They found no overall difference, although the survival of patients with extensive disease was significantly longer in the group who received MER (12 versus 7 months median) [19]. Cohen et al. have reported their experience with thymosin [4], in which all patients treated on high-dose CMC (CTX + MTX + CCNU) regimens at their institution (including the alternating, sequential approach), were randomly allocated to receive, during induction, thymosin at 20 mg/m^2 twice a week, thymosin at 60 mg/m^2 twice a week, or no immunotherapy. There was no effect on response rate, but the median survival was 8−9 months for the 0 or low dose thymosin groups and 14 months for high-dose thymosin. Interpretation of this study is clouded by the small numbers and heterogeneous patient populations involved, but thymosin is certainly worthy of further study.

Future Directions

After a period of "log-phase" growth and ferment, the therapy of small cell bronchogenic carcinoma has reached a plateau. Especially for patients with extensive disease, who make up 60%−75% of the total, new approaches will be necessary to increase the CR rate above the 20%−30% range. These might involve: (1) alternation with a noncross-resistant regimen based on the individual patient's response, rather than the same fixed schedule for all patients; (2) initial therapy with "cell cycle specific" drugs to capitalize on the tumor's high initial growth fraction; (3) local radiation therapy when feasible to sites of major previous involvement, in patients with major response to chemotherapy; and (4) the use of hemibody radiation therapy. Each will be discussed briefly.

After two courses of high-dose, intermittent therapy (about 6 weeks), most investigators have found that maximal response has been achieved with a single chemotherapeutic regimen [5, 39]. Those in CR may benefit from continuation of the same regimen, but patients who have achieved only a partial response at 6 weeks may benefit from *selective* administration of a mutually noncross-resistant combination.

Small-cell carcinoma has a high initial growth fraction in most patients [26, 32]. Since depression of the thymidine labeling index after chemotherapy appears to be a concomitant of tumor response [10, 25], it may be much better to administer "cell cycle specific" agents first, and "cell cycle non specific" agents as the subsequent regimen.

The current SWOG study attempts to utilize both of these approaches, in patients with extensive disease. Patients with CR clinically after 6 weeks will receive continued therapy with their initial induction regimen. Those with partial response or stable disease will be "crossed-over" to the mutually noncross-resistant regimen. For initial induction, a "cell cycle specific" regimen including MTX and VP-16 is being compared to a "cell cycle nonspecific" regimen including ADR and CTX, VCR is given in both regimens for a total of 6 weeks.

Although no apparent advantage has been demonstrated for the addition of chest radiotherapy to all patients with extensive disease versus expected results from chemotherapy alone [28], it may benefit selected patients, in particular those with CR. Among five patients with extensive disease who achieved CR in a recent study from our institution [27], four relapsed initially in the chest as an isolated site. Cohen et al. observed similar "chest only" relapse in 5 of 9 patients with extensive disease who relapsed from CR [6]. In neither study was chest radiation given prior to relapse.

Finally, Salazar has described exciting preliminary experience with upper hemibody irradiation in a single dose of 600–800 rads, delivered over several hours with a 10 MeV linear accelerator [36]. After observing responses of tumor masses in a number of patients with advanced, refractory lung cancer of various histologies, Salazar and Creech have initiated a pilot study in ECOG of chemotherapy followed by 600 rads of upper hemibody irradiation, followed by intensive, high dose local radiation therapy, then further chemotherapy. Some patients with extensive small cell carcinoma appear to have had partial responses converted to CR (Salazar 1979, personal communication). The toxicity of this approach is, however, quite formidable, and more pilot work needs to be done before its value can be assessed in large-scale, comparative trials.

References

1. Abeloff MD, Ettinger DS, Khouri N (1979) Intensive induction therapy for small cell carcinoma of the lung (SCC). Proc Am Assoc Cancer Res Proc Am Soc Clin Oncol 20: 326
2. Broder LE, Selawry OS, Johnson MK (1979) Treatment of small cell carcinoma (SCC) of the lung utilizing mutually non-cross resistant chemotherapy regimens. Proc Am Assoc Cancer Res Proc Am Soc Clin Oncol 20: 278
3. Cohen MH, Broder LE, Fossieck BE Jr (1977) Combination chemotherapy with vincristine, adriamycin, and procarbazine in previously treated patients with small cell carcinoma. Cancer Treat Rep 61: 485–487
4. Cohen MH, Chretien PB, Ihde DC, Fossieck BE Thymosin fraction V and intensive combination chemotherapy. Prolonging the survival of patients with small-cell lung cancer. JAMA 241: 1813–1815
5. Cohen MH, Creaven PJ, Fossieck BE, Broder LE (1977) Intensive chemotherapy of small cell bronchogenic carcinoma. Cancer Treat Rep 61: 349–354

6. Cohen MH, Ihde DC, Bunn PA Jr (1979) Cyclic alternating combination chemotherapy for small cell bronchogenic carcinoma. Cancer Treat Rep 63:163–170

7. Cohen M, Ihde D, Fossieck B (1977) Intensive chemotherapy of small cell bronchogenic carcinoma. Proc Am Assoc Cancer Res Proc Am Soc Clin Oncol 18:286

8. Creech RH, Seydel HG, Mietlowski O (1979) Radiation therapy and chemotherapy of localized small cell carcinoma of the lung. Proc Am Assoc Cancer Res Proc Am Soc Clin Oncol 20:313

9. Dombernowsky P, Hansen HH, Sorensen S, Osterlind K (1979) Sequential versus non-sequential combination chemotherapy using 6 drugs in advanced small cell carcinoma. Proc Am Assoc Cancer Res Proc Am Soc Clin Oncol 20:277

10. Durie B, Vaught L, Salmon S (1977) Prognostic significance of tritiated thymidine labeling index in multiple myeloma and acute myeloid leukemia. Proc Am Assoc Cancer Res Proc Am Soc Clin Oncol 18:80

11. Deleted in production

12. Einhorn LH, Bond WH, Hornback N, Joe B-T (1978) Long-term results of combined-modality treatment of small cell carcinoma of the lung. Semin Oncol 5:309–313

13. Feld R, Pringle J, Evans WK (1979) Combined modality treatment of small cell carcinoma of the lung (SCC). Proc Am Assoc Cancer Res Proc Am Soc Clin Oncol 20:312

14. Greco FA, Einhorn LH, Richardson RL, Oldham RK (1978) Small cell lung cancer: Progress and perspectives. Semin Oncol 5:323–335

15. Greco FA, Richardson RL, Snell JD (1979) Small cell lung cancer. Complete remission and improved survival. Am J Med 66:625–630

16. Hande KR, Greco FA, Fer MF (1979) Combination chemotherapy plus high dose methotrexate for extensive stage small cell lung cancer. Proc Am Assoc Cancer Res Proc Am Soc Clin Oncol 20:90

17. Hansen HH, Dombernowsky P, Hansen HS, Rorth M (1979) Chemotherapy versus chemotherapy plus radiotherapy in regional small-cell carcinoma of the lung. A randomized trial. Proc Am Assoc Cancer Res Proc Am Soc Clin Oncol 20:277

18. Jackson DV jr, Richards F, Muss HB (1979) Immunotherapy of small cell carcinoma of the lung (SCC): A randomized study. Proc Am Assoc Cancer Res Proc Am Soc Clin Oncol 20:367

19. Johnson RE, Brereton HD, Kent CH (1978) "Total" therapy for small cell carcinoma of the lung. Ann Thorac Surg 25:510–515

20. Kanne RC, Cashdollar MR, Porter P, Beiler DD (1979) Alternating drug combinations in small cell bronchogenic carcinoma (SCBC: A randomized trial. Proc Am Assoc Cancer Res Proc Soc Clin Oncol 20:406

21. Deleted in production

22. Krauss S, Perez C (1979) Treatment of localized undifferentiated small cell lung carcinoma (SCLS) with radiation therapy (RT) with or without combination chemotherapy with cyclophosphamide, adriamycin and dimethyltriazenoimidazole carboximide. Proc Am Assoc Cancer Res Proc Am Soc Clin Oncol 20:316

23. Deleted in production

24. Livingston RB (1978) Treatment of small cell carcinoma: evolution and future directions. Semin Oncol 5:299–308

25. Livingston RB (1977) Clinical applications of cell kinetics. Ann Rev Pharmacol Toxicol 17:529–543

26. Livingston RB, Ambus U, George SL (1974) In vitro determination of thymidine ^{3}H labeling index in human solid tumors. Cancer Res 24:1376–1380

27. Livingston RB, Mira J, Haas C, Heilbrun L (to be published) Unexpected toxicity of combined modality therapy for small cell carcinoma. A southwest oncology group study. Int J Radiol Oncol Biol Phys

28. Livingston RB, Moore TN, Heilbrun L (1978) Small-cell carcinoma of the lung: Combined chemotherapy and radiation. A southwest oncology group study. Ann Intern Med 88:194–199

29. McCracken J, White J, Reed R (1978) Combination chemotherapy, radiotherapy, and immunotherapy for oat cell carcinoma of the lung. Proc Am Assoc Cancer Res Proc Am Soc Clin Oncol 19:395
30. Deleted in production
31. Mountain CF (1977) Assessment of the role of surgery for control of lung cancer. Ann Thorac Surg 24:365
32. Muggia FM, Krezoski SK, Hansen HH (1974) Cell kinetic studies in patients with small-cell carcinoma of the lung. Cancer 34:1683–1690
33. Natale R, Hilaris B, Golbey R, Wittes R (1979) Induction chemotherapy in small cell carcinoma of the lung. Proc Am Assoc Cancer Res Proc Am Soc Clin Oncol 20:343
34. Deleted in production
35. Deleted in production
36. Salazar OM, Rubin P, Keller B, Scarantino C (1978) Systemic (half body) radiation therapy: response and toxicity. Int J Radiat Oncol Biol Phys 4:937–950
37. Skarin AT, Greene H, Canellos GP (1979) High dose methotrexate with citrovorum factor rescue alternating with combination chemotherapy in small cell lung cancer. Proc Am Assoc Cancer Res Proc Am Soc Clin Oncol 20:328
38. Stevens E, Einhorn L, Rohn R (1974) Treatment of limited small cell lung cancer. Proc Am Assoc Cancer Res Proc Am Soc Clin Oncol 20:435
39. Trauth C, Livingston RB (to be published) Patterns of response, relapse, and longterm survival in small cell carcinoma of the lung: A southwest oncology group study
40. Valdivieso M, Cabanillas F, Bedikian AY (1979) Intensive induction chemotherapy of small cell lung cancer with ECHO: E = Epipodophyllotoxin VP-16, C = Cytoxan, H = Hydroxydaunorubicin, O = Oncovin. Proc Am Assoc Cancer Res Proc Am Soc Clin Oncol 20:383
41. Vogelzang NJ, Trowbridge RA, Theologides A (1979) Four drug chemotherapy of small cell carcinoma of the lung compared to two drug therapy. Proc Am Assoc Cancer Res Proc Am Soc Clin Oncol 20:385
42. Weiss RB (1978) Small-cell carcinoma of the lung: therapeutic management. Ann Intern Med 88:522–531

Combination Chemotherapy of Head and Neck Cancer in the United States*

R. E. Wittes

Solid Tumor Service, Department of Medicine, Memorial-Sloan-Kettering Cancer Center, 1275 York Avenue, USA – New York, NY 10021

Introduction

In 1973 Bertino and co-workers [3] reviewed the chemotherapy of head and neck cancer. They concluded that "several agents are effective in the treatment of epidermoid cancers of the head and neck. The time is ripe for the development of effective drug combinations and programs utilizing chemotherapy, radiation therapy, and surgery in the treatment of these difficult neoplasms." During the six years that have elapsed since those words were written, oncologists have been working busily along these very lines. In doing so, they have been spurred on by several factors: a resurgence of interest in methotrexate, particularly in high dose with leucovorin rescue; the identification of cis-diammine-dichloroplatinum (II) as an agent with significant activity in these tumors; and, perhaps most important, the climate of general optimism surrounding the combined-modality approach to human solid tumors. In this review we shall examine the general directions of systemic drug therapy for epidermoid carcinoma of the head and neck (ECHN) in the United States over the past few years. We shall not deal with intra-arterial chemotherapy or with the combination of single drugs and radiotherapy, both of which have been reviewed in detail elsewhere [3, 9, 20, 27].

The Single Agent Background

Most oncologists have held to the premise that effective combinations of drugs are most likely to result from the simultaneous or sequential administration of single agents which are themselves active. Table 1 shows the several drugs which have been regarded as active against ECHN. The list includes representatives of the several major classes of antineoplastic agents: alkylating agents, antimetabolites, antibiotics, and plant alkaloids. All except bleomycin have significant myelotoxicity when used clinically, and five of them have the potential for producing severe gastrointestinal ulceration. The largely overlapping nature of the toxicities of the individual agents has been a major obstacle to the development of effective combinations, since it has proved very difficult to combine these drugs without seriously compromising the doses of each.

* Supported in part by NIH grants CA-08748 and CA-08526

Table 1. Drugs with activity in head and neck cancer

Drug	Evaluable cases	Response rate (%)
Methotrexate (qw or biw)	100	50
Methotrexate (monthly courses)	107	29
Hydroxyurea	18	39
Cyclophosphamide	77	36
Vinblastine	35	29
Adriamycin	34	23
5-Fluorouracil	118	15
Bleomycin	298	18

Data are from references [3, 9, 20]

Clearly the greatest experience is with methotrexate. This agent has been given singly in an almost bewildering variety of doses and schedules. As has been previously noted [3, 20], weekly or twice-weekly administration appears more effective than loading courses or daily administration. Response rates have varied widely from study to study, in part probably because of differences in patient selection and criteria of response, but also very possibly because of real differences in the activity of certain schedules of this cycle-active agent. Since the original observation by Goldin and co-workers, that the therapeutic index of methotrexate is enhanced in mouse model systems by the administration of leucovorin, clinical investigators have been examining whether a corresponding phenomenon exists in human tumors in general and in ECHN in particular. Although Goldin's observations are 25 years old, interest in this area continues to increase. Table 2 shows most of the phase II studies in the United States which have employed methotrexate and leucovorin. As time has passed, the trend has been toward increasing doses of methotrexate [24, 42, 46], aggressive hydration and alkalinization of the urine to avert the nephrotoxicity that otherwise occurs commonly at high methotrexate doses [24, 45], and, in some cases, more frequent administration of the drug [46, 62]. With the more widespread use of assays for methotrexate in plasma, some centers are tailoring the leucovorin-rescue schedules of individual patients around the kinetics of disappearance of methotrexate from plasma [24, 46].

The methotrexate-leucovorin system is admittedly a complex one; to describe a given regimen completely, one must specify the dose, route, schedule, and duration of administration of both agents, as well as the temporal relation between the two. With so many variables, therefore, it is not surprising that, after 20 or more years of clinical experience, there is no unanimity among inestigators on the optimal regimen. The 11 entries in Table 2 represent the study of ten distinct regimens; in four of the ten, the number of patients studied is ten or fewer.

Even more fundamentally, no conclusive evidence is available that high doses of methotrexate with leucovorin are more efficacious than conventional doses, with or without leucovorin (Table 3). In a multiinstitutional randomized trial, Levitt et al. [34] were unable to demonstrate a statistically significant increase in response rate with moderately high doses of methotrexate and leucovorin over that achieved with methotrexate alone; the toxicity of the combination, however, appeared to be less than with methotrexate alone. Preliminary analysis of an ECOG trial [16] shows no differences among the three treatments tested. Early results of an Australian study [68]

Table 2. High-dose methotrexate with leucovorin in head and neck cancer

Author [ref]	Methotrexate	Rescue at	Leucovorin	Patients	CR	PR	RR (%)	MDR (mo.)
Lefkowitz et al. [32]	1–3 mg/kg × 24 h	24 h	6 mg IM q 12 h × 6 doses	18	0	4	22	–
Capizzi et al. [7]	240 mg/m² × 24 h q 4 d	24 h	75 mg IV × 12 h; 12 mg IM q 6 h × 4 doses	PT 13 PU 8	0 0	8 5	62 63	4 NA
Tarpley et al. [61]	240 mg/m² × 24 h q 4 d	24 h	75 mg IV × 12 h; 12 mg IM q 6 h × 4 doses	PU 30	0	23	76	NA
Pitman and Frei [46]	1–7.5 g/m² bolus with hyd, alk	24 h	10 mg/m² IV-p.o. q 6 h × 12 doses	PT 17	0	14	82	–
Kirkwood et al. [30]	1–7.5 g/m² bolus with hyd, alk	24 h	10 mg/m² IV-p.o. q 6 h × 12 doses	PU 19	0	10	53	NA
Khandekar and Wolff [28]	500 mg/m² × 24 h with escalation to 4 g/m² max (M preceded by V)	30 h	? q 4 h p.o. × 7 doses	PT 20	4	9	65	5+
Goldberg et al. [19]	50 mg/m² bolus; then 1500 mg/m² × 36 h	36 h	25 mg/m² IV bolus; 200 mg/m² q 12 h; 25 mg/m² IM q 6 h × 6	PT 5 PU 5	0 0	0 4	0 80	– NA
Ohnuma et al. [42]	100–250 mg/kg × 6 h qw	8 h	12 mg IM or IV q 6 h × 12 doses	PT 10	0	4	40	⎫ ⎬ 1–3 +
	1–4 g/m² × 1 h with hyd, alk	24 h	15 mg IV; then 15 mg p.o. q 6 h × 11 doses	PT 9	0	2	22	⎭
Isacoff et al. [24]	50–100 mg/kg × 4 h with escalation; hyd, alk (V given during infusion)	8 h	40 mg/m² IV; 15 mg q 6 h × 11 with escalation if M clearance is decreased	PT 7	0	3	43	3
Buechler et al. [6]	15 mg/kg × 24 h q 3 w c/s BCG	24 h	9 mg IM q 6 h × 6 doses	PT 23	2	4	26	3
Taylor et al. [62]	60 mg/m² IM q 6 h × 4 d 1, 5, 9 with escalation	6 h	40 mg p.o. q 6 h × 2 doses; 10 mg q 6 h × 2 doses	PU 17	–	–	–	NA

Table 3. Methotrexate in head and neck cancer — randomized trials comparing high and low dose schedules

Author [ref]	Treatment plan	Patients	RR(%)	MDR (mo)
Levitt et al. [34]	1) M 80 mg/m^2 × 30 h q 2 w with esc to tox	16	44	3
	2) M 240−360 mg/m^2 × 36−42 h with esc to 1080 mg/m^2 with L 40 mg/m^2 IV bolus; 25 mg/m^2 p.o. q 6 h × 4 doses	25	60	3
DeConti et al. [16]	1) M 40 mg/m^2 IV qw		Overall RR 24%, MDR 50 days; no significant differences among the three arms	
	2) M 240 mg/m^2 IV with L 25 mg q 6 h × 8 doses q 2 w			
	3) M and L as in (B) plus C 500 mg/m^2 IV and Ara-C 300 mg/m^2 IV q 2 w			
Woods et al. [68]	1) M 50 mg/m^2 bolus L 15 mg p.o. q 6 h × 12 doses	11	45	
	2) M 500 mg/m^2 bolus L as in (A)	16	31	2
	3) M 5000 mg/m^2 bolus L as in (A)	12	50	
Kirkwood et al. [29]	1) M 40−200 mg/m^2 biw L 50 mg/m^2 IV single dose	18	61	3
	2) M 1−7.5 g/m^2 × 24 h qw L 10 mg/m^2 IV-p.o. q 6 h × 12 doses	16	50	3

involving three doses of methotrexate varying over a 100-fold range show no obvious differences among the treatments. Kirkwood et al. [29] have recently reported the preliminary results of a trial comparing weekly high-dose methotrexate with leucovorin to a twice-weekly escalating regimen of methotrexate at much lower doses, each of which is followed by a single intravenous bolus of leucovorin at 24 h. No apparent differences in activity of the two regimens have emerged and the low-dose regimen seems significantly less toxic.

In summary, there is no good evidence that, above a dose of 40−50 mg/m^2 every week, the response rate increases with increasing dose of methotrexate in ECHN. This, of course, is not to say that such a relationship does not exist; it may mean simply that studies to date have not been designed with enough power to detect such differences. Alternatively, those high-dose methotrexate regimens, which might actually be superior to lower doses, may not have been subjected to adequate comparative trials. It is quite clear, however, that the dose and schedule modifications which have been investigated over the past several years have not increased the dismally short response durations that are produced by methotrexate or by the other single agents in common use in ECHN. The brevity of the responses more than anything else serves to limit severely the utility of methotrexate by any dose and schedule in the palliation of the

Table 4. DDP in head and neck cancer

Author [ref]	Dose and schedule	Patients	CR	PR	RR (%)	MDR (mo)
Wittes et al. [65]	3 mg/kg bolus q3w with hyd, osm diur	PT 26	2	6	31	4
Wittes et al. [66]	120 mg/m² bolus q3w hyd, osm diur	PU 22	1	8	40	NA
Panettiere et al. [43]	50 mg/m² d 1,8 q4w	PT 21	0	8	38	–
Jacobs et al. [25]	80 mg/m² × 24 h hyd q4w	PT 18	1	6	39	–
Sako et al. [55]	120 mg/m² bolus q3w hyd, osm diur	PT 15	2	3	33	5
	20 mg/m² bolus qd × 5 doses q3w	PT 15	1	3	27	
Salem et al. [56]	5 mg/m² bolus; then 20 mg/m² × 24 h qd × 5 days	PT 4	0	1	–	–
Randolph and Wittes [52]	40 mg/m² bolus q w	PT 13	1	3	31	2.5

patient with advanced disease, recurrent after radiation and/or surgery. Identification of the optimal methotrexate regimen, however, remains important even if response durations are short, since the drug is in increasing use as a preoperative or preradiation adjuvant [30, 61], a subject to which we shall return later.

DDP has substantial activity in ECNH (Table 4). In striking contrast to the variability of response rates in the methotrexate trials, these results are remarkable for their uniformity over a rather impressive number of dose and schedule modifications. In the one study that addressed the question of schedule dependency, none was found [55]. It seems certain that intensive hydration, with or without diuretic administration, protects against dose-limiting nephrotoxicity. The nature of the dose-response curve for DDP in ECNH has not been defined. There is no good evidence that the previously untreated patient is much more responsive to DDP than the patient who has already failed radiation and/or surgery [65, 66]. DDP, however, is by itself no more the solution to the head and neck cancer problem than is methotrexate; response durations are diappointingly short, and palliation of the late-stage patient often remains elusive.

Combination Chemotherapy

Since the last comprehensive reviews of the chemotherapy of head and neck cancer [9, 20], interest in combinations of drugs has burgeoned. Table 5 lists the various two-drug combinations which have been studied in the United States. Many of these involve very small numbers of patients, and useful conclusions are often impossible. As might be expected from its lack of clinically significant myelotoxicity, bleomycin has been a favorite for combination with other agents. In the studies involving previously treated

Table 5. Two-drug combinations in head and neck cancer

Author [ref]	Treatment	Patients	CR	PR	RR (%)	MDR (mo)
Cortes et al. [14]	A 20−25 mg/m²/d × 3 IV B 15−20 mg/m²/d × 5 IV	8	0	4	50	3
Mosher et al. [40]	B 15−30 mg IV biw or IM in 5-day courses M 240 mg/m² × 36 h − L during the week off B	4	0	2	50	−
Lokich and Frei [37]	B 10−15 ⎱ mg/m² IV biw M 15−25 ⎰	5	1	3	80	4
Yagoda et al. [69]	B 15 mg ⎱ IV q4−14d M 15 mg/m² ⎰	15	3	5	53	3+
Moseley et al. [39]	CCNU 100−130 mg/m² po d 1 B 0.5 mg/kg IM or IV biw starting day 8 Recycle q6w	7	0	3	43	3
Wittes et al. [64]	P 2 mg/kg IV q3w B 0.25 mg/kg/d IV to tox	24	0	3	13	3
Bianco et al. [4]	P 30 mg/m² d 1−3 B 15 mg/m² d 3, 10, 17 Recycle q3w	7	0	1	14	1
Pitman et al. [48]	1. P 80 mg/m² × 24 h q2w × 2 then M 3 g/m² × 1 h qw × 4 − L	9	0	6	67	−
	2. M 3 g/m² × 1 h qw × 4 − L then P 80 mg/m² × 24 h q2w × 2	11	0	6	55	−
Bonomi et al. [5]	A 50 ⎱ mg/m² IV P 50 ⎰	16	1	5	37	4.5
Randolph et al. [51]	P 3 mg/kg IV d 1 B 0.25 mg/kg IV d 3 B 0.25 mg/kg/d CIVI d 3−10	PT 12 PU 21	0 4	4 11	33 71	− NA
Hong et al. [22, 23]	P 3 mg/kg IV d 1 B 0.25 mg/kg IV d 3 B 0.25 mg/kg/d CIVI d 3−10	PU 39	8	22	76	NA

patients, most of the response rates fall well within the range one might expect from conventional methotrexate alone, and those which are higher involve too few patients to be meaningful.

Certain individual features of some of these trials are of interest. Pitman et al. [48] are currently comparing two DDP-methotrexate combinations differing only in the sequence of administration of these two drugs. Their preliminary results confirm a high order of activity for both single drugs, but they also show that the two are difficult to give in combination. DDP-induced toxicity, involving both marrow and kidneys, significantly compromised the subsequent administration of methotrexate and seemed to result in an increased incidence of methotrexate toxicity when this agent followed

DDP. Further results of this trial will be important, since these two drugs are probably the most active currently available for ECHN. Others [8, 66] have also found these two agents difficult to administer together with acceptable toxicity.

High doses of DDP (120 mg/m^2) have been combined with bleomycin by continuous intravenous infusion in two independently executed trials [22, 51]. When this regimen was used as initial therapy, a high order of activity was demonstrated in both trials. The same regimen seemed less active in previously treated patients, although numbers were small [51]. Previously untreated patients seemed more responsive to DDP + bleomycin than to DDP alone [51, 66], though the difference is not statistically significant, perhaps because of the small sample sizes. The potential contribution of the bleomycin infusion is difficult to assess without reliable activity studies of bleomycin infusion alone in ECNH. The scanty data which are available (two partial responses of II cases, 18%, [31]) were obtained in a very sick group of patients with poor performance status and they cannot be assumed representative of the drug's activity in a less symptomatic population without further study.

Many three- and four-drug combinations including DDP, and bleomycin and/or methotrexate have been studied (Table 6). The addition of high-dose methotrexate to DDP and bleomycin as initial therapy does not seem to increase the antitumor activity of DDP and bleomycin but has resulted in an increase in toxicity [8, 16, 26, 66]. In a population of patients most of whom failed prior therapy, Kaplan et al. [26] have observed that relatively low doses of DDP, methotrexate, and bleomycin produce responses in 29 (63%) of 46 evaluable patients; when the 12 excluded cases are restored, however, the response rate falls to 50%. Despite the modest doses of drugs in this study, 24% of patients developed WBC < 2 000. Caradonna et al. [8], employing higher doses of DDP, were able to achieve good objective responses in 79% of their patient population, but only at the expense of rather severe toxicity; treatment had to be curtailed in four patients because of leucopenia or nephrotoxicity. A feature of all these studies is the brevity of the remissions; except for those achieving CR in the trial of Kaplan et al., these combinations have not increased the durability of remissions over what can be achieved, often with less toxicity, by the use of single agents.

By no means all the combinations of interest have included DDP or high-dose methotrexate. Some of these trials (Table 7), particularly those involving combinations of bleomycin and CMF [13, 21], appear to have somewhat higher rates of response than one might expect from single agent treatment, but all these studies are uncontrolled. Moreover, effects on duration of response are incompletely described and more follow-up is necessary. Investigators from the M.D. Anderson Hospital have examined the effects of a series of combinations [35, 54] originally designed for lung cancer; the activity of these regimens has been disappointing in ECHN, especially since toxicity has been impressive. The subsequent use of sequential drug administration by this group [36, 41] does not seem to have effected a significant increase in either rate or duration of remission. Costanzi et al. [15] have employed short bleomycin infusions followed, after a 24-h delay, by pulses of low-dose methotrexate or hydroxyurea; this regimen, the motivation for which was based on kinetic data obtained in human epidermoid carcinoma, has yielded results which are not different from methotrexate and bleomycin given without regard to niceties of scheduling (Table 5), and, as always, remissions are very short.

There has been much work on the combination of chemotherapy, mostly with single agents, and radiotherapy [9, 20]. Recently, investigators have been administering

Table 6. Three and four-drug regimens containing DDP and bleomycin and/or methotrexate

Author [ref]	Treatment	Patients	CR	PR	RR (%)	MDR (mo)
Kaplan et al. [26]	B 10 mg IM qw M 40 mg/m² IM d 1, 15 P 50 mg/m² IV d 4 Repeat q3w	46	8	21	63	CR 11 mo PR 5 mo
Leone and Ohnuma [33]	P ⎱ ML ⎰ doses not given B	PT 24 PU 8	1 3	5 4	25 88	2 NA
Caradonna et al. [8]	B 15 mg/m² d 1 M 20 mg/m² d 1 P 120 mg/m² d 2	14	2	9	79	3–4
Wittes et al. [66]	M 50 mg/m² IV bolus 　d 1; then M 1500 　mg/m² × 36 h − L P 120 mg/m² IV d 4 B 10 mg/m² IV bolus d 6; B 10 mg/m²/d CIVI d6–14	PU 8	0	4	50	NA
Elias et al. [18]	P 100 mg/m² IV d 1; B 15 mg/m² IV d 5 　15 mg/m²/d CIVI × 5 M 50 mg/m² IV bolus; 　1500 g/m² × 36 h − L d 　11–13 as tolerated	PT 11 PU 22	0 4	6 12	55 73	– NA
Baker and AlSarraf [2]	P 100 mg/m² IV d 1 V 1 mg IV d 2.5 B 30 mg/d CIVI d 2–5	10	1	4	50	–
Amer et al. [1]	V 0.5 mg/m² d 1,4 B 30 mg/d CIVI d 1–4 P 100–120 mg/m² IV d 6	16	0	6	38	2+
Bianco et al. [4]	M 500 mg/m² × 24 h d 1 − L V 1 mg/m² IV q 12 h × 2, d 1 P 40 mg/m² IV d 8 q3w with escalation of M	7	0	0	0	–
Wittes et al. [66]	M 40 mg/m² IV d 1 Vb 7 mg/m² IV d 1 B 20 mg/m² IV d 1 　20 mg/m²/d CIVI d 1–4 P 100 mg/m² IV d 5	PU 21	0	10	48	NA

combinations of drugs simultaneously with radiotherapy (Table 8). The seminal study of Clifford and colleagues [11, 12] from the Royal Marsden Hospital, while uncontrolled, appears to have yielded a higher proportion of complete regressions than one might anticipate from radiation alone in patients with such advanced disease. Survival at 50 months seems to be about double that of a historical control group (57% versus 22%) matches for stage. Although the design of this trial will not permit

Table 7. Other drug combinations

Author [ref]	Drugs	Patients	CR	PR	RR (%)	MDR (mo)
Cortes et al. [13]	BCMF	26	7	8	58	3–12
Holoye et al. [21]	BCMF	22	4	9	59	–
	BCMFV	22	8	3	48	–
	BCM	13	0	4	31	–
	BCF	8	0	1	13	–
	BMF	7	0	1	14	–
Bianco et al. [4]	BCMF	9	0	1	11	2
Costanzi et al. [15]	BM-BH	17	0	10	59	2
Livingston et al. [35]	CVB + methyl-CCNU	21	0	6	29	–
Richman et al. [54]	BAVN + CCNU with and without BCG	34	3	12	44	4
Livingston et al. [35]	CVB → M → A + methyl-CCNU (sequential)	28	5	7	43	6
Murphy et al. [41]	CAVB → M → CA (sequential)	19	2	3	26	–
Dowell et al. [17]	CMFV	10	0	2	20	–
	CMFV + Pred	12	0	6	50	–
Presant et al. [49, 50]	BCNU + AC	19	0	6	32	6
Ratkin et al. [53]	BVM	PT 14	0	6	43	4.7 +
		PU 7	0	5	71	NA
Wittes et al. [67]	CAMB	26	0	9	35	2.5

Table 8. Combination chemotherapy and concurrent radiotherapy

Author [ref]	Drugs	Radiation (rads)	Total	CR
Clifford [11, 12]	VBM	6000–6500	76	52
Petrovich et al. [44]	1) None	6500	11	1
	Versus			
	2) VM	6500	12	3
Smith et al. [60]	BAF	Not stated	36	20
Seagren et al. [57]	CB	5400	18	10
Silverberg et al. [59]	CVB	7000–7500	15	3

definitive conclusions, the results are sufficiently promising to warrant further exploration of this general approach. Most of the studies in progress are too recent to allow any firm conclusion (Table 8). Such simultaneous combined-modality treatment has clearly produced much greater local toxicity than radiation therapy alone. Whether such combinations will produce selective tumor cell kill at acceptable levels of normal tissue toxicity is the major unanswered question at present.

Initial Chemotherapy

The use of chemotherapy as a preoperative or preradiation adjuvant in advanced (stage III, IV), previously untreated patients has become rather widespread over the last two or three years in the United States. The basis for this approach is the assumption that drugs will be more effective if given before local therapies have caused perturbations in the local physiology of the primary tumor. As we have previously noted, the evidence to support this supposition is not at all compelling. Nevertheless, many investigators have used this approach with methotrexate [7, 19, 30, 61, 66], or DDP, either alone [66] or in combination [18, 22, 33, 51, 66], as well as with other combinations [21, 53]. Response rates with regimens used in this fashion are generally high, though not always much higher than the same regimen produces in previously treated patients [7, 18, 30, 46, 65, 66]. It has proved possible to carry through with surgery and/or radiation therapy after such chemotherapy without any obvious increase in the morbidity from either. In patients who undergo major resections after initial chemotherapy, the surgical specimen almost always contains viable-appearing tumor, even after rather striking responses to the drugs; occasionally, no tumor can be identified in the specimen. Shapshay et al. [58] have described an apparent increase in the tumor's content of keratin following response to DDP + bleomycin, and have speculated that the drugs may induce differentiation of the malignant cells.

No such study from a single institution has been designed in controlled fashion because of the limited numbers of patients available even to the largest institutions. In the interpretation of any adjuvant trial, proper controls are critical. The National Cancer Institute has recently coordinated the formulation and activation of a multi-institutional large-scale cooperative study, the purpose of which is to assess the role of initial and maintenance chemotherapy in prolonging the disease-free interval following primary treatment and total survival. Specifically, operable stage III and IV patients with ECHN at selected primary sites in the oral cavity and larynx are randomized among three treatment arms: 1) Surgery, followed by postoperative radiation; 2) Initial treatment with DDP + bleomycin, followed in 3 weeks by 1); 3) Arm 2) followed by 6 months of adjuvant therapy with 24-h infusions of DDP given at monthly intervals [25], in the hope of reducing the appreciable incidence of distant failure [38] in this advanced group of patients.

If the expected accession of approximately 300 patients can be realized, this trial will be capable of answering important questions concerning the validity of many of our current assumptions concerning proper directions in head and neck cancer treatment. In any event, the formation of a large scale trial, national in scope, certainly represents a salutary sign for the future of head and neck clinical trials in the United States.

Abbreviations used in Tables

A, adriamycin; alk, alkalinization; ARA-C, cytosine arabinoside; B, bleomycin; C, cyclophosphamide; CIVI, continuous intravenous infusion; CR, complete response; esc, escalation; F, fluorouracil; H, hydroxyurea; hyd, hydration; L, leucovorin; M, methotrexate; MDR, median duration of remission; N, nitrogen mustard; NA, not applicable; osm diur, osmotic diuresis; P, cis-diamminedichloroplatinum (II); PR, partial response; Pred, prednisone; PT, previously treated; PU, previously untreated; PR, response rate; V, vincristine; Vb, vinblastine.

References

1. Amer M, Izbicki R, Al-Sarraf M (1978) Combination of high-dose cis-platinum, oncovin, and bleomycin in treatment of patients with advanced head and neck cancer. Proc Am Soc Clin Oncol 19: 312
2. Baker L, Al-Sarraf M (1979) Comparative trial of cisplatinum, oncovin, and bleomycin versus methotrexate in patients with advanced epidermoid carcinoma of the head and neck. Proc Am Assoc Cancer Res 20: 202
3. Bertino JR, Mosher MB, Deconti RC (1973) Chemotherapy of cancer of the head and neck. Cancer 31: 1141–1149
4. Bianco A, Taylor SG IV, Reich S, Merrill JM, Dewys WD (1979) Combination chemotherapy pilot studies in head and neck squamous cell cancer. Cancer Treat Rep 63: 158–159
5. Bonomi PD, Slayton RE, Wolter J (1978) Phase II trial of adriamycin and cis-dichloro-diammineplatinum (II) in squamous cell, ovarian, and testicular carcinomas. Cancer Treat Rep 62: 1211–1213
6. Buechler M, Mukherji B, Chasin W, Nathanson L (1979) High-dose methotrexate with and without BCG therapy in advanced head and neck malignancy. Cancer 43: 1095–1100
7. Capizzi RL, Deconti RC, Marsh JC, Bertino JR (1970) Methotrexate therapy of head and neck cancer: improvement in therapeutic index by use of leucovorin "rescue". Cancer Res 30: 1782–1788
8. Caradonna R, Paladine W, Goldstein J, Ruckdeschel J, Hillinger S, Horton J (1978) Combination chemotherapy with high-dose cis-diamminedichloroplatinum (II), metho-trexate, and bleomycin for epidermoid carcinoma of the head and neck. Proc Am Soc Clin Oncol 19: 401
9. Carter SK (1977) The chemotherapy of head and neck cancer. Semin Oncol 4: 413–424
10. Chretien P, Lipson SD, Makuch R, Ketcham A (1979) Adjuvant methotrexate in operable head and neck squamous carcinoma: follow-up report of a feasibility trial. Abstract in Proceedings of the 25th Meeting, Society of Head and Neck Surgeons, Pittsburgh, Pa
11. Clifford P (1979) Synchronous multiple drug chemotherapy and radiotherapy in the treatment of advanced (stage III and IV) squamous cell carcinoma of the head and neck. Proc Am Assoc Cancer Res 20: 83
12. Clifford P, O'Connor AD, Durden-Smith J, Hollis BA, Edwards W, Dalley VM (1978) Synchronous multiple drug chemotherapy and radiotherapy for advanced (stage III and IV) squamous carcinoma of the head and neck. Antibiot Chemother 24: 60–72
13. Cortes EP, Amin VC, Attie J, Eisenbud L, Khafif R, Wolk D, Arel I, Sciubba J, Akbiyik N (1979) Combination of low-dose bleomycin followed by cyclophosphamide, methotrexate, and 5-flurururacil for advanced head and neck cancer. Proc Am Soc Clin Oncol 20: 259
14. Cortes EP, Shedd D, Albert DJ, Ohnuma T, Hreshchyshyn M (1972) Adriamycin and bleomycin in advanced cancer. Proc Am Assoc Cancer Res 13: 86
15. Costanzi JJ, Loukas D, Gagliano R, Griffiths C, Barranco S (1976) Intravenous bleomycin infusion as a potential synchronizing agent in human disseminated malignancies: a preliminary report. Cancer 38: 1503–1506
16. Deconti RC (1976) Phase III comparison of methotrexate with leucovorin versus methotrexate alone versus a combination of methotrexate plus leucovorin, cyclophos-phamide, and cytosine arabinoside in head and neck cancer. Proc Am Soc Clin Oncol 17: 248
17. Dowell KE, Armstrong DM, Aust JB, Cruz AB (1975) Systemic chemotherapy of advanced head and neck malignancies. Cancer 35: 1116–1120
18. Elias EG, Chretien P, Monnard E, Khan T, Bouchelle W, Wiernik P, Lipson S, Hande K, Zentai T (1979) Chemotherapy prior to local therapy in advanced squamous cell carcinoma of the head and neck. Cancer 43: 1025–1031

19. Goldberg N, Chretien P, Elias EG, Hande K, Chabner B, Myers C (1977) Preoperative high-dose methotrexate – a well-tolerated regimen in head and neck cancer. Proc Am Soc Clin Oncol 18: 292
20. Goldsmith MA, Carter SK (1975) The integration of chemotherapy into a combined modality appraoch to cancer therapy. V. Squamous cell cancer of the head and neck. Cancer Treat Rev 2: 137–158
21. Holoye PY, Byers RM, Gard DA, Goepfert H, Guillamondequi O, Jesse R (1978) Combination chemotherapy of head and neck cancer. Cancer 42: 1661–1669
22. Hong WK, Bhutani R, Shapshay S, Craft ML, Ucmakli A, Snow MN, Vaughan C, Strong S (1978) Induction chemotherapy of advanced unresectable head and neck cancer with cis-diamminedichloroplatinum (II) (DDP) and bleomycin. Proc Am Soc Clin Oncol 19: 321
23. Hong WK, Shapshay SM, Bhutani R, Craft ML, Ucmakli A, Yamaguchi KT, Vaughan CW, Strong MS (to be published) Induction chemotherapy in advanced squamous head and neck carcinoma with high-dose cis-platinum and bleomycin infusion. Cancer
24. Isacoff WH, Eilber F, Tabbarah H, Klein P, Dollinger M, Lemkin S, Sheehy P, Cone L, Rosenbloom B, Sieger L, Block J (1978) Phase II clinical trial with high-dose methotrexate therapy and citrovorum factor rescue. Cancer Treat Rep 62: 1295–1304
25. Jacobs C, Bertino J, Goffinet D, Fee W, Goode RL (1978) 24-hour infusion of cis-platinum in head and neck cancers. Cancer 42: 2135–2140
26. Kaplan BH, Vogl SE, Chiuten D, Lanham R, Wollner D (1979) Chemotherapy of advanced cancer of the head and neck with methotrexate, bleomycin, and cis-diamminedichloroplatinum in combination. Proc Am Soc Clin Oncol 20: 384
27. Khandekar JD, Dewys WD (1978) Chemoimmunotherapy of head and neck cancer. Am J Surg 135: 688–695
28. Khandekar J, Wolff A (1977) A clinical trial of high dose methotrexate with leucovorin "rescue" in advanced epidermoid carcinoma of the head and neck. Proc Am Soc Clin Oncol 18: 281
29. Kirkwood JM, Ervin T, Pitman S, Miller D, Weichselbaum R, Canellos G (1979) Twice-weekly low-dose methotrexate-leucovorin versus weekly high-dose methotrexate-leucovorin for advanced squamous carcinoma of the head and neck. Proc Am Soc Clin Oncol 20: 314
30. Kirkwood J, Miller D, Pitman S, Canellos G, Frei E (1978) Initial high-dose methotrexate-leucovorin in advanced squamous cell carcinoma of the head and neck. Proc Am Soc Clin Oncol 19: 398
31. Krakoff IH, Cvitkovic E, Currie V, Yeh S, Lamonte C (1977) Clinical pharmacologic and therapeutic studies of bleomycin given by continuous infusion. Cancer 40: 2027–2037
32. Lefkowitz E, Papac R, Bertino J (1967) Head and neck cancer III. Toxicity of 24 h infusions of methotrexate (NSC-740) and protection by leucovorin (NSC-3590) in patients with epidermoid carcinoma. Cancer Chemother Rep 51: 305–311
33. Leone L, Ohnuma T (1979) Combined high-dose methotrexate rescue, bleomycin, and cis-platinum for untreated stage III and localized stage IV for advanced squamous carcinoma of the head and neck. Proc Am Soc Clin Oncol 20: 374
34. Levitt M, Mosher MB, Deconti RC, Farber LR, Skeel RT, Marsh JC, Mitchell MS, Papac RJ, Thomas ED, Bertino JR (1973) Improved therapeutic index of methotrexate and leucovorin "rescue". Cancer Res 33: 1729–1734
35. Livingston RB, Einhorn LH, Bodey GP, Burgess MA, Freireich E, Gottlieb J (1975) COMB (Cyclophosphamide, oncovin, methyl-CCNU, and bleomycin): A four-drug combination in solid tumors. Cancer 36: 327–332
36. Livingston RB, Einhorn LH, Burgess MA, Gottlieb JA (1976) Sequential combination chemotherapy for advanced recurrent squamous carcinoma of the head and neck. Cancer Treat Rep 60: 103–105
37. Lokich J, Frei E III (1974) Phase II study of concurrent methotrexate and bleomycin chemotherapy. Cancer Res 34: 2240–2242

38. Merino OR, Lundberg RD, Fletcher GH (1977) An analysis of distant metastases from squamous cell carcinoma of the upper respiratory and digestive tracts. Cancer 40: 145–151
39. Moseley HS, Sasaki T, McConnell DB, Merhoff G, Wilson WL, Grage TB, Weiss AJ, Fletcher WS (1976) A randomized pilot study comparing two regimens in the treatment of squamous cell carcinoma. J Surg Oncol 8: 35–42
40. Mosher MB, Deconti RC, Bertino JR (1972) Bleomycin therapy in advanced Hodgkin's disease and epidermoid cancers. Cancer 30: 56–60
41. Murphy WK, Livingston RB, Gehan E, Bodey GP (1977) Sequential chemotherapy in the treatment of cancer of the head and neck. Proc Am Assoc Cancer Res 18: 190
42. Ohnuma T, Biller H, Kopel S, Holland JF (1978) High-dose methotrexate and leucovorin in patients with head and neck cancer. Proc Am Soc Clin Oncol 19: 350
43. Panettiere FJ, Lane M, Lehane D (1978) Effectiveness of a new outpatient program utilizing CACP in the chemotherapy of advanced epidermoid head and neck tumors. A SWOG study. Proc Am Soc Clin Oncol 19: 410
44. Petrovich Z, Block J, Barton R, Casciato R, Hittle R, Rice D, Jose L (1979) Treatment of stage IV carcinoma of the head and neck with radiotherapy and chemotherapy and radiotherapy combination. Proc Am Soc Clin Oncol 20: 422
45. Pitman SW, Frei E III (1977) Weekly methotrexate – calcium leucovorin rescue: effect of alkalinization on nephrotoxicity; pharmacokinetics in the CNS; and use in CNS non-Hodgkin's lymphoma. Cancer Treat Rep 61: 695–701
46. Pitman S, Frei E III (1977) Weekly methotrexate-citrovorum with alkalinization: tumor response in a phase II study. Proc Am Assoc Cancer Res 18: 124
47. Pitman SW, Miller D, Weichselbaum R (1978) Initial adjuvant therapy in advanced squamous cell carcinoma of the head and neck employing weekly high-dose methotrexate with leucovorin rescue. Laryngoscope 88: 632–638
48. Pitman SW, Minor DR, Papac R, Knopf T, Lowenthal I, Nystrom S, Bertino JR (1979) Sequential methotrexate-leucovorin and cis-platinum in head and neck cancer. Proc Am Soc Clin Oncol 20: 419
49. Presant CA, Kolhouse JF, Klahr C (1976) Adriamycin, 1,3-bis(2-chlorethyl)-1-nitrosourea (BCNU-NSC 409462), and cyclophosphamide in refractory adeno carcinoma of the breast and other tumors. Cancer 37: 620–628
50. Presant C, Ratkin G, Klahr C (1977) Adriamycin, BCNU, and cyclophosphamide in head and neck cancer. Proc Am Soc Clin Oncol 18: 281
51. Randolph VL, Vallejo A, Spiro RH, Shah J, Strong EW, Huvos A, Wittes RE (1978) Combination therapy of advanced head and neck cancer: induction of remissions with diamminedichloroplatinum (II), bleomycin, and radiation therapy. Cancer 41: 460–467
52. Randolph VL, Wittes RE (1978) Weekly administration of cis-diamminedichloroplatinum (II) without hydration or osmotic diuresis. Eur J Cancer 14: 753–756
53. Ratkin GA, Brown C, Ogura J (1978) Combination chemotherapy in head and neck cancer. Proc Am Soc Clin Oncol 19: 330
54. Richman SP, Livingston RB, Gutterman J, Suen J, Hersh E (1976) Chemotherapy vs chemoimmunotherapy of head and neck cancer. Report of a randomized study. Cancer Treat Rep 60: 535–539
55. Sako K, Razack MS, Kalnins I (1978) Chemotherapy for advanced and recurrent squamous cell carcinoma of the head and neck with high and low dose cis-diamminedichloroplatinum. Am J Surg 136: 529–533
56. Salem P, Hall SW, Benjamin RS, Murphy WK, Wharton JT, Bodey GP (1978) Clinical phase I-II study of cis-dichlorodiammineplatinum (II) given by continuous IV infusion. Cancer Treat Rep 62: 1553–1555
57. Seagren S, Byfield J, Nahum A, Bone R (1979) Concurrent cyclophosphamide, bleomycin, and ionizing radiation in advanced squamous carcinoma of the head and neck. Proc Am Soc Clin Oncol 20: 324

58. Shapshay SM, Hong WK, Incze JS, Yamaguchi K, Bhutani R, Vaughan CW, Strong MS (1978) Histopathologic findings after cis-platinum-bleomycin therapy in advanced previously untreated head and neck carcinoma. Am J Surg 136: 534–538

59. Silverberg IJ, Philips TL, Friedman MA, Fu KA (1978) A phase I study of radiotherapy and multidrug chemotherapy in advanced head and neck cancer. Proc Am Soc Clin Oncol 19: 345

60. Smith BL, Franz JL, Mira JG, Gates GA, Sapp J, Cruz AB Jr (1979) Simultaneous combination radiotherapy and multidrug chemotherapy for Stage III and Stage IV squamous carcinoma of the head and neck. Proc Am Soc Clin Oncol 20: 394

61. Tarpley JL, Chretien P, Alexander JC Jr, Hoye RC, Block J, Ketcham AS (1975) High-dose methotrexate as a preoperative adjuvant in the treatment of epidermoid carcinoma of the head and neck. A feasibility study andd clinical trial. Am J Surg 130: 481–486

62. Taylor SG, Bytell D, Sisson G (1977) Methotrexate with leucovorin as an adjuvant to surgery and radiotherapy in locally advanced squamous carcinoma of the head and neck. Proc Am Soc Clin Oncol 18: 346

63. Turrisi AT, Rosenzweig M, Von Hoff D, Muggia F (1978) The role of bleomycin in the treatment of advanced head and neck cancer. In: Bleomycin: Current Status and New Developments. Academic Press, New York, NY, pp 151–163

64. Wittes RE, Brescia F, Young CW, Magill GB, Golbey RB, Krakoff IH (1975) Combination chemotherapy with cis-diamminedichloroplatinum (II) and bleomycin in tumors of the head and neck. Oncology 32: 202–207

65. Wittes RE, Cvitkovic E, Shah J, Gerold F, Strong EW (1977) Cis-dichloro-diammineplatinum (II) in the treatment of epidermoid carcinoma of the head and neck. Cancer Treat Rep 61: 359–366

66. Wittes RE, Heller K, Randolph V, Howard J, Vallejo A, Farr H, Harrold C, Gerold F, Shah J, Spiro R, Strong EW (to be published) Platinum-based chemotherapy as initial treatment in advanced head and neck cancer. Cancer Treat Rep

67. Wittes RE, Spiro RH, Shah J, Gerold F, Koven B, Strong EW (1977) Chemotherapy of head and neck cancer: combination treatment with cyclophosphamide, adriamycin, methotrexate, and bleomycin. Med Pediatr Oncol 3: 301–309

68. Woods RL, Tattersall MHN, Sullivan J (1979) A randomized study of three doses of methotrexate in patients with advanced squamous cell cancer of the head and neck. Proc Am Assoc Cancer Res 20: 262

69. Yagoda A, Lippman A, Winn RJ, Schulman P, Cohen FB (1975) Combination chemotherapy with bleomycin and methotrexate in patients with advanced epidermoid carcinoma. Proc Am Assoc Cancer Res 16: 247

High-Dose Methotrexate and Cis-Platinum in the Treatment of Recurrent Head and Neck Cancer*

C. Jacobs

Division of Medical Oncology, Room C005, Stanford University Medical Center, USA − Stanford, CA 94305

Chemotherapy has had only a limited role in the treatment of recurrent squamous cell cancer of the head and neck. Methotrexate (MTX), the most extensively studied drug, produces 30%−50% response rates. Most of these responses, however, are of short duration [1]. Although response rates with high-dose MTX with leucovorin rescue (LR) have not been shown to be superior to those with conventional doses of MTX [5, 12], the relative lack of hematologic toxicity with the high-dose regimen [13, 14] may be advantageous when MTX is combined with other chemotherapeutic agents. Cis-diamminedichloroplatinum (CP) gives response rates comparable to MTX [11, 17], but appears to produce longer durations of response. Since the advent of mannitol diuresis [4, 10] and the administration of the drug by 24-h infusion [11], renal toxicity has been minimal.

The goal of combination chemotherapy is to achieve a higher response rate without added toxicity. Combinations of drugs have shown increased responses compared to single agents in a variety of cancers. However, in patients with recurrent head and neck cancers, the therapeutic impact of combination chemotherapy has been small [2, 7, 16]. The purpose of this investigation is to determine if combination chemotherapy with CP and weekly high-dose MTX is superior to single agent CP without increased toxicity. The results of patients treated with MTX-CP in a pilot study and interim report of a controlled trial of CP versus MTX-CP will be presented.

Materials and Methods

Between April 1977 and May 1978, 27 patients with recurrent head and neck squamous cell carcinoma entered the study at Stanford University. Five patients were treated with MTX-CP in a pilot study. In the randomized study 12 patients have been treated with MTX-CP and ten with CP. Pretreatment evaluation consisted of history and physical exam, blood counts, blood urea nitrogen, creatinine, creatinine clearance, urinalysis, liver function tests, chest X ray, audiogram, and selected scintiscans if indicated. Blood counts, creatinine, and urinalysis were repeated twice during each CP

* This study was supported by National Cancer Institute, National Institute of Health, Grant CA 05838 and a gift from the Bristol-Myers Company. The author thanks Michael Friedman, MD, for his contribution of clinical material

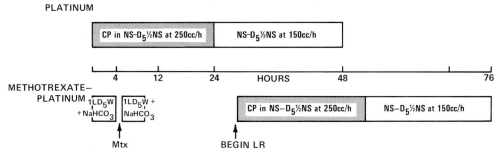

Fig. 1. Treatment schema

cycle and weekly during each MTX-CP cycle. Creatinine clearance and audiogram were repeated prior to each cycle.

Ten patients were treated with CP as a single agent at a dose of 80 mg/m^2. CP was delivered by 24-h infusion as previously described [11] with one-sixth of the total dose administered in 1 liter of NS alternating with D_5 $^1/_2$ NS every 4 h (Fig. 1). This was followed by 24 h of fluid at 150 cc/h. Potassium chloride and/or Lasix were added as necessary. CP was repeated every 3 weeks and patients received from one to six courses.

Seventeen patients received MTX-CP (Fig. 1). The patients were prehydrated with 1 liter of fluid and sodium bicarbonate until urine was alkaline. MTX was infused over 30 min followed at 24 h by 25 mg leucovorin orally every 6 h for 16 doses. Also at 24 h following MTX, the patient began a 24-h infusion of CP at 80 mg/m^2 as described above. The weekly dose of MTX was 250 mg/m^2. A CP dose of 80 mg/m^2 was given every 3 weeks. Patients received from one to seven courses.

Response was evaluated every 3 weeks by an otolaryngologist, a radiotherapist, and a medical oncologist. Only measurable cancers were used to determine complete or partial responses ($\geq$ 50% in all sites). Duration of response was calculated from the date of onset of tumor reduction to progression.

Results

Pilot Study

Five patients were initially treated with MTX-CP in a pilot study. All were treated for locally recurrent disease. Two patients had partial responses lasting 4 and 6.5 months. There was no mucositis, ototoxicity, renal toxicity, or thrombocytopenia. Two patients had mild neutropenia. Vomiting occurred in all patients.

Randomized Study

Twenty-two patients have been treated thus far in the randomized study. The patient's characteristics are presented in Table 1. The majority of patients were men, and the mean age was 44 in the CP group and 54 in the MTX-CP group. The average Karnofsky status was 60 in the CP group and 78 in the MTX-CP group. All patients

Table 1. Characteristics of patient population

	Platinum	Methotrexate − Platinum
Total	10	12
Sex		
Male	9	10
Female	1	2
Age		
Mean	44	54
Range	(19−70)	(39−67)
Karnofsky status		
Mean	60	78
Range	(40−90)	(60−90)
Site of disease		
Local	7	8
Distant	3	4
Primary site		
Oral cavity	2	3
Oropharynx	4	2
Larynx	2	3
Nasopharynx	2	3
Hypopharynx	1	
Maxillary sinus		1
Prior treament		
Radiotherapy	10	10
Surgery	8	8
Chemotherapy	4	1
No. of courses of chemotherapy		
Mean	2.2	2.8
Range	(1−6)	(1−6)
% Calculated dose (mean)		
CP	86%	96%
MTX		63%

had prior treatment with radiotherapy and/or surgery, and approximately 70% were treated for local recurrences. The mean number of courses of chemotherapy given was 2.2 in the CP group and 2.8 in the MTX-CP group, with a range of one to six courses. The mean percent calculated dose that was delivered in the CP group was 86%, and in the MTX-CP group was 96% CP, 63% MTX.

As shown in Table 2, one patient treated with CP had a biopsy-proven complete response that lasted 7 months. Three patients in the MTX-CP group have had partial responses lasting 1.5, 4, and 5+ months. One of these patients had cryosurgery of residual disease and is now free of disease.

As shown in Table 3, the hematologic toxicity has been greater in the MTX-CP group. Fifty-eight percent of the patients experienced leukopenia with four having a total white blood cell count of less than 3 000/mm^2. Two patients had infections, one fatal. Forty-two percent of the patients developed thrombocytopenia and one patient had

Table 2. Therapeutic results

	Platinum		Methotrexate − Platinum	
	No. patients	Duration (months)	No. patients	Mean duration (months)
CR	1 (10%)	7	−	−
PR	−	−	3 (25%)	1.5, 4.5$^+$

Table 3. Toxicity incurred in randomized study

	Platinum	Methotrexate − Platinum
Hematolic		
WBC 3,000−3,500/mm^3	1 (10%)	3 (58%)
1,000−2,900/mm^3	−	4
Platelets		
50,000−100,000/mm^3	−	3 (42%)
< 50,000/mm^3	−	2
Hemoglobin ↓ 2−3 gm%	3 (40%)	4 (50%)
↓ 3−5 gm%	1	2
Creatinine ≥ 2 mg%	−	−
Ototoxicity	−	1 (8%)
Gastrointestinal[a] − grade 1	4 (40%)	−
2	3 (30%)	8 (67%)
3	3 (30%)	4 (33%)
Mucositis	−	2 (17%)

[a] grade 1, slight nausea
grade 2, nausea + occasional vomiting
grade 3, vomit 1−3 times per day

bleeding from the base of the tongue. Only one patient had leukopenia in the CP group, but there were three mild infections. No patient had thrombocytopenia. A normochromic, normocytic anemia was common in both groups.
There was no significant renal toxicity (creatinine ≥ 2 mg%) in either group. Ototoxicity occurred in one patient in the MTX-CP group with a 30 dB loss at 8 000 Hz. No patient had subjective hearing loss. Vomiting occurred on the day of treatment only (grade 2−3) in 60% of patients in the CP group and all patients in the MTX-CP group. One patient discontinued therapy due to vomiting. Forty percent of patients in the CP group had nausea only. There were two episodes of mucositis in the MTX-CP group. No patient developed neurologic changes, alopecia, or an allergic reaction.

Discussion

Palliation of recurrent cancer of the head and neck is only rarely achieved with single agents, not only because of low response rates, but also because of the short duration of response [1]. Although combination chemotherapy has been shown to be superior to single agents in several other amlignancies, it has not been beneficial in recurrent head and neck cancers [1]. We combined the two most active single agents, CP and MTX, in a small pilot and, encouraged by the response and toxicity, have begun a randomized study comparing MTX + CP to CP alone.

In the pilot study two of five patients had partial responses. However, the randomized study to date has been discouraging with only one CR (10%) in the CP group and three PRs (25%) in the MTX-CP group. Although the numbers of patients are too small to compare the groups as yet, there is concern about the overall poor response in comparison to other reports of CP or high-dose MTX alone [5, 11−13, 17]. One reason may be the strict criteria of a PR ($\geq$ 50% by three observers, including a radiotherapist, oncologist, and otolaryngologist) in a disease which is often difficult to measure. Three patients in the CP group and five in the MTX-CP group had PR of less than 50%. A second reason may be that no patient was excluded from analysis although three patients were unevaluable due to early deaths.

Weekly high-dose MTX (at 250 mg/m^2) with LR can safely be added to CP without causing dose-reduction of CP. Although both drugs are potentially nephrotoxic [3, 6, 8, 9], the addition of MTX to CP did not increase nephrotoxocity. However, there has been more hematologic toxicity in the MTX-CP group with 58% developing leukopenia and 42% developing thrombocytopenia as compared to a 10% incidence of leukopenia and no thrombocytopenia in the CP group.

Pitman [15] has treated patients with CP (80 mg/m^2) and MTX (3 g/m^2) in a sequential manner and noted a 60% PR. Patients had significant compromise of MTX dose following CP due to nephrotoxicity and myelosuppression. In our study, using the same dose of CP and a lower dose of MTX, the hematologic toxicity is greater in combination, but 96% of CP and 63% of MTX dose has been delivered. We have observed no added renal toxicity. As yet our response rates as a single agent or in combination are much lower. However, more patients must be studied in this randomized study before any conclusions can be made.

References

1. Bertino JR, Boston B, Capizzi RL (1975) The role of chemotherapy in the management of cancer of the head and neck, a review. Cancer 36: 752−758
2. Bertino JR, Mosher MB, Deconti RC (1973) Chemotherapy of cancer of the head and neck. Cancer 31: 1141−1149
3. Condit PT, Changes RE, Joel W (1969) Renal toxicity of methotreaxate. Cancer 23: 126−131
4. Cvitkovic E, Spaulding J, Bethune V, Martin J, Whitmore WF (1977) Improvement of cis-dichlorodiammine platinum: therapeutic index in an animal model. Cancer 39: 1357−1361
5. Deconti RC (1976) Phase III comparison of methotrexate with leucovorin rescue vs. methotrexate alone vs. a combination of methotrexate plus leucovorin, cyclophosphamide and cytosine arabinoside in head and neck cancer. Proc Am Assoc Cancer Res Proc Am Soc Clin Oncol 17: 248
6. Deconti RC, Toftness BR, Lange RC, Creasey WA (1973) Clinical and pharmacologic studies with cis-diamminedichloroplatinum (II). Cancer Res 33: 1310−1315
7. Dowell KE, Armstrong DM, Aust JB, Cruz AB (1975) Systemic chemotherapy of advanced head and neck malignancies. Cancer 35: 1116−1120

8. Drewinko B, Green C, Loo TL (1975) Combination chemotherapy in vitro with cis-dichlorodiammineplatinum (II). Cancer Treat Rep 60: 1619—1625
9. Gottlieb JA, Drewinko B (1975) Review of the current clinical status of platinum coordination complexes in cancer chemotherapy. Cancer Chemother Rep 59: 621—628
10. Hayes DM, Cvitkovic E, Golbey RB, Scheiner E (1977) High dose cisplatinum diammine dichloride. Cancer 39: 1372—1381
11. Jacobs C, Bertino JR, Goffinet DR, Fee WE 24-hr infusion of cis-platinum in head and neck cancers. Cancer 42: 2135—2140
12. Khandekar JD, Wolff A (1977) A clinical trial of high dose methotrexate with leucovorin rescue in advanced epidermoid carcinoma of the head and neck. Proc Am Assoc Cancer Res Proc Am Soc Clin Oncol 18: 281
13. Levitt M, Mosher MB, Deconti RC, Farber LA (1973) Improved therapeutic index of methotrexate with leucovorin rescue. Cancer Res 33: 1729—1734
14. Ohnuma T, Biller H, Kopel S, Holland JF (1978) High dose methotrexate and leucovorin in patients with head and neck cancer. Proc Am Assoc Cancer Res Proc Am Soc Clin Oncol 19: 350
15. Pitman SW, Minor DR, Papac R, Knopf T, Lowenthal I, Nystrom S, Bertino JR (1979) Sequential methotrexateleucovorin (MTX-LCV) and cis-platinum in head and neck cancer. Proc Am Assoc Cancer Res Proc Am Soc Clin Oncol 20: 419
16. Wittes RE, Brescia F, Young CW, Magill GB Combination chemotherapy with cis-diamminedichloroplatinum (II) and bleomycin in tumors of the head and neck. Oncology 32: 202—207
17. Wittes RE, Cvitkovic E, Shah J, Gerold FP (1977) Cis-dichlorodiammineplatinum (II) in the treatment of epidermoid carcinoma of the head and neck. Cancer Treat Rep 61: 359—366

Current Strategy in the Chemotherapy of Advanced Breast Cancer

H. L. Davis

Wisconsin Clinical Cancer Center, Department of Human Oncology, University of Wisconsin, 600 Highland Avenue, USA – Madison, WI 53792

Three decades of active treatment research have produced some important conclusions which may serve as a guide to future attempts to circumvent the inevitably fatal outcome portended by the appearance of dissemination.

The first milestone was the demonstration of high initial response rates for combination chemotherapy [35, 47]. The brief duration of response and meager impact of survival of single agent therapy has been thoroughly reviewed in several publications [30, 98]. Thus the potential for improvement in duration of response and survival with highly active combinations has preoccupied clinical investigators during the 1970s.

The second milestone was the demonstration of a high degree of correlation of the presence of steroid hormone receptors with response to endocrine therapy [67]. The many previous studies in this area were based on empiricism and clinical insights into patient characteristics that were predictive for response, e.g., disease free interval, menopausal age, and dominant site of metastases [84]. The ability to determine steroid hormone receptors has further led to opportunities to combine the two modalities of endocrine and cytotoxic therapy.

The active drug development program of the NCI has produced numerous new anticancer agents during this period. Since most patients have been exposed to one or more combinations as treatment early in the course of their disseminated disease, the population of patients suitable for testing of a new agent now is a truly different one from that employed in the past.

The Impact of Combination Therapy

Table 1 documents selected instances of the impact of combination therapy on rate and duration of response and, in a few cases, survival. As background to Table 1 it might be well to document briefly some examples of survival experience with endocrine treatment of breast cancer. The examples quoted are generally from the precombination chemotherapy era to avoid the potential survival gain from active secondary therapy. The response to castration in premenopausal patients averaged about 30% with mean durations of response of 10−25 months and average survival of 32 months in responders and 8−9 months in nonresponders [93]. Major endocrine ablative

Table 1. Response and survival with single agents and combinations

Author [ref.]	Study design	CR + PR (%)	Duration of response (months)	Survival (months)	Comments
Baker [16]	a. Cyclophosphamide + 5 fluorouracil + vincristine	44	6.4	11.25	
	b. Sequential 5-fluorouracil, cyclophosphamide, vincristine	53	8.0	13.9	
Ahmann [2]	a. Adriamycin	50	5	20 (mean)	
	b. Cyclophosphamide + 5-fluorouracil + prednisone	59	9 +	18	
	c. b + vincristine	46	9 +	18	
	d. Adriamycin + methotrexate	38	6	36	
	e. Ifosfamide	20	4	22	
	f. MeCCNU	5	2	13	
Canellos [29]	a. Cyclophosphamide + methotrexate + 5-fluorouracil	53	6.2	Longer survival with combination	
	b. L-Phenylalanine mustard	20	3.0		
Chlebowski [31]	a. Pooled sequential therapy	27	–	Survival comparable	Combination better only in patients with liver metastases
	b. Combination therapy results (Southeast Oncology Group + Western Cancer Study Group)	43	–		
Ansfield [93]	a. 5-Fluorouracil, repeated loading courses	23	10	29, responders 26, stable 9, progression	Survival calculated from dissemination
Central Oncology Group-Ansfield [14]	a. 5-Fluorouracil loading, weekly maintenance	35	4	22	No significant difference in response or survival
	b. 5-Fluorouracil weekly	25	6	13	
	c. 5-Fluorouracil nontoxic schedule	17	3	14	
	d. 5-Fluorouracil oral	20	2.5	14	

Table 1 (continued)

Author [ref.]	Study design	CR + PR (%)	Duration of response (months)	Survival (months)	Comments
Mouridsen [70]	a. Oral cyclophosphamide	25	7	–	Survival could not be compared
	b. Cyclophosphamide + methotrexate + 5-Fluorouracil + vincristine + Prednisone	63	13	–	
Smalley [89]	a. Cytoxan + methotrexate + 5-fluorouracil vincristine + prednisone-simultaneous	46	7	12	25% each arm dead in 15 wks, 25% lived > 75 weeks
	b. Same combination intermittent	27	8.5	12	
	c. Sequential 5-fluorouracil, methotrexate, cyclophosphamide vincristine, prednisone	18	4	6	
Nemoto [73]	a. Adriamycin	38	7.6	17	Each regimen followed sequentially by the remaining arms on progression
	b. Adrenalectomy	35	9.2	13.9	
	c. Cytoxan + 5-fluorouracil + prednisone	43	21.3	21.5	
Hoogstraten [54]	a. Adriamycin	39	4	11	Response to crossover reduced (overall 28% with adriamycin 21%)
	b. Cyclophosphamide + methotrexate + 5-Fluorouracil + vincristine + Prednisone – weekly continuous	59	8	14	
	c. Same – intermittent	40	10	14	

procedures likewise gave response rates of approximately 30% overall and variable periods of survival ranging from 15−40 months for responding patients [92].

Classical additive therapy with estrogens produced responses of 31%−37% in two large series with average survival of 16.5 months overall and 27 months for responding patients [11]. Androgens were somewhat less successful in several trials [11, 33, 91] producing 15%−21% responses and average survivals of 10−12 months and extension to 19 months in responding cases [33].

These figures illustrate a baseline experience only. It is of interest that the average age of the AMA series estrogen-treated patients was 63 and the corresponding age for those treated with androgens 51 [11].

Survival experience in this era was correlated with disease free interval, number and sites of metastases, and menopausal age. Patients with dominant local recurrence did best with median survivals of 22 months; osseous dominant disease was intermediate (∼ 16 months), and visceral dominant disease had the shortest median suvival (∼ 10 months) [44]. A subset of patients with CNS, lymphangitic pulmonary metastases, and symptomatic liver metastases were identified as "dire" with survival of 4−6 months [36]. More recent trials of single agent chemotherapy cannot be evaluated easily for survival experience in view of effective secondary therapy. Note that Table 1 illustrates the difficulties in analyzing survival data that is influenced by multiple variables. Certainly the *initial* response rate is to combination chemotherapy higher in all studies. The *total* response rate may be similar when responses to successive treatments are pooled as in Baker's study [16]. The effect on survival is less clear as illustrated by the combined experience of the Southeast Oncology Group and the Western Cancer Study Group [31]. Survival was improved significantly only in the patients with liver metastases. The previous observations of Smalley [89] suggested that combination chemotherapy conferred a survival benefit on approximately 50% of the patients; 25% died within 4 months and 25% survived for more than 19 months regardless of regimen. Thus one might conclude the impact of combination programs on long-term survival is minimal at this time [94].

Nevertheless combination programs remain of great interest. The addition of adriamycin has led to a respectable gain in rate and duration of response; in some studies, though, survival gain is difficult to demonstrate. Table 2 illustrates some effective combinations employing this agent, which is undoubtedly the most active single agent available [98]. These studies represent a selection of randomized studies reported.

Again the conclusion is the same, the addition of adriamycin results in a small gain and little or no survival advantage. Moreover two studies employing fixed crossovers to delay or circumvent resistance have shown little advantage for this strategy [6, 24]. A major problem may be the limitation of total dose imposed with adriamycin therapy [76]. Two new approaches have recently been published in abstract form. The first is "super CMF"-adriamycin piloted at the Sidney Farber Cancer Center [51]. In this regimen methotrexate is given at a dose of 3.0 gm/m^2 on days 1 and 8 followed by citrovorum rescue rather than the conventional 40 mg/m^2. On day 29 adriamycin is given at a dose of $70−90 \text{ mg/m}^2$ resulting in 7-week cycles. The overall response rate is 73% with 32% complete remissions. The remissions seem durable to date with a median follow-up of 13.5 months.

The concept of late intensification is being tested at Mt. Sinai Hospital [79] based on animal work by Norton and Simon [75]. This is a promising approach which is additionally being tested in Milan in postmenopausal stage II patients [22]. A further

H. L. Davis

Table 2. Randomized trials of adriamycin containing combinations

Author [ref.]	Study design	CR + PR (%)	Duration of response	Survival	Comments
Tranum [100]	a. Adriamycin + cyclophosphamide	42	37 wk	70 wk	No significant difference
	b. Same + 5 fluorouracil	45	42 wk	70 wk	
	c. Adriamycin followed by cyclophosphamide + methotrexate + 5 fluorouracil + vincristine + prednisone	44	39 wk	70 wk	
Bull [26]	a. Cyclophosphamide + adriamycin + 5-fluorouracil	82	11 mo	27.2 mo	Difference not significant
	b. Cyclophosphamide + methotrexate + 5-fluorouracil	62	9 mo	17 mo	
Smalley [88]	a. Cyclophosphamide + adriamycin + 5-flourouracil	64	32 wk	–	Difference significant $p = 0.005$
	b. Cyclophosphamide + methotrexate + 5-fluorouracil + vincristine + prednisone	37	22 wk	–	
Muss [72]	a. Cyclophosphamide + adriamycin + 5-fluorouracil + vincristine + prednisone	58	15 mo	33 mo	Difference not significant
	b. Cyclophosphamide + methotrexate + 5-fluorouracil + vincristine + prednisone	57	13 mo	20 mo	

interesting trial is providing intensive local and systemic treatment for first recurrence. Patients are rendered clinically free of disease and then subjected to 2 years of intense chemoimmunotherapy [21]. Fifty-two perecent of "stage IV NED patients" are relapse-free at 39 months, compared to a matched group of historical controls with only 12% clinically free of disease.

The Resurrection of Endocrine Therapy
and the Potential for Combined Endocrine/Cytotoxic Treatment

Prior to 1967 endocrine therapy for breast cancer was on a strictly empirical basis, with clinical variables guiding the selection of patients and their subsequent management [84]. In 1967 a series of provocative experiments showing significant uptake of radiolabeled estradiol in estrogen-sensitive target tissues [58] culminated in the demonstration of cytoplasmic estrogen receptor protein ("estrophilin") [46]. It became apparent that the presence of absence of estrogen receptor protein in breast tumors had relevance as a predictive variable in the response to hormonal manipulations. In several large reviews it was shown that 50%–70% of receptor positive patients demonstrated objective responses to virtually all hormonal manipulations whether ablative or additive; conversely less than 10% of receptor negative patients responded [67]. Subsequent observations were extended to the presence of progesterone receptor (PGR) [68] and the quantitative level of estrogen receptor [53]. Moreover, the response to corticosteroid therapy is superior in estrogen receptor positive (ER+) patients [67].

A number of clinical correlations have emerged. It should be possible to compare endocrine versus cytotoxic therapy in ER+ patients. Because of the difficulty in obtaining receptor determinations in recurrent metastatic disease it will be difficult to classify a randomly selected sample. A randomized comparison of endocrine versus combination cytotoxic chemotherapy resulted in a clear preference for chemotherapy [80]. However, there was a subset of patients with predominately local recurrence who fared equally well on tamoxifen or cytotoxic therapy.

Another issue that has recently arisen is the comparative efficacy of chemotherapy in the ER+ versus the ER− (estrogen receptor negative) patient. Lippman [63] and Allegra [8] have presented preliminary evidence of a high response rate in ER− patients with a conversely low response rate in ER+ patients, especially ER+ and GPR+ (34 of 45 CR + PR in ER− patients versus 3 of 25 CR + PR in those ER+ and 21 of 24 CR + PR in ER− PGR-patients). This has not been universally observed and there are recent studies showing either no difference [23] or improved response rates in ER+ patients [59]. These conflicting observations not withstanding, the combination of aggressive cytotoxic chemotherapy and hormonal manipulations remains of theoretical and practical interest.

A selection of recently published work is shown in Table 3. Note that these studies show a mixture of regimens comparing ablative endocrine approaches with or without supplementary chemotherapy and chemotherapy alone versus endocrine therapy plus chemotherapy. "Endocrine therapy" includes prednisone. The results of combined oophorectomy with chemotherapy suggest modest improvement over either modality alone [25, 39]. Since the response rate to initial oophorectomy is low in Ahmann's and Falkson's study there was considerable early attrition in the castration group, although the chemotherapy programs were able to salvage some castration failures. This early

Table 3. Comparison of endocrine therapy or chemotherapy versus the combined approach

Author [ref.]	Study design	Results	Comments
Falkson [39]	Oophorectomy-delayed cyclophosphamide Oophorectomy + cyclophosphamide	18% 5-yr survival 33% 5-yr survival	Non-randomized study
Ahmann [5]	Oophorectomy → cyclophosphamide + 5-fluorouracil + prednisone on progression Oophorectomy + cyclophosphamide + 5-fluorouracil + prednisone	7/26 CR + PR 10/26 CR + PR	Median survival 88 weeks Median survival 131 weeks
Falkson [41]	Oophorectomy Oophorectomy + cyclophosphamide Oophorectomy + cyclophosphamide + methotrexate + 5-fluorouracil + vincristine + prednisone	17% CR + PR 65% CR + PR 63% CR + PR	Median survival slightly longer with combined approach
Brunner [25]	Cyclophosphamide + methotrexate + 5-fluorouracil + vincristine + prednisone	43% CR + PR	Duration response 7.8 mo survival 13.2
	Oophorectomy + cyclophosphamide + 5-fluorouracil + vincristine + prednisone	74% CR + PR	Duration response 9.5 mo survival 19.5 mo
	Cyclophosphamide + methotrexate + 5-fluorouracil + vincristine + prednisone	54% CR + PR	Duration 10.6 mo survival 19.2 mo
	Cyclophosphamide + methotrexate + 5-fluorouracil + vincristine + prednisone + stilbesterol	63% CR + PR	Duration 8.4 mo survival 27.7 mo
	Cyclophosphamide + methotrexate + 5-fluorouracil + vincristine + prednisone	63% CR + PR	Duration 10.0 mo survival 22.8 mo
	Cyclophosphamide + methotrexate + 5-fluorouracil + vincristine + prednisone + medroxyprogesterone	53% CR + PR	Duration 8.9 mo survival 18.1 mo
Heuson [52]	Adriamycin + vincristine alternating with cyclophosphamide + methotrexate + 5-fluorouracil + continuous tamoxifen	73% CR + PR	Phase II EORTC trial
Tormey [95]	Adriamycin + dibromodulcitol Adriamycin + dibromodulcitol + tamoxifen	36% CR + PR 64% CR + PR	Randomized — results striking in patients < age 50
Glick [45]	Tamoxifen Cyclophosphamide + methotrexate + 5-fluorouracil + tamoxifen added if stable at 12 weeks	50% response to tamoxifen	All patients ER + or unknown cyclophosphamide + methotrexate + 5-fluorouracil was not additive

Reference	Treatment	Response	Comment
Morgan [69]	Tamoxifen Cyclophosphamide + methotrexate + 5-fluorouracil added at 12 weeks for responders	38% response to tamoxifen responses continued with added CMF	Duration responses longer with added + cyclophosphamide + methotrexate + 5-fluorouracil
Eagen [43]	Cyclophosphamide + 5-fluorouracil + prednisone Cyclophosphamide + 5-fluorouracil + prednisone + calusterone	57% response 50% response	Calusterone not additive
Lloyd [64]	Low dose adriamycin + cyclophosphamide Same + calusterone	53% response 65% response	Duration 11.5 mo survival 13.5 mo Duration 21.5 mo survival 23.5 mo
Cocconi [32]	Cyclophosphamide + methotrexate + 5-fluorouracil Cyclophosphamide + methotrexate + 5-fluorouracil + tamoxifen	41% response 72% response	Duration 39 weeks Duration 52 weeks
Ramirez [82]	Cyclophosphamide + methotrexate + 5-fluorouracil + vincristine Cyclophosphamide + methotrexate + 5-fluorouracil + vincristine + prednisone	44% response 62% response	No significant difference In survival
Band [18]	Cyclophosphamide + methotrexate + 5-fluorouracil Cyclophosphamide + methotrexate + 5-fluorouracil + prednisone	48% response 63% response	Duration 21 weeks Duration 34 weeks
Tormey [97]	Cyclophosphamide + methotrexate + 5-fluorouracil + prednisone maintenance Cyclophosphamide + methotrexate + 5-fluorouracil + prednisone + fluoxymesterone maintenance	5.9 mo to progression 11.1 mo to progression	Maintenance study to Band's study above Added fluoxymesterone prolonged time to progression – not survival
Rosner [83]	Cyclophosphamide + 5-fluorouracil Cyclophosphamide + 5-fluorouracil Cyclophosphamide + methotrexate + 5-fluorouracil + vincristine + prednisone	33% response 42% response 41% response	Length of response similar = 8.5 mo

progression group in Ahmann's study had a median survival of only 22 weeks compared to 105 weeks for those patients with more indolent disease who could receive benefit from salvage chemotherapy [5]. Brunner's study likewise favored the combined approach over chemotherapy alone utilizing the CMFVP regimen containing prednisone [25].

The additive programs represent a mixture of results that illustrate the heterogeneity of this group of patients. Conflicting results abound although the tendency favors the combined use of added hormonal therapy. This even extends to the use of prednisone with both negative and positive results in the published series.

These studies, however, provide a golden opportunity for investigators since the cytoplasmic hormone receptor status of the primary tumor is being determined with increasing frequency at the time of mastectomy. The ER+ subset may respond equally well to an initial endocrine approach followed by chemotherapy upon failure. In this situation chemotherapy may not be additive as an initial approach as suggested by Glick's study [45]. In addition there is increasing evidence that prolonged hormonal therapy may result in ER depletion or select out ER- subpopulations of cells. Conversely prolonged initial chemotherapy may select out ER+ cell populations which conceivably could result in improved results with secondary hormonal therapy [9].

Overall Implications of These Study

No matter what the treatment sequence it would appear disseminated breast cancer is invariably fatal. Long-term suvivors are reported in favorable patients treated predominately with endocrine therapy or chemotherapy. A recent analysis of the fate of clinical complete remissions by Decker [37] further suggest that virtually all patients in complete remission will relapse within a year if chemotherapy is discontinued.

Even though these observations are rather grim there is some evidence of improved survival using current treatment modalities. Bonnadonna has recently published a provocative review on overall survival of a large series of breast cancer patients treated primarily and secondarily with the then best available therapy [22]. There has been a steady improvement in the proportion of patients surviving at 1–3 years after first relapse and this is most marked in patients receiving initial combination chemotherapy versus endocrine therapy. Patients relapsing on the current controlled adjuvant trial of CMF versus observation demonstrate a 3 year survival of 51%–57% when treated with modern combination programs versus 16%–29% when treated initially with endocrine maneuvers.

The Search for Effective Secondary Combination Programs
Aimed at Patients Relapsing After Adjuvant Chemotherapy

Even though chemotherapy or endocrine manipulations do not seem curative for recurrent breast cancer, successful therapy provides major palliative benefit for some patients.

Table 4 illustrates some recent efforts in this regard. Those programs specifically utilized after failure of adjuvant therapy are so identified; the remainder are

Table 4. Combination programs active as second line treatment

Author [ref.]	Study design	Results	Comments
Bonnadonna [22]	Cyclophosphamide + methotrexate + 5-fluorouracil after observation	53% response	
	Cyclophosphide + methotrexate + 5-fluorouracil after cyclophosphamide + methotrexate + 5-fluorouracil-adjuvant	12.5% response	
	Adriamycin + vincristine after cyclophosphamide + methotrexate + 5-fluorouracil adjuvant	39% response	
Tormey [95]	Adriamycin + dibromodulcitol	36% response	All patient had prior chemotherapy for advanced disease
	Adriamycin + dibromodulcitol + tamoxifen	64% response	
Tisman [99]	High dose methotrexate followed by 5-fluorouracil 2 hours later and citrovorum rescue	40% response	All had prior combination adjuvant therapy
Marcus [66]	5-Fluorouracil + vincristine + adriamycin + mitomycin C	62% response	All patients has failed adjuvant cyclophosphamide + methotrexate + 5-fluorouracil or L-phenylalanine mustard
Yap [103]	Sequential L-asparaginase + methotrexate	30% response	5/17 with prior methotrexate responded all patients failed prior adriamycin combinations
Rosner [83]	Adriamycin + cyclophosphamide	33% response	Tertiary therapy after cyclophosphamide + methotrexate + 5-fluorouracil + vincristine + prednisone failure

combination programs active after failure of initial treatment. The most promising combinations would seem to contain adriamycin [98], although the promise of cycle active programs is considerable [51]. More information regarding these and other salvage programs will undoubtedly accrue as the various ongoing adjuvant trials mature and more relapses occur.

New Drug Investigations in Breast Cancer

In spite of the modest advances to date, there remains a critical need for new active agents. Moreover a special concern is the development of less myelosuppressive agents and agents devoid of other limiting organ toxicities. Table 5 demonstrates the current "drugs of choice" tested in the time frame through adriamycin.

The current problems in testing new agents are considerable. Some of the problems are shown below, in a list concerning factors to be considered in phase II trials: Today's phase II patients are likely to have been exposed to at least two active combinations of the agents displayed in Table 5 and frequently at least one trial of endocrine therapy. As an illustration, the early trials of hexamethylmelamine done by the CDEP (Central Drug Evaluation Program) demonstrated activity [102]. The patients in this group represented a mixture who received only single agent chemotherapy and/or hormonal therapy. More recent investigations have been carried out by the Southwest Oncology Group and the Southeast Oncology Group where only minimal activity was demonstrated in a population that had failed initial combination programs [38, 60]. Thus, the real activity of hexamethylmelamine remains unsettled. A realistic conclusion would be that it is inactive as a third live single agent. Hexamethylmelamine has been successfully combined with vincristine and methotrexate, however, as

Table 5. Most active single agents in advanced breast cancer

Drug	Activity (CR + PR/Eval.)	Rating
Alkylating agents		
CTX	182/529	++
HN_2	32/92	+
TSPA	53/307	+
L-PAM	20/86	+
CLB	11/54	+
Antimetabolites		
5FU	324/1263	++
FUDR	50/169	++
MTX	120/356	++
Vinca alkaloids		
VCR	47/226	+
VLB	19/95	++
Antibiotics		
ADR	67/193	++
Mito C	41/110	++

a second line combination [65]. Thus, single illustration demonstrates the difficulty in precisely characterizing the activity of new agents.

Table 6 lists those drugs tested that have recently activity in one or more trials. Table 7 lists the drugs that have shown little or no activity. The drugs listed in Table 6 include several, in addition to hexamethylmelamine, which require modifying statements. High-dose methotrexate has not received a comparative trial to conventional doses. The "Super CMF" progam may indeed yield a high response rate but the CMF portion is interspersed with high-dose adriamycin. It is thus unclear what portion provides the improvement. Ifosfamide [27] and ftorafur [50] have not added substantially when substituted for cytoxan and 5-fluorouracil in the 5-FU, adriamycin + cytoxam regimen. Vindesine is myelosuppressive and may not be a good substitute for vincristine although further trials are indicated [90]. The continuous infusion of vinblastine [104] is of interest as is the early phase II activity of m-AMSA [62]. The agents in Table 1 are mostly inactive. The cis-platinum story is early, however, and this agent should not be discarded without further trial in view of its relative lack of myelosuppression [86]. Finally, the steroid coupled alkylators remain of interest; there are limited efforts in progress to develop new compounds with enhanced receptor binding and experimental antitumor activity [71].

Conclusion

Clearly a major goal of breast cancer treatment is to develop optimum chemotherapy and/or hormonal manipulations to improve the long-term prognosis of primary treatment [22].

Table 6. Factors to be considered in phase II trials

I	The Tumor Burden
	− Dominant Site of Mestastases
	− # of Sites
II	Organ Fuction
	− Marrow
	− Liver
	− Renal
III	Performance Status
	− a clinical summation of Effects of I and II
IV	Prior Therapy
	− Radiotherapy
	− Hormonal manipulations
	− Combination chemotherapy
	− Prior phase II trials
	− Prior adjuvant therapy
V	Other Clinical Parameters
	− Estrogen receptor status
	− Menopausal age
	− Disease free interval

Table 7. Agents receiving recent phase II testing and showing activity in one or more trials

Agents	Level of activity	Comments	Reference
Dibromodulcitol (DBD)	+ − + +	Some activity in all trials	[12, 96]
Hexamethylmelamine (HMM)	+	Disputed activity 14/56 in broad	[38, 102]
		Phase II-2/55 + 0/19 in recent trials	
High-dose methotrexate (HDMTX)	+ − + +	Modest single agent activity	[57]
Sequential L-asparaginase/methotrexate	+ +	30% response in priot MTX failures	[103]
Ifosfamide	+ − + +	4/20 + 9/22 in two trials	[1, 40]
Ftorafur	+	4/9 PR as single agent	[15]
Vindesine	+	5/18 PR-little prior treament	[90]
Vinblastine (infusion)	+	5-day infusion 8/19 PR	[104]
m-AMSA	+	3/22 PR	[62]

Levels of Activity:
  + +, definite
  +, hints of activity
  −, no activity
  NE, not evaluable

Table 8. Agents showing marginal or no activity in recent phase II trials

Agent	Level of activity	Comments incl. PR/eval.	Reference
Dianhydrogalactitol	–	1/55 Mayo + SWOG	[4, 55]
Piperazinedione	–	3/58-SWOG	[78]
ICRF-159	–	0/14-Mayo	[4]
Cis-Platinum diaminedichloride	+	Hints of activity at high dose	[49]
Yoshi 864	–	0/16 COG	[10]
Phenestrin	+	5/46-ECOG	[19]
Estradiol mustard	+	"Hints"	[Cooperative Breast Group, unpublished work]
Estramustine phosphate	+	2/34-EORTC	[48]
VP 16–213	–	5/120 pooled	[85]
VM-26	NE	2/22 pooled	[85]
Maytansine	NE	Hints of activity	[20, 28]
Chromomycin A₃	–	2/48-SWOG	[87]
Rubidazone	–	2 negative studies including comparison with adriamycin	[56, 61]
Bleomycin	+	2/24 } ECOG study	[17]
Streptozotocin	+	2/20 } ECOG study	[17]
Triazinate	+		[74]
Pyrazofurin	–		[74]
2 Anhydro 2' Arabinosylflurocytidine	–	1/17-EORTC	[7]
5-Azacytidine	–	1/38-SWOG + COG	[10, 81]
Cyclocytidine	–	1/36-SWOG	[77]
Cytembena	–	2 negative studies	[3, 42]

Our current efforts in chemotherapy have resulted in modest gains in survival for the intermediate subset of patients who would have rapidly failed hormonal and single agent sequential approches [89, 94]. These efforts represent a major achievement in palliation but not in cure. Intensive treatment both locoregional and systemic for the first recurrence represents an approach of interest for this limited group of patients [21]. Defining a "favorable" subset of patients by hormone receptors and clinical characteristics and using an aggressive chemotherapy-endocrine therapy approach likewise seems a desirable goal in treatment research. The "dire group" may provide a population targeted to the most intensive efforts possible. Phase II testing remains of interest but investigators may have to enlarge and expand on the current criteria of objective response. Careful attention to the "stable disease" category, particularly for length of stability, may be a valuable approach with these heavily pretreated patients.

Clearly advanced breast cancer remains a major therapeutic challenge. We have traveled only a part of the journey that remains a frustrating one. The achievements to date are considerable and there is hope that these will provide the foundation to achieve the endpoint; the cure of advanced breast cancer.

References

1. Ahmann DL, Bisel HF, Hahn RG (1974) Phase II clinical trial of isophosphamide (NSC 109724) in patients with advanced breast cancer. Cancer Chemother Rep 58: 861–865
2. Ahmann DL, Bisel HF, Hahn RG, Eagen RT, Edmonson JH, Steinfeld JL, Tormey DC, Taylor WF (1975) An analysis of multiple drug programs in the treatment of patients with advanced breast cancer utilizing 5-fluorouracil, cyclophosphamide and prednisone with or without vincristine. Cancer 36: 1925–1935
3. Ahmann DL, Bisel HF, Eagan RT, Edmonson JH, Hahn RG, O'Connell MJ, Frytak S (1976) Phase II evaluation of VP16-213 (NSC 141540) and cytembena (NSC 104801) in patients with advanced breast cancer. Cancer Treat Rep 60: 633–635
4. Ahmann DL, O'Connell MJ, Bisel HF, Edmonson JH, Hahn RG, Frytak S (1977) Phase II study of dianhydrogalactical and ICRF 159 in patients with advanced breast cancer previously exposed to cytotoxic chemotherapy. Cancer Treat Rep 61: 81–87
5. Ahmann DL, O'Connell MJ, Hahn RG, Bisel HF, Lee RA, Edmonson JH (1977) An evaluation of early or deleayed adjuvant chemotherapy in premenopausal patients with advanced breast cancer undergoing oophorectomy. N Engl J Med 297: 356–360
6. Ahmann DL, O'Fallon J, O'Connell MJ, Bisel HF, Hahn RG, Frytak S, Edmonson JH, Rubin J, Ingle JN, Kvols LK (1978) Evaluation of a fixed alternating treatment in patients with advanced breast cancer. Cancer Clin Trials 1: 219–226
7. Alberto P, Gangji D, Kenis Y, Brugarolas A, Clarysse A, Sylvester R (1977) Phase II study of anhydro-ara-5-fluorocytodine (AAFC). Proc Am Assoc Cancer Res Proc Am Soc Clin Oncol 18: 231
8. Allegra JC, Lippman ME, Thompson EB, Simon R, Barlock A, Green L, Huff KK, Do HMT, Aitken SC, Warren R (1978) Association between steroid hormone receptors and response rate to cytotoxic chemotherapy in metastatic breast cancer. Cancer Treat Rep 62: 1281–1286
9. Allegra JC, Barlock A, Huff KK, Lippman ME (1979) Changes in multiple or sequential estrogen receptor (ER) determinations in breast cancer. Proc Am Assoc Cancer Res Proc Am Soc Clin Oncol 20: 321
10. Altman SJ, Metter GE, Nealon TF, Weiss AJ, Ramirez G, Madden RE, Fletcher WS, Strawith JG, Multhauf PM (1978) Yoshi 864 (1-propanol, 3,3^1-imindoi-, dimethanesul-

fonate [ester], hydrochloride): A phase II study in solid tumors. Cancer Treat Rep 62: 389–395

11. American Medical Association Council on Drugs (1960) Androgens and estrogens in the treatment of disseminated mammary carcinoma. Retrospective study of nine hundred forty-four patients. JAMA 172: 1271–1283

12. Andrews NC, Weiss AJ, Wilson WL, Nealon T (1974) Phase II study of dibromidulcital (NSC 104800). Cancer Chemother Rep 58: 653–660

13. Ansfield FJ, Ramirez G, Mackman S, Bryan GT, Curreri AR (1969) A ten year study of 5-FU in disseminated breast cancer with clinical results and survival times. Cancer Res 29: 1062–1066

14. Ansfield FJ, Klotz J, Nealon T, Ramirez G, Minton J, Hill G, Wilson W, Davis HL, Cornell G (1977) A phase III study comparing the clinical utility of four regimens of 5-fluorouracil. A preliminary report. Cancer 39: 34–40

15. Ansfield FJ, Kallas G, Singson J, Uy B (1979) Phase I–II clinical studies with IV and oral ftorafur-A preliminary report. Proc Am Assoc Cancer Res Proc Am Soc Clin Oncol 20: 349

16. Baker LH, Vaughin CB, Al-Sarraf M, Reed ML, Vaitkevicius VK (1974) Evaluation of combination vs sequential cytotoxic chemotherapy in the treatment of advanced breast cancer. Cancer 33: 513–518

17. Band PR, Canellos GP, Sears M, Isreal L, Pocock SJ (1977) Phase II trial with bleomycin, CCNU and streptozotocin in patients with metastatic cancer of the breast. Cancer Treat Rep 61: 325–328

18. Band PR, Tormey DC, Bauer M (1977) for the ECOG, Induction chemotherapy and maintenance chemo-hormonotherapy in metastatic breast cancer. Proc Am Assoc Cancer Res 18: 228

19. Bennett JM, Frank J, Sears M, Lagakos SW, Horton J, Colsky J, Hall TC (1978) A phase II study of phenestrin (NSC 104469). Med Pediatr Oncol 4: 241–246

20. Blum RM, Kahlert T (1978) Maytansine: A phase I study of an ANSA macrolide with antitumor activity. Cancer Treat Rep 62: 435–438

21. Blumenschein GR, Buzdar AV, Hortobagyi GN, Tashima CK (1979) Update on the adjuvant chemoimmunotherapy of stage IV NED breast cancer. Proc Am Assoc Cancer Res Proc Am Soc Clin Oncol 20: 368

22. Bonnadonna G, Valagussa P, Rossi A, Zucali R, Tancini G, Bajetta E, Brambilla C, de Lena M, di Fronzo G, Banfi A, Rilke F, Veronesi U (1978) Are surgical adjuvant trials altering the course of breast cancer? Semin Oncol 5: 450–464

23. Bonnadonna G, di Fronzo G, Tancini G (1979) Estrogen receptors and response to chemotherapy in advanced and early breast cancer. Proc Am Assoc Cancer Res Proc Am Soc Clin Oncol 20: 359

24. Brambilla C, Valagussa P, Bonnadonne G (1978) Sequential combination chemotherapy in advanced breast cancer. Cancer Chemother Pharmacol 1: 35–39

25. Brunner KW, Sonntag RW, Alberto P, Senn HJ, Martz G, Obrecht P, Maurice P (1977) Combined chemo and hormonal therapy in advanced breast cancer. Cancer 39: 2923–2933

26. Bull JM, Tormey DC, Li SH, Carbone PP, Falkson G, Blom J, Perlin E, Simon R (1978) A randomized comparative trial of adriamycin versus methotrexate in combination drug therapy. Cancer 41: 1649–1657

27. Buzdar AV, Legha SS, Tashima CK, Yap HY, Hortobagyi GW, Hersh EM, Blumenschein GR, Bodey GP (1979) Ifosfamide versus cyclophosphamide in combination drug therapy for metastatic breast cancer. Cancer Treat Rep 63: 115–120

28. Cabanillas F, Rodriguez V, Hall SW, Burgess MA, Bodey GP, Freireich EJ (1978) Phase I study of maytansine using a 3 day schedule. Cancer Treat Rep 62: 425–433

29. Canellos GP, Pocock SJ, Taylor SG, Sears ME, Klassen DJ, Band PR (1976) Combination chemotherapy for metastatic breast carcinoma: prospective comparison of multiple drug therapy with L-phenylalamine mustard. Cancer 38: 1882–1886

30. Carter SK (1972) Single and combination nonhormonal chemotherapy in breast cancer. Cancer 30: 1543−1555

31. Chlebowski R, Smalley R, Weiner J, Irwin L, Bartolucci A, Bateman J (1979) Combination (COMB) vs sequential single agent (SEQ) chemotherapy in advanced breast cancer: relationship between survival and metastatic site. Proc Am Assoc Cancer Res Proc Am Soc Clin Oncol 20: 436

32. Cocconi G, de Lisi V, Boni C, Amadori D, Poletti T, Bertusi M (1979) Chemotherapy (CMF) vs combination of hormonal and chemotherapy (CMF plus tamoxifen) in metastatic breast cancer. Proc Am Assoc Cancer Res Proc Soc Clin Oncol 20: 302

33. Cooperative Breast Cancer Group (1964) Testosterone propionate therapy in breast cancer. JAMA 188: 1069−1972

34. Deleted in production

35. Cooper RG (1969) Combination chemotherapy in hormone resistant breast cancer. Proc Am Assoc Cancer Res 10: 15

36. Cutler SJ, Asire AJ, Taylor SG III (1969) Classification of patients with disseminated cancer of the breast. Cancer 24: 861−869

37. Decker DA, Ahmann DL, Bisel HF, Edmonson JH, Hahn RG, O'Fallon JR (1979) Characterization and analysis of complete regressions to chemotherapy in metastatic breast cancer. Proc Am Assoc Cancer Res Proc Soc Clin Oncol 20: 241

38. Denefrio JM, Vogel CL (1978) Phase II study of hexamethylmelamine in women with advanced breast cancer refractory to standard cytotoxic therapy. Cancer Treat Rep 62: 173−175

39. Falkson G (1972) An annotation on the treatment of disseminated breast cancer in premenopausal women. S Afr J Surg 10: 41−44

40. Falkson G, Falkson HC (1976) Further experience with isophosphimide. Cancer Treat Rep 60: 955−957

41. Falkson G, Falkson HC, Leone L, Glidewell O, Weinberg V, Holland JF (1978) Improved remission rates and duration in premenopausal women with metastatic breast cancer. A cancer and leukemia group B study. Proc Am Assoc Cancer Res 19: 416

42. Falkson HC, Falkson G (1976) Phase II trial of cytembena in patients with advanced ovarian and breast cancer. Cancer Treat Rep 60: 1655−1658

43. Eagen RT, Ahmann DL, Edmonson JH, Hahn RG, Bisel HF (1975) Controlled evaluation of the combination of adriamycin (NSC 123127) vincristine (NSC 675514) and methotrexate (NSC 740) in patients with disseminated breast cancer. Cancer Chemother Rep (Part 3) 6: 339−342

44. Escher GC, Kaufman RJ (1963) Advanced breast carcinoma-factors influencing survival. Acta UICC 19: 1039−1043

45. Glick J, Creech R, Holroyde C, Karpf M, Torri S, Varano M (1978) Tamoxifen (TAM) plus CMF for metastatic breast cancer. Prc Am Assoc Cancer Res 19: 354

46. Gorski J, Toft DO, Skymala G, Smith D, Notides A (1968) Hormone receptors: studies on the interaction of estrogen with the uterus. Recent Prog Horm Res 24: 45−80

47. Greenspan EM (1966) Combination cytotoxic chemotherapy in advanced disseminated breast carcinoma. J M Sinai Hosp NY 33: 1−27

48. Groupe Europeen du Cancer du Sein (1969) Essai clinique du phenol bis (2-chloro-ethyl)carbamate d'oestradiol daus le cancer mammaire en phase avancee. Eur J Cancer 5: 1

49. Hakes TB, Wittes JT, Wittes RE, Knapper WH (1979) Cis-diaminedichloroplatinum II (DDP) in breast cancer − high versus low dose. Proc Am Assoc Cancer Res Proc Am Soc Clin Oncol 20: 304

50. Hortobagyi GN, Gutterman JU, Blumenschein GR, Buzdar A, Burgess MA, Richman SP, Tashima CK, Schwaz M, Hersh EM (1978) Chemoimmunotherapy of advanced breast cancer with BCG. In: Terry WD, Windhorst D (eds) Immunotherapy of cancer: present status of trials in man. Raven Press, New York, pp 655−663

51. Henderson IC, Canellas GP, Blum RH, Skarin AT, Mayer RJ, Parker LM, Frei E III (1979) Prolonged disease free survival in advanced breast cancer (BC) treated with "super CMF"-adriamycin: an alternating regimen employing high dose methrotrexate (*M*) with citrovorum (CF) rescue. Proc Am Assoc Cancer Res Proc Am Soc Clin Oncol 20:327
52. Heuson JC (1976) Current overview of EORTA clinical trials with tamoxifen. Cancer Treat Rep 60:1463–1466
53. Heuson JC, Longeval E, Mattheiem WH, Deboel MC, Sylvester RJ, Leclercq G (1979) Significance of quantitative assessment of estrogen receptors for endocrine therapy in advanced breast cancer. Cancer 39:1971–1977
54. Hoogstraten B, George SL, Samal B, Rivkin SE, Costanzi JJ, Bonnet JF, Thigpen T, Braine H (1976) Combination chemotherapy and adriamycin in patients with advanced breast cancer. A Southwest Oncology Group Study. Cancer 38:13–20
55. Hoogstraten B, O'Bryan R, Jones S (1978) 1,2:5,6-dianhydrogalactitol in advanced breast cancer. Cancer Treat Rep 62:841–842
56. Ingle JN, Ahmann DL, Bisel HF, Rubin J, Kvols LK (1979) Randomized phase II trial of rubidazone (RUBI) and adriamycin (ADR) in women with advanced breast cancer. Proc Am Assoc Cancer Res Proc Am Soc Clin Oncol 20:427
57. Isacoff WH, Eilber F, Tabbarah H, Klein P, Dollinger M, Lemkin S, Sheeley P, Cone L, Rosenbloom B, Sieger L, Block JB (1978) Phase II clinical trial with high-dose methotrexate therapy and citrovorum factor rescue. Cancer Treat Rep 62:1295–1304
58. Jensen EV, Jacobson HI (1960) Fate of steroid estrogens in target tissues. In: Pincus G, Vollmer EP (eds) Biological activities of steroids in relation to cancer. New York, Academic Press, pp 161–178
59. Kiang DT, Frenning DH, Goldman AI, Ascensao VF, Kennedy BJ (1978) Estrogen receptors and responses to chemotherapy and hormonal therapy in advanced breast cancer. N Engl J Med 299:1330–1334
60. Leite C (1978) Hexamethylmelamine (HEX) with or without pyridoxine (PYR) in refactory breast cancer. Proc Am Assoc Cancer Res Proc Am Soc Clin Oncol 19:392
61. Legha SS, Benjamin RS, Buzdar AV, Hortobagyi GN, Blumenschein GR (1979) Rubidazone in metastatic breast cancer. Cancer Treat Rep 63:135–136
62. Legha SS, Bodey GP, Keating MJ, Blumenschein GR, Hortobagyi GN, Buzdar AV, McCredie K, Freireich EJ (1979) Early clinical evaluation of acridnylamino-methane-sulfon-m anisidide (AMSA) in patients with advanced breast cancer and acute leukemia. Proc Am Assoc Cancer Res Proc Am Soc Clin Oncol 20:416
63. Lippman ME, Allegra JC, Thompson EB, Simon R, Barlock A, Green L, Huff KK, Do HMT, Aitken SC, Warren R (1978) The relation between estrogen receptors and response rate to cytotoxic chemotherapy in metastatic breast cancer. N Engl J Med 298:1223–1228
64. Lloyd RE, Jones SE, Salmon SE (1979) Comparative trial of low-dose adriamycin plus cyclophosphamide with or without additive hormonal therapy in advanced breast cancer. Cancer 40:60–65
65. Longacre D, Donavan M, Paladine W, Cunningham T, Sponzo R (1977) Hexamethyl-melamine, vincristine and methotrexate chemotherapy in advanced neoplasms. Cancer Treat Rep 61:919–922
66. Marcus F, Friedmann MA, Hammers R, Phillips T, Resser K (1979) 5FU + oncovin + adriamycin + mitomycin C (FOAM): An effective new therapy for metastatic breast cancer patients – even those who have failed CMF. Proc Am Assoc Cancer Res Proc Am Soc Clin Oncol 20:306
67. McGuire WL, Carbone PP, Sears ME, Escher GE (1975) Estrogen receptors in human breast cancer: An overview. In: McGuire WL, Carbone PP, Vollmer EP (eds) Estrogen receptors in human breast cancer. Raven Press, New York, pp 1–7

68. McGuire WL (1978) Hormone receptors: Their role in predicting prognosis and response to endocrine therapy. Semin Oncol 5: 428–433

69. Morgan LR, Posey LE, Krementz ET, Hawley W, Beasley RW (1977) Tamoxifen plus CMF for advanced breast cancer. Proc Am Assoc Cancer Res 18: 308

70. Mouridsen HT, Palshof T, Brahm M, Rahbek I (1977) Evaluation of single-drug versus multiple-drug chemotherapy in the treatment of advanced breast cancer. Cancer Treat Rep 61: 47–50

71. Muggia FM, Lippman M, Heuson JC (1978) Reports from the workshop on the use of steroids as carriers of cytotoxic agents in breast cancer. Cancer Treat Rep 62: 1239–1268

72. Muss HB, White DR, Richards F II, Cooper MR, Stuart JJ, Jackson DV, Rhyne L, Spurr CL (1978) Adriamycin versus methotrexate in five drug combination chemotherapy for advanced breast cancer: A randomized trial. Cancer 42: 2141–2148

73. Nemoto T, Rosner D, Diaz R, Dao T, Sponzo R, Cunningham T, Horton J, Simon R (1978) Combination chemotherapy for metastatic breast cancer. Comparison of multiple drug therapy with 5-fluorouracil, cytoxan and prednisone with adriamycin or adrenalectomy. Cancer 41: 2073–2077

74. Nichols WC, Kvols LK, Ingle JN, Edmonson JH, Ahmann DL, Rubin J, O'Connell MJ (1978) Phase II study of triazinate and pyrayofurin in patients with advanced breast cancer previously exposed to cytotoxic chemotherapy. Cancer Treat Rep 62: 837–839

75. Norton L, Simon R (1977) Tumor size, sensitivity to therapy and design of treatment schedules. Cancer Treat Rep 61: 1307–1317

76. I'Bryan RM, Baker LJ, Gottlieb JE, Rivikin SE, Balcerzak SP, Grumet GN, Salmon SE, Moon TE, Hoogstraten B (1977) Dose response evaluation of adriamycin in human neoplasia. Cancer 39: 1490–1498

77. O'Bryan RM, Baker L, Whitecar J, Salmon S, Vaughn C, Hoogstraten B (1978) Cyclocytidine in breast cancer. Cancer Treat Rep 62: 455–456

78. Palmer RL, Samal BA, Vaughn CB, Tranum BL (1977) Phase II evaluation of piperazinedione in metastatic breast carcinoma. Cancer Treat Rep 61: 1711–1712

79. Perloff M, Norton L, Holland JF (1979) Treatment of advanced breast cancer with a novel cyclophosphamide (C), methotrexate (M), 5-fluorouracil (F), vincristine (V), and prednisone (P) regimen. Proc Am Assoc Cancer Res Proc Am Soc Clin Oncol 20: 343

80. Priestman T, Baum M, Jones V, Forbes J (1977) Comparative trial of endocrine versus cytotoxic treatment in advanced breast cancer. Br Med J 1: 1248–1250

81. Quagliana JM, O'Bryan RM, Baker L, Gottlieb J, Morrison F, Eyre HJ, Tucker WG, Costanzi J (1977) Phase II study of 5-azacytidine in solid tumors. Cancer Treat Rep 61: 51–54

82. Ramirez G, Klotz J, Strawitz JG, Wilson WL, Cornell GN, Madden RE, Minton JP, Central Oncology Group (1975) Combination chemotherapy in breast cancer: A randomized study of 4 versus 5 drugs. Oncology 23: 101–108

83. Rosner R, Nemoto T (1979) An alternate strategy for combination chemotherapy of metastatic breast cancer. Proc Am Assoc Cancer Res Proc Am Soc Clin Oncol 20: 310

84. Rozencweig M, Heuson JC (1975) Breast cancer: Prognostic factors and clinical evaluation. In: Staquet MJ (ed) Cancer therapy. Prognostic factors and criteria of response. Raven Press, New York, pp 139–183

85. Rozencweig M, von Hoff DD, Henney JE, Muggia FM (1977) VM 26 + VP 16-213: A comparative analysis. Cancer 40: 334–342

86. Rozencweig M, von Hoff DD, Slavik M, Muggia FM (1977) Cis-diaminedichloroplatinum II – A new anticancer drug. Ann Intern Med 86: 803–812

87. Samal B, Jones S, Brownlee RW, Morrison F, Hoogstraten B, Caoili E, Baker L (1978) Chromomycin A_3 for advanced breast cancer: A Southwest Oncology Group Study. Cancer Treat Rep 62: 19–22

88. Smalley RV, Carpenter J, Bartolucci A, Vogel C, Krauss S (1977) A comparison of cyclophosphamide, adriamycin, 5-fluorouracil, vincristine, prednisone (CMFVP) in patients with metastatic breast cancer. Cancer 40: 625−632
89. Smalley RV, Murphy S, Huguley CM jr, Bartolucci A (1976) Combination versus sequential five-drug chemotherapy in metastatic carcinoma of the breast. Cancer Res 36: 3911−3916
90. Smith IE, Hedley DW, Powles TJ, McElwain TJ (1978) Vindesine: A phase II study in the treatment of breast cancer, malignant melanoma and other tumors. Cancer Treat Rep 62: 1427−1433
91. Stoll BA (1972) Androgen, corticosteroid and progestin therapy. In: Stoll BA (ed) Endocrine therapy in malignant disease. Saunders, London, pp 165−191
92. Stoll BA (1972) Major endocrine ablation and cytotoxic therapy. In: Stoll BA (ed) Endocrine therapy in malignant disease. Saunders, London, pp 193−214
93. Taylor SG II (1962) Endocrine ablation in disseminated mammary carcinoma. Surg Gynecol Obstet 115: 443−448
94. Tormey DC, Carbone PP, Band P (1977) Breast cancer survival in single and combination chemotherapy trials since 1968. Proc Am Assoc Cancer Res 18: 64
95. Tormey DC, Falkson H, Falkson G, Davis TE (1978) Evaluation of chemotherapy and tamoxifen in breast cancer. Proc Am Assoc Cancer Res 19: 34
96. Tormey DC, Falkson G, Perlin E, Bull J, Blom J, Lippman ME (1976) Evaluation of an intermittent schedule of dibromodulcitol in breast cancer. Cancer Treat Rep 60: 1593−1596
97. Tormey DC, Gelman R, Band P, Falkson G (1979) Impact of chemohormonal therapy upon maintenance in advanced breast cancer. Proc Am Assoc Cancer Res Proc Am Soc Clin Oncol 20: 356
98. Tormey DC, Neifeld JP (1977) Chemotherapeutic approaches to disseminated disease. In: Stoll BA (ed) Breast cancer management − early and late. Heinemann, London, pp 117−131
99. Tisman G, Isacoff WH, Drakes T (1979) Salvage of breast cancer adjuvant treatment failures with high dose methotrexate and 5FU. Proc Am Assoc Cancer Res Proc Am Soc Clin Oncol 20: 140
100. Tranum B, Hoogstraten B, Kennedy A, Vaughn A, Samal B, Thigpen T, Rivkin S, Smith F, Palmer RL, Costanzi J, Tucker W, Wilson H, Maloney TR (1978) Adriamycin in combination for the treatment of breast cancer. Cancer 41: 2078−2083
101. Weiss AJ, Metter GE, Nealon TF, Keenan JP, Ramirez G, Swaminathan A, Fletcher WS, Moss SE, Manthai RW (1977) Phase II study of 5-azacytidine in solid tumors. Cancer Treat Rep 61: 55−58
102. Wilson WL, Bisel HF, Cole D, Rochlin DB, Ramirez G, Madden RE (1970) Prolonged low dose administration of hexamethylmelamine (NSC 13875). Cancer 25: 568−570
103. Yap HY, Benjamin RS, Blumenschein GR, Hortobagyi GN, Taskima CK, Buzdar AU, Bodey GP (1979) Phase II study with sequential L-asparaginase and methotrexate in advanced refractory breast cancer. Cancer Treat Rep 63: 77−83
104. Yap HY, Blumenschein GR, Hortobagyi GN, Tashima CK, Loo TL (1979) Continuous 5-day infusion vinblastine (VLB) in the treatment of refractory advanced breast cancer. Proc Am Assoc Cancer Res Proc Am Soc Clin Oncol 20: 334

Recent Advances in Chemotherapy for Advanced Breast Cancer

T. Wada, H. Koyama, and T. Terasawa

Department of Surgery, The Center for Adult Diseases, Osaka 1-3-3., Nakamichi, Higashinariku, J − Osaka 537

Abstract

Current status of chemotherapy for advanced breast cancer in Japan was reviewed with special reference to some recent studies of special interest. As for single drug chemotherapy, cyclophosphamide (CTX) and 5-fluorouracil (5-FU) were used most commonly. Ftorafur, (N_1-[2′-tetrahydrofuryl]-5-fluorouracil), a cytotoxic agent which was under clinical trial until recently, showed more favorable results than these conventional agents, averaging a 36% response rate and 5.7 months duration of response, an. Tamoxifen, a new antiestrogenic agent, also showed encouraging results with a 36% response rate and 9.7 months duration of response. As for combination chemotherapy, higher response rates were observed in regimens including CTX, 5-FU, and adriamycin (ADR): 50% in a combination of CTX and 5-FU, 70% in a combination of CTX, 5-FU, ADR and methotrexate (MTX). Intra-arterial infusion chemotherapy produced prominent effects in locoregional lesions with a response rate of 82%. It is useful as a preoperative procedure for locally advanced breast cancer.

Introduction

The incidence of breast cancer in Japan had been one of the lowest in the world. Japanese women with breast cancer had shown better prognosis [12] than the patients in European and American countries where the incidence of this cancer is high. As the Japanese have become used to the westernized mode of life, however, the recent incidence of breast cancer has increased rapidly. This phenomenon suggests the possibility of higher malignancy and more frequent dissemination of breast cancer than before. On the basis of these circumstances, chemotherapy as a systemic treatment for breast cancer has come to be considered of importance.

Chemotherapy was performed for inoperable advanced breast cancer with a single agent before, but in recent years multiple-drug treatments are being attempted. With both treatments, better clinical results have been obtained in breast cancer than in other solid tumors. Furthermore, chemotherapy as a part of a multidisciplinary treatment has been performed in conjunction with other treatments, such as surgery and endocrine therapy. One of the examples of the multidisciplinary treatment is

Table 1. Effect of chemotherapeutic agents on advanced breast cancer

Agents	No. patients	No. responders (%)	Source
CTX	213	75[a] (35)	Jap. Soc. for Breast Cancer [6]
5-FU	87	29[a] (33)	Jap. Soc. for Breast Cancer [6]
MMC	69	17[a] (25)	Jap. Soc. for Breast Cancer [6]
FT	40	18[a] (45)	Jap. Soc. for Breast Cancer [6]
ADR	35	10[a] (29)	Jap. Soc. for Breast Cancer [6]
ACM	39	8[b] (21)	OKA, S. [13]

ACM, Aclacinomycin A; ADR, Adriamycin; CTX, Cyclophosphamide; 5-FU, 5-Fluorouracil; FT, Ftorafur; MMC, Mitomycin C
[a] Criteria of Japan Society for Cancer Therapy
[b] Criteria of Karnosfky

surgical adjuvant chemotherapy, which has been demonstrated to be definitely effective in several controlled studies.

This report describes the current status of chemotherapy for advanced breast cancer in Japan, and presents three points that are recently drawing attention in this field, i.e., efficacy of tetrahydrofuryl fluorouracil (FT), tamoxifen, and intra-arterial infusion chemotherapy for the management of patients with advanced breast cancer.

Single Drug Chemotherapy

Table 1 summarizes the clinical results of single drug chemotherapy in the 88 institutions compiled by the Japan Society for Breast Cancer [6] in 1977, and also the data from several publications (Kubol K, personal communication) [4, 13, 14].

Thirty-five per cent of patients responded to CTX which was most frequently used for breast cancer chemotherapy and was administered orally daily. 5-Fluorouracil (5-FU) and mitomycin C (MMC) ranked second in terms of clinical use and were given intravenously, continuously, or intermittently: 33% and 25% of patients responded to these drugs, respectively.

The response rate to FT was 45% and demonstrated the highes effectiveness. Although the series of these patients in this study are still small, FT is getting to be one of the most popular chemotherapeutic agents in the treatment of advanced breast cancer.

Adriamycin (ADR), which is an anthracycline antibiotic, showed response in 29% of patients. Aclacinomycin A (ACM), another anthracycline derivative under phase I and II studies, showed response in 21%. At present, many institutions are conducting clinical trials with both agents in Japan.

Combination Chemotherapy

Response rates by combination chemotherapy are shown in Table 2. Experience in multiple-drug treatments for advanced breast cancer is still in an early stage. There are few established regimens for multiple-drug treatments, and most investigators treat

Table 2. Effect of combination chemotherapy or advanced breast cancer

Regimens	No. patients	No. responders (%)	Source
MMC + CTX	26	19[a] (35)	Sakai, K [14]
5-FU + CTX	36	18[b] (50)	Jap. Soc. for Breast Cancer [6]
MMC + 5-FU	16	2[b] (13)	Jap. Soc. for Breast Cancer [6]
MMC + 5-FU + CTX	47	13[b] (28)	Jap. Soc. for Breast Cancer [6]
MFC	43	12[b] (28)	Jap. Soc. for Breast Cancer [6]
FAMT	25	9[b] (36)	Jap. Soc. for Breast Cancer [6]
CAMF	30	21[a] (70)	Kubo, K. [10]
VEMFAH	6	6[a] (100)	Hoshino, A. [4]

CTX, Cyclophospamide; 5-Fu, 5-fluorouracil; MMC, Mitomycin C; MFC, MMC + 5-FU + Cytosine Arabinoside; FAMT, 5-FU + CTX + MMC + Chromomycin A 3; CAMF, CTX + Adriamycin + Methotrexate + 5-FU; VEMFAH, Vincristine + CTX + Methotrexate + 5-FU + Adriamycin + Prednisone
[a] UICC, Criteria
[b] Criteria of Japan Society for Cancer Therapy

patients with their own individual combination and dosage schedule. Table 2 lists the combinations of drugs regardless of the dosage schedule.

The response rate in a combination of CTX and 5-FU was 50%. It is a considerable improvement of effectiveness as compared with the rates when CTS and 5-FU are given singely (35% and 33%, respectively, in Table 1).

Two of the established regimens in combination chemotherapy are MFC (MMC 4 mg + 5-FU 500 mg + cytosine arabinoside 40 mg/50 kg IV once or twice weekly) and FAMT (5-FU 500 mg + CTX 200 mg + MMC 2 mg + chromomycin A_3 0.5 mg/50 kg IV once or twice weekly), and their response rates have been 28% and 36%, respectively. The other popular regimen is a combination of MMC, 5-FU, and CTX. The response rate, however, was only 13%. Kubo (personal communication) reported recently that CAMF (CTX + ADR + methotrexate + 5-FU) produced response in as many as 70% of the patients in his personal series. Hoshino et al. [4] reported that six patients in his series all responded favorably to six-drug treatment (VEMFAH). According to the data in Table 2, regimens containing CTX, 5-FU, and ADR were highly effective, but those with MMC were not as highly effective.

Some Recent Studies of Special Interest

Some comments will be made concering those agents and their method of administration which have been coming into notice recently.

Ftorafur (N_1-[2'-tetrahydrofuryl]-5-fluorouracil) − FT

This chemotherapeutic agent is a masked compound, and is inactive in vitro. It is converted to 5-FU and other active substances in the liver. Since the cytotoxic action of

Table 3. Effect of ftorafur, cumulative data from 24 Japanese reports

Route of administration	Cumulative number of patients	Responders (%)	Daily dose	Interval to onset of response (weeks)	Duration of response (months)	Leukopenia (< 3,000) (%)	Thrombo-cytopenia (< 70,000) (%)
Oral	120	37	400~1200 mg	4.5[a]	4.7	3.3	4.0
Suppository	44	39	1~2 g	3.1	6.2	6.8	4.0
Intravenous	26	27	800 mg	3.6	–	4.0	0
Total	190	36		3.5	5.7		

[a] Based on the evaluable data in 9, 20, and 6 patients, respectively; Criteria see text

this agent is time-dependent, Kimura [8] tried to administer it orally to patients and Konda [7] intrarectally. Their results indicated that 5-FU or other active metabolites were identified rapidly in the blood after oral or intrarectal as well as intravenous administration of FT. The blood level of these metabolites remained high for a longer time than in intravenous administration. For this reason, clinical experiences with intermittently intravenous massive dose administration of FT have been few and consecutive oral or intrarectal use has been predominant in Japan.

Table 3 summarizes the cumulative efficacy of FT in patients with breast cancer reported in 24 references. Because of different evaluation criteria for efficacy in each report, in Table 3 the clinical results corresponding to complete or partial responses of the UICC criteria are regarded as responders. Overall response was 36%. In terms of response rate, oral and intrarectal administration exhibited better results than by intravenous administration. After initiation of intrarectal administration, patients responded more rapidly and longer than by other routes. When FT was given intrarectally to patients, the dose of this agent was greater than that by other routes. This is supposed to have led to better results by this route.

FT produced mild gastrointestinal troubles such as nausea and anorexia in 40% of patients. But leukopenia and thrombocytopenia were observed in only 3%−7%.

The effect of FT in patients having prior therapy with other agents is whown in Table 4 [5, 7]. FT was revealed to be considerably effective in patients who had been resistant to other therapy.

Tamoxifen

Since 1976 clinical trials with an antiestrogenic agent, tamoxifen, have been conducted. Table 5 pools the recent results of its use as reported by four authors [3, 15, 17, 19]. Tamoxifen was effective in 26%−36% of patients and was also characterized by its considerably prolonged effect, as long as 6.6−13.8 months.

The Hanshin Breast Cancer Research Group [3] showed that 42% of postmenopausal patients responded to tamoxifen as compared with 18% of premenopausal patients. There was significant difference ($p < 0.05$) between both groups in efficacy. In our personal series [17], 62% of patients whose tumors were estrogen receptor positive responded to it as compared with only 7% of patients with estrogen receptor negative tumors, and a significant difference ($p < 0.05$) between both groups in response rate was observed.

Table 4. Effect of ftorafur (oral) and prior therapy

	Prior therapy		Source
	No	yes	
Response rate	6/12	11/32	Konda, C. et al. [7]
	4/10	5/9	Ishida, T. et al. [5]
Total	10/22	16/41	
	(48%)	(39%)	

Table 5. Effect of tamoxifen

No. patients	No. responders (%)	Daily dose	Interval to onset of response (weeks)	Duration of response (months)	Source
72	25[a] (35)	20~40 mg	9.4	9.7	Hanshin Breast Cancer Research Group [3]
42	12[a] (29)	20~40 mg	7.8	13.8	Wada, T. et al. [17]
42	15[b] (36)	20~40 mg	6.8	9.3	Yoshida, M. [19]
23	6[a] (26)	20 mg	–	6.6	Tanaka, M. et al. [15]

[a] UICC criteria
[b] Author's criteria

Ten per cent of patients treated with tamoxifen showed slight gastrointestinal troubles; however, it did not produce marrow depression, hepatic damage, renal failure, or hypercalcemia. Thirteen per cent of premenopausal patients manifested amenorrhea after treatment with tamoxifen.

Since tamoxifen produces slight side effects, shows an effect for a long time, and can be administered orally to outpatients, this agent will presumably play an important role in the treatment of breast cancer.

Intra-arterial Infusion Chemotherapy

Since the middle of 1960s, intra-arterial infusion chemotherapy has been performed for patients with locally advanced breast cancer. Since then, after various modifications [9], the method has been adopted by many institutions. The data pooled by the Japan Society for Breast Cancer [6] in 1977 showed that this method was effective in 17 (59%) of 29 patients. MMC, 5-FU, ADR, MMC + 5-FU, and ADR + 5-FU were used. Among these agents ADR + 5-FU showed the highest response of 80% [8, 10], and MMC + 5-FU, the next highest of 58% [7, 12].

Infusion chemotherapy in our institution [16] consists of continuous infusion of 5-FU and intermittent infusion of MMC via canulation to the internal mammary artery and subclavian artery fo 2−4 weeks. This infusion chemotherapy reduces not only tumor size but metastatic foci in axillary, parasternal, and supraclavicular lymph nodes. Consequently, this treatment is useful for preoperative local management prior to radical mastectomy for locally advanced breast cancer such as T_3N_{2-3}, T_4N_{2-3} without distant metastases.

We treated 33 patients with locally advanced breast cancer with this method. Table 6 shows the effect of this treatment according to agents. We confirmed a response rate of 82% with a combination of continuous infusion of 5-FU and intermittent MMC. Recently attempts were made to administer an anthracycline antibiotic, adriamycin, or aclacinomycin A intermittently. The former was found to be satisfactorily effective, whereas the latter showed only a slight effect. Before or after infusion chemotherapy, patients underwent surgical ablation, radical mastectomy, and adjuvant chemotherapy. Five-year survival was 62% for patients receiving this multidisciplinary treatment. The five-year survival is calculated to be 35% for these patients, if they had received conventional treatment instead of intra-arterial infusion chemotherapy. This estimation is based on the 5-year survival data by the breast cancer survey of UICC. This indicates that intra-arterial infusion chemotherapy was successful not only for local management but also for improvement of survival in locally advanced breast cancer.

Table 6. Effect of intra-arterial infusion chemotherapy for locally advanced breast cancer

Agents	No. patients	Clinical response[a]				Total dose (average)
		CR	PR	NC	PD	
Mitomycin C +	28	5	18	5	0	51 mg
5-fluorouracil	(100%)	(18%)	(64%)	(18%)		6.5 g
Adriamycin	2	1	1	0	0	145 mg
Aclacinomycin A	3	0	0	3	0	335 mg

[a] UICC criteria

Discussion

Mutliple-drug treatment and massive dose administration of anticancer drugs are the most acceptable methods to enhance the effects of chemotherapy. Carter [2] and Carbone [1] suggest that combination chemotherapy consisting of two and more anticancer drugs which show different modes of action is preferable in obtaining better clinical results. There are probably no clinical views which are opposed to the iea that combination chemotherapy with confirmed anticancer drugs will be predominant in the future treatment of breast cancer. Before the choice of drugs and dosage, however, we must take into consideration the peculiarities of Japanese patients whith breast cancer. Nemoto et al. [12] pointed out that the incidence of breast cancer in Japan was lower than that in the United States and the prognosis of the former was better than that of the latter. Japanese weigh less than the Europeans and Americans. The former are considered to tolerate these drugs poorly, because dose of chemotherapeutic agents described in reports from western countries leads frequently to overdose even when calculated per square meter. Consequently, it should be cautioned that aggressive chemotherapy produces serious toxicity in Japanese patients. Favorable effectiveness and mild toxicity have been obtained by single drug chemotherapy which has been performed to date. Therefore, single agent treatment for a prolonged period should be given sonsideration was well as multiple-agent combination chemotherapy.

FT, a masked compound of 5-FU, can be administered orally or intrarectally to patients. It is easy to use, has only slight toxicity and produces results comparable to other active agents. Nakano et al. [11] reported that FT suppository administration to patients with gastric, colo-rectal, and breast cancers showed response rate of 30%, 19%, and 33% respectively. It thus showed good effect with slight toxicity. It has not been reported to date that FT induces any secondary cancer, like leukemia, which alkylating agents occasionally do. Therefore, patients will be able to complete FT therapy for a prolonged period. FT is expected to have utility value in the field of long-term adjuvant chemotherapy.

Tamoxifen showed from 26% to 36% in response rate. This meant that tamoxifen showed effect equal to other anticancer agents, for example, 20% for testosterone propionate, 40% for fluoxymesterone. Tamoxifen has the advantages of few side effects and prolonged duration of response. Tamoxifen was more effective in postmenopausal patients than in premenopausal patients in Japanese series, as was also reported by Ward [18] for western series.

Intra-arterial infusion chemotherapy allows administration of a far higher concentration of anticancer agents to the local lesion than systemic chemotherapy. When locoregional lesions are inoperable because of their extensiveness, systemic chemotherapy is inadequate and the addition of local intra-arterial chemotherapy is indicated. As Japanese patients with breast cancer characteristically show less dissemination in spite of the extensive locoregional foci, or else show a slow rate of progress of the disseminated lesions, intra-arterial chemotherapy would be often effective. Another significance of this treatment is that it may be used also as a screening test for the cytotoxic effects of compounds. A more suitable choice of anticancer drugs and dosage in this method might produce better clinical results. In cancer therapy the combination of better management of local tumor foci and systemic treatments is considered of utmost importance.

References

1. Carbone PP (1977) Chemotherapy of disseminated breast cancer. Cancer 39: 2916–2922
2. Carter SK (1976) Integration of chemotherapy into combined modality treatment of solid tumor. VII. Adenocarcinoma of the breast. Cancer Treat Rev 3: 141–174
3. Hanshin Breast Cancer Research Group (1980) Evaluation of tamoxifen for advanced and metastatic breast cancer. Clin Endocrinol 28: 425–436
4. Hoshino A, Nagura E, Osugi J (1978) Effect of multiple combination chemotherapy with vincristine, endoxan, methotrexate, 5-fluorouracil, adriamycin and prednisolone (VEMFAH) for advanced breast cancer. Cancer Chemother 5: 215–222
5. Ishida T (1975) Clincial studies on oral administration of N_1-[2′-tetrahydrofuryl]-5-fluoro-uracil for recurrent breast cancer. Cancer Chemother 1: 999–1003
6. Japan Society for Breast Cancer (1978) Chemotherapy for advanced and metastatic breast cancer. J Jpn Soc Cancer Ther 13: 103–108
7. Konda C (1975) Studies on oral and rectal use of N_1-[2′-tetrahydrofuryl]-5-fluorouracil in cancer chemotherapy. IRYO 29: 612–621
8. Konda C, Kuamoka S, Kimura K (1973) Chemotherapy of cancer with oral administration of N_1-[2′-furanidyl]-5-fluorouracil (FT-207). Jpn J Cancer Clin 19: 495–499
9. Koyama H, Wada T, Takahashi Y, Iwanaga T, Aoki Y, Wada A, Terasawa T, Kosaki G (1975) Intra-arterial infusion chemotherapy as a preoperative treatment of locally advanced breast cancer. Cancer 36: 1603–1612
10. Deleted in production
11. Nakano Y, Taguchi T (1975) Chemotherapy of cancer with suppository administration of FT-207. Cancer Chemother 2: 799–806
12. Nemoto T, Koyama H, Dao T (1977) Difference in breast cancer between Japan and the United States. J Natl Cancer Inst 59: 193–197
13. Oka S (1978) A review of clinical studies on aclacinomycin A − phase I and preliminary phase II evaluation of ACM. Sci Rep Res Inst Tohoku Univ −C 25: 37–49
14. Sakai K (1969) Breast cancer and chemotherapy. Surg Ther 21: 207–212
15. Tanaka M, Abe K, Ohnami S, Adachi I, Yamaguchi K, Miyakawa S (1978) Tamoxifen in advanced breast cancer: response rate, effect of pituitary hormone reserve and binding affinity to estrogen receptor. Jpn J Clin Oncol 8: 141–148
16. Terasawa T, Koyama H (1975) Intra-arterial infusion therapy for breast cancer. Operation 26: 67–71
17. Wada T, Koyama H, Takahashi Y, Nishizawa Y, Iwanaga T, Aoki Y, Terasawa T (to be published) Tamoxifen therapy in locally advanced and recurrent breast cancer. J Jpn Soc Cancer Ther
18. Ward HWC (1975) Antiestrogens in treatment of breast cancer. Br Med J 2: 500
19. Yoshida M (1978) Hormone therapy for breast cancer. Cancer Chemother 5: 69–76

The Current Status of Adjuvant Chemotherapy in Breast Cancer

S. K. Carter

Northern California Cancer Program, P. O. Box 10144, USA – Palo Alto, CA 94303

Breast cancer is in the forefront of the combined modality strategy involving the use of chemotherapy. No matter what effective local control therapy is utilized, metastatic relapse remains the major cause of treatment failure and ultimate demise. The histologic status of axillary lymph nodes is the most potent prognostic variable for this metastatic failure. In women with positive axillary nodes the median time to relapse is 3 years and slightly less than 25% will be disease free at 10 years. This compares to an approximate 75% relapse-free rate for women with negative nodes at 10 years. Where four or more nodes are found to be positive the ten-year relapse rate ranges from 83.6%–86.2%, with total survival being 13.4%–25.6% [11, 18].

Experimentally it has been shown that cytotoxic chemotherapy kills by first order kinetics and that smaller tumor cell burdens are more responsive to drug kill than are larger masses [15]. Chemotherapy, effective against clinically evident metastatic disease, should be even more effective against microscopic foci of tumor cells. Therefore, it is hypothesized that adjuvant drug treatment should be able to sterilize microscopic residual disease and turn what would be a failure with surgery only into a cure with combined modality treatment.

What still remains to be determined is what level of drug activity in advanced disease will predict for the total cell kill theoretically required to achieve cure [8]. What also has not been fully established is the predictability of the transplantable murine tumor models that form the experimental basis of the combined modality strategy.

Two major groups have taken the lead in adjuvant breast cancer trials. These are the National Surgical Adjuvant Breast Project (NSABP) and the Instituto Tumori in Milan (NCI, Milan). Between them they have completed and initiated eight protocols involving long-term use of chemotherapy (Table 1).

In 1972 the National Cancer Institute launched a large-scale controlled trial of the use of chemotherapy as an adjuvant to surgical operation in women in whom cancer had already spread. This study was carried out by NSABP, headed by Dr. Bernard Fisher. Half of the women were given L-phenylalanine mustard (L-PAM) after radical mastectomy and half were given a placebo [10]. Treatment failures occurred in 22% of 108 patients receiving placebo and 9.3% of 103 women given L-PAM. This difference was only statistically significant for premenopausal women and continued follow-up has shown no meaningful difference for women who are postmenopausal.

A follow-up of the NSABP data [9] has shown that at 48 months of follow-up the percentage of treatment failures overall is 48% in 169 placebo and 40% in 179 L-PAM patients with the p value being 0.02 (Table 2).

Table 1. Adjuvant trials of NSABP and NCI, Milan

I. NSABP trials

Pre- and postmenopausal status

1. R ⟨ L-PAM
         Placebo

2. R ⟨ L-PAM
         L-PAM + 5-FU

3. R ⟨ L-PAM + 5-FU
         L-PAM + 5-FU + MTX

4. R ⟨ L-PAM + 5-FU
         L-PAM + 5-FU + tamoxifen

5. R ⟨ L-PAM + 5-FU
         L-PAM + 5-FU + C. parvum

II. NCI, Milan trials

1. Pre- and postmenopausal
    R ⟨ CMF (12 cycles)
         Control

2. Premenopausal
    R ⟨ CMF (12 cycles)
         CMF (6 cycles)

3. Postmenopausal
    R ⟨ CMFP (6 cycles) → Adriamycin + vincristine (4 cycles)
         Same but with escalating doses

Table 2. Data according to menopausal status in NSABP L-PAM trial

Age	No. of patients	% Treatment failure	p
≤ 49 Placebo: L-PAM	60	55.0	0.005
	59	34.0	
≥ 50 Placebo: L-PAM	109	45.0	0.290
	120	43.0	

Table 3. Four year relapse free survival in CMF adjuvant study as of 1. Feb. 1979 [10]. Percentage 4 year relapse free survival

Status	Control	CMF	p Value
All patients	47.3	63.1	0.0001
1 node +	58.0	76.7	0.02
2−3 nodes +	47.3	67.1	0.01
≥ 4 nodes +	35.2	44.8	0.03
Premenopausal			
All patients	43.4	70.0	0.00002
1 node +	52.2	80.9	0.01
2−3 nodes +	49.3	84.2	0.0005
≥ 4 nodes +	26.7	45.4	0.005
Postmenopausal			
All patients	51.7	56.5	0.22
1 node +	63.2	72.0	0.24
2−3 nodes +	45.4	53.0	0.10
≥ 4 nodes +	43.6	46.2	0.23

The only situation in which the L-PAM is statistically significantly superior to placebo is with premenopausal patients with one to three positive nodes. In 31 patients the failure rate is 44% with placebo as opposed to 13% with L-PAM in 32 patients at 4 years ($p = 0.005$).

The first CMF adjuvant study was initiated on 1 June 1973 [2, 3, 5]. Patients with primary tumors staged as $T_{1b}-T_{2b}-T_{3b}$ or T_4 by the UICC TNM international classification were not considered eligible for inclusion in the protocol. Also excluded were those with N_2 or N_3 lesions which meant meant either nodes fixed to one another or to other structures or supraclavicular; infraclavicular nodes, or edema of the arm. After mastectomy randomization was to CMF begun within four weeks of surgery or to no further treatment.

As of 1 February 1979 [4], the clinical benefit in terms of relapse-free survival of adjuvant CMF overall in 207 CMF treated women remains highly significant as compared to the 179 controls ($p = 0.0001$) (Table 3). This benefit is seen exclusively in premenopausal women.

The CMF data are clearly positive in premenopausal women but not of much benefit in postmenopausal patients. When the L-PAM data and the CMF data are put together with earlier single course thio-tepa data of the NSABP [11] (Table 4), an enigma is seen. All are negative in postmenopausal women and a dichotomy exists in premenopausal women. A single course of thio-tepa is of value for the subset of ≥ 4+ nodes but not for the better risk group of 1−3+ nodes. The more aggressive 18 months of L-PAM is of value for the 1−3+ nodes but not for the ≥ 4+ nodes. CMF is effective for both subsets. Since CMF is more effective in advanced disease this is encouraging for advanced disease activity being predictive for adjuvant effect.

As breast cancer is a hormone responsive tumor, hormonal modifications related to drug administration may have therapeutic relevance. Chemotherapy, especially with alkylating agents, is known to produce a high incidence of ovarian failure. The incidence of amenorrhea in premenopausal women given CMF and its relationship with relapse-free survival (RFS) are reported in Table 5. In the course of CMF therapy

Table 4. The enigma of adjuvant chemotherapy results. Statistically significant positive results in critical subsets

Regimen	Follow up	Premenopausal		Postmenopausal	
		1–3 +	> 4	1–3 +	> 4
Thio-tepa One course	> 10 years	No	Yes RFS OS	No	No
L-PAM 18 months	> 4 years	Yes RFS	No	No	No
CMF 12 cycles	> 4 years	Yes RFS OS	Yes RFS OS	No	No

RFS, Relapse-free survival; OS, Overall survival

Table 5. CMF-induced amenorrhea in premenopausal patients. Incidence and relation to relapse-free survival

	Total	≤ 40 years	> 40 years
Incidence of amenorrhea	58/81 (71.6%)	14/33 (42.4%)	44/48 (91.6%)
Reversible amenorrhea	8/58 (13.8%)	6/14 (42.9%)	2/44 (4.5%)
4-year RFS			
With CMF amenorrhea	73.3%	54.7%[a]	80.9%[b]
Without amenorrhea	56.2%	50.7%[a]	75.0%[b]

[a] p, 0.26
[b] p, 0.43

71.6% of menstruating women developed amenorrhea defined as absence of menstrual periods for a minimum of 3 months. This finding was more frequent in the age group older than 40 years (91.6%). Furthermore, in this group CMF-induced amenorrhea was rarely reversible (4.5%). On the contrary, in 42.9% of women 40 years old or younger, normal menstrual function was resumed after temporary amenorrhea. In both age groups, however, the presence or absence of amenorrhea failed to influence significantly the RFS. Furthermore the 4-year RFS was 58.3% for reversible and 76.9% for nonreversible amenorrhea. Also this difference was not statistically significant ($p = 0.28$). Finally, therapeutic ovariectomy was also effective in women relapsing after surgery plus CMF, and this occurred irrespective of CMF-induced amenorrhea [4]. All above-mentioned results seem to exclude that drug-induced ovarian suppression played an essential role in the therapeutic effectiveness of adjuvant CMF.

Myelosuppression was the most common toxic effect of CMF. However, severe myelosuppression associated with infection and hemorrhagic complications never occurred. Gastrointestinal disturbances and stomatitis were mild to moderate in degree. Various degrees of hair loss were fairly common, but complete alopecia was observed in less than 10%.

As far as late toxic signs are concerned, neither chronic organ damage nor increased incidence of second cancers have so far been observed. In particular chronic liver damage secondary to methotrexate administration was not evident. In the first CMF study three women in the control group and four women in the CMF group developed a second solid tumor other than breast carcinoma. No acute leukemia has been observed.

The second CMF adjuvant program was initiated on 12 September 1975. In this study women were randomized to receive either 12 or 6 cycles of CMF within 2−4 weeks from radical mastectomy. Postmenopausal women were withdrawn after the analysis of the first CMF study revealed a lack of meaningful effect for the regimen in this subset. The trial was continued only in premenopausal patients and was closed on 31 May 1978. With analysis allowing actuarial projection of relapse-free survival for 3 years no difference has been seen between 6 and 12 cycles of CMF in premenopausal women.

The current Milan trial is based on a hypothesis published by Norten and Simon [14]. This hypothesis can be summarized as follows: (1) Human tumors grew in a Gompertzian fashion. For such growth the growth fraction of the tumor cells is maximum at the time of initiation of growth, while the growth rate is smallest for both tiny and very large tumors. The maximum growth rate occurs when the tumor is about 37% of its limiting size, which is the inflection point of the growth curve: (2) The maximum sensitivity to chemotherapy is at the inflection point and is less for very small and very large sized tumors. If this hypothesis is correct it would be best to give moderately intensive drug therapy initially (tumor above its inflection point), and when complete remission is achieved intensify the treatment. This late intensification would be required since the small residual tumor would be below the infection point and less sensitive.

In the current Milan trial for postmenopausal women, one group receives six cycles of CMF plus prednisone (CMFP) followed by four cycles of adriamycin plus vincristine (AV). A second group receives the sequential CMFP and AV beginning with lower doses, which progressively increase toward a maximum at the last cycle. To avoid excessive toxicity prednisone and vincristine are not intensified.

A Swiss cooperative group called OSAKO has studied a chemoimmunotherapy adjuvant regimen in both node-negative and node-positive women after mastectomy [16]. The chemotherapy consisted of a completely oral regimen of chlorambucil, methotrexate, 5-fluorouracil, and prednisone for 6 months at low doses followed by 18 months of BCG therapy. This study now has a nearly 3 year follow-up time and the analysis to data shows that the recurrence rate was significantly reduced only in node-negative women. In this subset the relapse rate is 5.1% in the chemoimmunotherapy group as compared to 19.7% in the control ($p = 0.02$). In node-positive patients the relapse rates are 22.4% in the treated group and 33.3% in the control ($p = 0.2$).

Current controlled protocols are on-going in the United States cooperative groups (Table 6) and in several cancer centers (Table 7). In addition some cancer centers are undertaking single arm studies relating to historical controls (Table 8). While some preliminary reports are available [1, 6, 12, 19], it is still too early to make any meaningful interpretation, especially since none, with any data to report, have a

Table 6. Selected list of recent surgical adjuvant breast trials in US cooperative groups

Group	Randomization
Southwest Oncology Group	Surgery + CMFVP vs Surgery + L-PAM
Eastern Cooperative Oncology Group	*Premenopausal* Surgery + CMF vs Surgery + CMFP *Postmenopausal* (< 65 years) Surgery vs Surgery + CMFP vs Surgery + CMFP + tamoxifen *Postmenopausal* (≥ 65 years) Surgery vs Surgery + tamoxifen
Cancer and leukemia Group B	Surgery + CMF vs Surgery + CMF + MER vs Surgery + CMFVP
Central Oncology Group	Surgery + L-PAM vs Surgery + CMFV
Southeastern Group	Surgery + CMF (6 cycles) vs Surgery + radiation + CMF (6 cycles) vs Surgery + CMF (12 cycles)

surgery-only control. With longer analysis it is now obvious the L-PAM alone is a poor control for postmenopausal women and studies which use this as a control will be particularly difficult to interpret.

The varying regimens currently in use in all the adjuvant studies currently on-going in terms of either patient accrual or continuing analysis are shown in Table 9. As can be seen a wide range of drug treatments are being used. There are 12 different drug regimens along with several chemohormonal and chemoimmunotherapy approaches. This mass of potential data will be complicated in analysis by the fact that there are internal variations of schedule, duration, intensity, patient selection, and data analysis techniques which will have to be taken into consideration.

Table 7. Selected list of a randomized single institution surgical adjuvant studies in the United States

Institution	Randomization
Mayo Clinic	Surgery + L-PAM vs Surgery + CFP vs Surgery + radiation + CFP
UCLA	Surgery + CMF vs Surgery + CMF + BCG + tumor cell vaccine
Cleveland Clinic	Surgery + CMF vs Surgery + CMF + tamoxifen vs Surgery + CMF + tamoxifen + BCG

Table 8. Selected list of single institution surgical adjuvant studies utilizing historical controls

Institution	Study regimen
M.D. Anderson	Surgery + FAC + BCG
University of Arizona	Surgery + adriamycin + cytoxan
Sidney Farber Cancer Institute	Surgery + adriamycin + cytoxan

It must be recognized that adjuvant trials are a long-term clinical experiment. It will take 10 years of follow-up before a definitive answer which will involve analyzing the trade off of overall survival with the toxic cost. The toxic cost will include the following: (1) The acute drug related morbidity and mortality, (2) the chronic toxicity in terms of organ damage, e.g., adriamycin cardiomyopathy, (3) the induction of second tumors, and (4) the psychosocial and economic cost. Relapse-free survival at 2 and 3 years after surgery is an early end point which can be either overly optimistic or overly pessimistic. The early actuarial projections of the L-PAM and CMF data indicated an improvement in postmenopausal women that failed to be confirmed by longer follow-up. On the other hand in Meakens [13] study of prophylactic castration and prednisone the early analysis was discouraging. Only with longer follow-up did the benefit in premenopausal women over the age of 45 become evident.

When should the results on an adjuvant study first be presented? It will not be practical to wait 10 years until a definitive answer is available. A reasonable compromise would appear to be when the median follow-up time is 24 months so that an actuarial projection of relapse-free survival can be made. What has to be understood by the scientific community is the limitations of such an analysis with the possibility that the ultimate answers may be different after 5 and 10 years of follow-up. Many postmenopausal women were treated with L-PAM after the initial study report. Many

Table 9. Selected list of combinations in adjuvant trials

	Group
I. *Non adriamycin containing*	
1. L-PAM	NSABP
2. L-PAM + 5-FU	NSABP
3. L-PAM + 5-FU + MTX	NSABP
4. Cytoxan + 5-FU + MTX (CMF)	Various
5. Chlorambucil + 5-FU + MTX ± prednisone (LMF)	OSAKO
6. Cytoxan + 5-FU + prednisone	Mayo Clinic
7. Cytoxan + 5-FU + MTX + prednisone	ECOG
8. Cytoxan + 5-FU + MTX + vincristine	COG
9. Cytoxan + 5-FU + MTX + vincristine + prednisone	Various
II. *Adriamacin containing combinations*	
1. Adriamycin + cytoxan	Various
2. Adriamycin + cytoxin + 5-FU (FAC)	M.D. Anderson
3. CMFP 6 cycles → adriamycin + vincristine (4 cycles)	NCI, Milan
III. *Hormone containing combinations*	
1. CMF + tamoxifen	Cleveland Clinic
2. CMF + prednisone + tamoxifen	ECOG
3. Tamoxifen	ECOG
4. L-PAM + 5-FU + tamoxifen	NSABP
IV. *Immunotherapy containing*	
1. CMF + BCG	UCLA
2. CMF + BCG + tumor cells	UCLA
3. CMF + tamoxifen + GCG	Case Western
4. LMF + BCG	OSAKO
5. FAC + BCG	M.D. Anderson
6. L-PAM + 5-FU + C. Parvum	NSABP

protocols switched to L-PAM controls, from surgery only controls, at the same time. Now that 4 year follow-up data are available it is clear that L-PAM alone for 18 months is not a valuable therapy in this clinical situation.

Another important aspect of primary breast cancer studies, including those with adjuvant drug, is the heterogeneity of the populations under study (Table 10) [7]. Within the mass of patients who present with a surgically approachable lesion are subsets with significantly different prognostic implications. A clinical result that fails to analyze these subsets is almost meaningless. These subsets are of such prognostic significance that some may require separate protocol approaches (Table 11). The tendency to present breast cancer data as a total number should be discouraged. Each subset of menopausal status, nodal status, and ER status should be presented separately.

Breast cancer has been a disease of shifting emphasis. For many years the essential strategy was to maximize local control equating that achievement with cure. Surgery was the major tool and it was extended as much as was deemed possible to accomplish that end. The apogee of this approach was the extended radical mastectomy. In recent years a complete shift in the emphasis has taken place. It is now recognized by most

Table 10. Current therapeutic options for Stage I–II breast cancer and critical subsets for analysis

Critical subsets	Therapeutic options

1. Menopausal status
   A. Pre
   B. Peri
   C. Post
	1. Minimal surgery plus high dose X ray
	   A. Excisional biopsy
	   B. Segmental resection
	   C. Quadrentectomy

2. Clinical stage (tumor size)	2. Total mastectomy
	   A. Without irradiation
	   B. With irradiation

3. Nodal status
   A. Negative
   B. 1–3 +
   C. ≥ 4 +
	3. Modified radical
	   Mastectomy ± Irradiation

4. Estrogen receptor status
   A. ≤ 3 Femtamol
   B. 3–10 Femtamol
   C. ≥ 10 Femtamol
	4. Axillary sampling in option 1 and 2

5. Tumor differentiation
   A. Well
   B. Moderate
   C. Poor
	5. Adjuvant chemotherapy ± Hormones

6. Location
   A. Outer
   B. Inner
	6. Prophylactic castration
	   A. Surgical
	   B. Radiation

that a major cause of failure after local control treatment is disseminated disease. Therefore local control, with optimal cosmesis, is now striven for. The scientific quest is now for how little can be done and still achieve the cure potential available with local control therapy.

Complicating all of this has been the utilization of chemotherapy as adjuvant treatment. Since metastatic failure is a critical problem a systemic therapy is being utilized in hopes that residual microscopic metastatic disease can be sterilized. The success of adjuvant drug treatment has not been as dramatic as some of the early reports indicated it might be. Still it has made a significant impact on relapse-free survival in premenopausal women and early analysis of some current studies are optimistic that this will be accomplished in postmenopausal women as well.

The success of adjuvant drug treatment has implications for the debate about optimal local control therapy. These implications impact in a variety of ways. In clinical situations where the cure situation with surgery and X ray only is poor, a more vigorous approach can now be contemplated within a clinical research setting. On the other hand, where the cure potential is better, a lesser surgical approach can be contemplated, since with sampling of axillary nodes, the poor prognosis subset can be separated out and given adjuvant drug treatment. In addition adjuvant chemotherapy has been shown to diminish local relapse and so may obviate the need for irradiation after surgery, which can only be justified in terms of diminished local failure.

Table 11. Protected protocol flow in stage II breast cancer with positive nodes

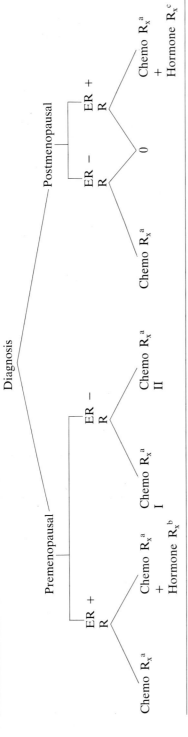

[a] Options: CMF 12 cycles, CMF 6 cycles, CMFP, CMFVP, CMFV, FAC, AC, LMF
[b] Oopherectomy or tamoxifen
[c] Tamoxifen or estrogens

References

1. Ahmann DL, Payne WS, Scanlon PW, O'Fallon JR, Bisel HF, Hahn RG, Edmonson JH, Ingle JN, Frytak S, O'Connell MJ, Rubin J (1978) Repeated adjuvant chemotherapy with phenylalanine mustard or 5-fluorouracil, cyclophosphamide, and prednisone with or without radiation, after mastectomy for breast cancer. Lancet 1: 983
2. Bonadonna G, Brusamolino E, Valagussa P, Rossi A, Brugnatelli L, Brambilla C, de Lena M, Tancini G, Bajetta E, Musumeci R, Veronesi U (1976) Combination chemotherapy as an adjuvant treatment in operable breast cancer. N Engl J Med 294: 405
3. Bonadonna G, Rossi A, Valagussa P, Banfi A, Veronesi U (1977) The CMF program for operable breast cancer with positive axillary nodes. Updated analysis on the disease-free interval site of relapse and drug tolerance. Cancer 39: 2904
4. Bonadonna G, Valagussa P, Rossi A, Tancini G, Bajetta E, Marchini S, Veronesi U (1979) CMF adjuvant chemotherapy in operable breast cancer. In: Salmon SE, Jones SE (eds) Adjuvant therapy of cancer II. Grune & Stratton New York
5. Bonadonna G, Valagussa P, Rossi A, Zucali R, Tancini G, Bajetta E, Brambilla C, de Lena M, di Fronzo G, Banfi A, Rilke F, Veronesi U (1978) Are surgical adjuvant trials altering the course of breast cancer? Semin Oncol 5: 450
6. Budzar AU, Blumenschein GR, Gutterman JU, Tashima CK, Hortobagyi GN, Smith TL, Campos LT, Wheeler WL, Hersh EM, Freireich EJ, Gehan EA (to be published) Postoperative adjuvant chemotherapy with 5-fluorouracil, adriamycin, cyclophosphamide and BCG. A follow-up report. JAMA
7. Carter SK (1978) Adjuvant chemotherapy in breast cancer: Critique and perspectives. Cancer Chemother Pharmacol 1: 187—197
8. Carter SK (1977) Correlation of chemotherapy activity in advanced disease with adjuvant results. In: Salmon SE, Jones SE (eds) Adjuvant therapy of cancer. North Holland Publishing, Amsterdam, pp 589—597
9. Fisher B (to be published) Breast cancer: Studies of the National Surgical Adjuvant Primary Breast Cancer Project (NSABP). In: Salmon SE, Jones SE (eds) Adjuvant therapy of cancer II. Grune & Stratton, New York
10. Fisher B, Carbone P, Economou S, Frelich R, Glass A, Lerner H, Redmond C, Zelen M, Band P, Katrych D, Wolmark N, Fisher ER (and other co-operative investigators) (1975) L-phenylalanine mustard (L-PAM) in the management of primary breast cancer. N Engl J Med 292: 117—122
11. Fisher B, Slack NH, Katrych D, Wolmark N (1975) Ten year follow-up results of patients with carcinoma of the breast in a cooperative clinical trial evaluating surgical adjuvant chemotherapy. Surg Gynecol Obstet 140: 528—534
12. Glucksberg H, Rivkin SE, Rasmussen S (to be published) Adjuvant chemotherapy for stage II breast cancer: A comparison of CMFVP versus L-PAM. In: Salmon SE, Jones SE (eds) Adjuvant therapy of cancer II. Grune & Stratton, New York
13. Meakin JW, Allt WEC, Beale FA, Brown TC, Bush RS, Clark RM, Fitzpatrick NV, Hawkins RDT, Jenkin JF, Pringle JF, Rider WD, Hayward JL, Bulbrook RD (1977) Ovarian irradiation and prednisone following surgery for carcinoma of the breast. In: Salmon SE, Jones SE (eds) Adjuvant therapy of cancer. Elsevier, Amsterdam, pp 95—100
14. Norton L, Simon R (1977) Tumor size, sensitivity to therapy, and design of treatment schedules. Cancer Treat Rep 61: 1307
15. Schabel FM (1975) Concepts for systemic treatment of micrometastases. Cancer 35: 15—24
16. Senn HJ, Jungi WF, Amgwerd R, Sprenger F, Hochueli R, Engelhart G, Heinz C, Wick A, Enderlin F, Creux G, Simeon B, Lanz R, Bigler R (1978) Adjuvant chemoimmunotherapy with LMF + BCG in node-negative and node-positive breast cancer patients. Antibiot Chemother 24: 213—228

17. Tancini G, Bajetta E, Marchini S, Valagussa P, Bonadonna G, Veronesi U (1979) Operable breast cancer with positive axillary nodes (N+): Results of 6 vs 12 cycles of adjuvant CMF in premenopausal women. Proc Am Assoc Cancer Res 20: 172
18. Valagussa P, Bonadonna G, Veronesi U (1978) Patterns of relapse and survival following radical mastectomy: Analysis of 716 consecutive patients. Cancer 41: 1170–1178
19. Wendt AG, Jones SE, Salmon SE, Giordano GF, Jackson RA, Miller RS, Heusinkveld RS, Moon TE (to be published) Adjuvant treatment of breast cancer with adriamycin-cy-clophosphamide with or without radiation therapy. In: Salmon SE, Jones SE (eds) Adjuvant therapy of cancer II. Grune & Stratton, New York

Recent Results in Cancer Research

Sponsored by the Swiss League against Cancer. Editor in Chief: P. Rentchnick, Genève